# CHILDHOOD OBESITY

## Prevention and Treatment

# CRC SERIES IN
# MODERN NUTRITION
## Edited by Ira Wolinsky and James F. Hickson, Jr.

### Published Titles

*Manganese in Health and Disease*, Dorothy J. Klimis-Tavantzis

*Nutrition and AIDS: Effects and Treatments*, Ronald R. Watson

*Nutrition Care for HIV-Positive Persons: A Manual for Individuals and Their Caregivers*,
Saroj M. Bahl and James F. Hickson, Jr.

*Calcium and Phosphorus in Health and Disease*, John J.B. Anderson and
Sanford C. Garner

## Edited by Ira Wolinsky

### Published Titles

*Handbook of Nutrition in the Aged*, Ronald R. Watson

*Practical Handbook of Nutrition in Clinical Practice*, Donald F. Kirby
and Stanley J. Dudrick

*Handbook of Dairy Foods and Nutrition*, Gregory D. Miller, Judith K. Jarvis,
and Lois D. McBean

*Advanced Nutrition: Macronutrients*, Carolyn D. Berdanier

*Childhood Nutrition*, Fima Lifschitz

*Nutrition and Health: Topics and Controversies*, Felix Bronner

*Nutrition and Cancer Prevention*, Ronald R. Watson and Siraj I. Mufti

*Nutritional Concerns of Women*, Ira Wolinsky and Dorothy J. Klimis-Tavantzis

*Nutrients and Gene Expression: Clinical Aspects*, Carolyn D. Berdanier

*Antioxidants and Disease Prevention*, Harinda S. Garewal

*Advanced Nutrition: Micronutrients*, Carolyn D. Berdanier

*Nutrition and Women's Cancers*, Barbara Pence and Dale M. Dunn

*Nutrients and Foods in AIDS*, Ronald R. Watson

*Nutrition: Chemistry and Biology, Second Edition*, Julian E. Spallholz,
L. Mallory Boylan, and Judy A. Driskell

*Melatonin in the Promotion of Health*, Ronald R. Watson

*Nutritional and Environmental Influences on the Eye*, Allen Taylor

*Laboratory Tests for the Assessment of Nutritional Status, Second Edition*,
H.E. Sauberlich

*Advanced Human Nutrition*, Robert E.C. Wildman and Denis M. Medeiros

*Handbook of Dairy Foods and Nutrition, Second Edition*, Gregory D. Miller,
Judith K. Jarvis, and Lois D. McBean

*Nutrition in Space Flight and Weightlessness Models*, Helen W. Lane
and Dale A. Schoeller

*Eating Disorders in Women and Children: Prevention, Stress Management, and Treatment,* Jacalyn J. Robert-McComb

*Childhood Obesity: Prevention and Treatment,* Jana Pařízková and Andrew Hills

*Alcohol and Substance Abuse in the Aging,* Ronald R. Watson

*Handbook of Nutrition and the Aged, Third Edition,* Ronald R. Watson

*Vegetables, Fruits, and Herbs in Health Promotion,* Ronald R. Watson

*Nutrition and AIDS, 2nd Edition,* Ronald R. Watson

## Forthcoming Titles

*Nutritional Anemias,* Usha Ramakrishnan

*Advances in Isotope Methods for the Analysis of Trace Elements in Man,* Malcolm Jackson and Nicola Lowe

*Handbook of Nutrition for Vegetarians,* Joan Sabate and Rosemary A. Ratzin-Tuner

*Tryptophan: Biochemicals and Health Implications,* Herschel Sidransky

*Handbook of Nutraceuticals and Functional Foods,* Robert E. C. Wildman

*The Mediterranean Diet,* Antonia L. Matalas, Antonios Zampelas, Vasilis Stavrinos, and Ira Wolinsky

*Handbook of Nutraceuticals and Nutritional Supplements and Pharmaceuticals,* Robert E. C. Wildman

*Inulin and Oligofructose: Functional Food Ingredients,* Marcel B. Roberfroid

*Micronutrients and HIV Infection,* Henrik Friis

*Nutrition Gene Interactions in Health and Disease,* Niama M. Moussa and Carolyn D. Berdanier

# CHILDHOOD OBESITY

## Prevention and Treatment

Jana Pařízková
Andrew Hills

**CRC Press**
**Boca Raton   London   New York   Washington, D.C.**

## Library of Congress Cataloging-in-Publication Data

Pařízková, Jana.
　　Childhood obesity : prevention and treatment / by Jana Pařízková, Andrew P. Hills.
　　　　p. cm.-- (CRC series in modern nutrition)
　　Includes bibliographical references and index.
　　ISBN 0-8493-8736-1 (alk. paper)
　　　1. Obesity in children. 2. Children--Nutrition. I. Hills, Andrew P. II. Title. III. Modern
nutrition (Boca Raton, Fla.)

　　RJ399.C6 P37 2000
　　618.92'398--dc21                                                                         00-031171

© 2001 by CRC Press LLC

No claim to original U.S. Government works
International Standard Book Number 0-8493-8736-1
Library of Congress Card Number 00-031171
Printed in the United States of America  1  2  3  4  5  6  7  8  9  0
Printed on acid-free paper

# *Series Preface for Modern Nutrition*

The CRC Series in Modern Nutrition is dedicated to providing the widest possible coverage of topics in nutrition. Nutrition is an interdisciplinary, interprofessional field par excellence. It is noted by its broad range and diversity. We trust the titles and authorship in this series will reflect that range and diversity

Published for a scholarly audience, the volumes in the CRC Series in Modern Nutrition are designed to explain, review, and explore present knowledge and recent rends, developments, and advances in nutrition.

As such, they will also appeal to the educated layman. The format for the series will vary with the needs of the author and the topic, including, but not limited to, edited volumes, monographs, handbooks, and text.

Contributors from any bona fide area of nutrition, including the controversial, are welcome.

We welcome the timely contribution of *Childhood Obesity: Prevention and Treatment*, authored by the well-known scientists Jana Pařízková and Andrew P. Hills. Although meant to be self contained, it may also serve as a companion volume to *Nutrition, Physical Activity, and Health in Early Life*, also authored by Jana Pařízková, and also published by CRC Press. Alone or together they provide a wealth of information about childhood.

# *Preface*

The worldwide epidemic of overweight and obesity in adults is now a major health problem for children and youth. While childhood obesity has existed since ancient times, there is increasing evidence that prevalence rates today are greater than ever before. This increase in fatness heightens the health risks for later periods of life but also has a substantial impact during the growing years.

Over the last decade more research has been devoted to this significant problem. There has been considerable effort devoted to the identification of suitable ways to prevent, treat, and manage the condition. However, numerous questions remain unanswered.

This volume summarizes many of the findings on obesity during growth with a particular focus on more recent knowledge and an appraisal of research on treatment and management. Most important, the volume addresses some potential solutions for the prevention of obesity in childhood. While the major focus of the book is children and adolescents, some reference is made to relevant research with adults. Significantly more research has been completed with the adult population; therefore, knowledge and understanding of practices with this group may have important consequences for children and adolescents. Readers are referred to data presented elsewhere, for example, in proceedings of previous International and European Congresses on Obesity.

A number of approaches to prevent, treat, and manage childhood obesity have been presented in the literature to date. The authors of this volume, however, believe that the prevention and management of obesity should be promoted with the incorporation of natural factors (appropriate nutrition and physical activity) to rectify energy imbalance and achieve a desirable body composition. This approach has a greater opportunity for success in earlier periods of life when obesity is not fully developed. These comments assume, of course, the absence of pathological conditions such as Cushing or Prader-Willi syndrome and others. Genetic anomalies with an impact on body fatness are quite rare in children; poor lifestyle behaviors are largely responsible for excess fatness in the majority of cases of obesity during childhood. As shown by some authors, even in such cases, an environmental intervention can have a significant impact and help to improve the situation for the child.[1] The management of an appropriate environment for an obese child requires a conscious and consistent arrangement of diet and physical activity that may be difficult for both the child and his/her family. Weight loss for an obese child or youth is not the sole aim in weight management, but rather, the overall improvement of the physiological, psychological, and social status of the individual.[2]

A significant restriction of food intake may be needed when the degree of obesity is excessive or morbid. Unfortunately, this scenario is necessary with an increasing number of children and adolescents. This trend may be the result of childhood obesity being underestimated and neglected as a health problem. The best way to manage obesity in the family, school, and the wider environment of the child is to be vigilant and help in the early detection and intervention to minimize excess deposition of fat. The optimal scenario in the management of childhood obesity is not to permit its development at all. Early interventions should be well planned, timely, and follow best practice guidelines to achieve the desired outcomes.

The aim of this volume is to cover a broad range of ideas and collect presently available information. However, definitive suggestions for the solution of childhood obesity would be premature. Knowledge in the individual areas of research has not been increasing at a similar pace. Further research and clinical experience will contribute more positively in the future.

# Authors

Jana Pařízková, M.D., Ph.D., D.Sc. is a Senior Scientist and Associate Professor at the Centre for the Management of Obesity 1st Medical Faculty, 3rd Department Internal Medicine, Charles University, in Prague, Czech Republic. She earned her medical degree from Charles University in 1956, where she graduated summa cum laude. She pursued her Ph.D. in medical physiology at the Institute of Physiology of the Czechoslovak Academy of Sciences in 1960, and received her Dr.Sc. in nutrition and metabolism in 1977. She was given a fellowship at the Laboratoire de Nutrition Humaine, Hopital Bichat in Paris, France for 1965 and 1966.

Dr. Pařízková's main research interests include body composition as related to dietary intake, physical performance and fitness, lipid metabolism variables, development of gross and fine motor skills, and physical activity regimes during the human life span, with a special focus on the growth and development periods. She has focused on the development of obesity during growth and cardiovascular risks later in life, and also health promotion and the reduction of health risks through nutritional and physical activity interventions. Another main area of research is obesity accompanied by metabolic and clinical problems as related to actual physical activity level and diet in all age categories.

Dr. Pařízková is the author of several monographs including "Development of Lean Body Mass and Depot Fat in Children" (1962); "Body Composition and Lipid Metabolism under Conditions of Various Physical Activity" (1974), which is in Czech and updated in English by Martinus Nijhoff, B.V. Medical Division (The Hague, 1977) and by Editora Guanabara Dois (Rio de Janeiro, 1982) as "Body Fat and Physical Fitness". In 1996 she published the monograph "Nutrition, Physical activity and Health in Early Life," CRC Press, USA. In addition, she co-authored and edited ten other monographs, including "Physical Fitness and Nutrition during Growth" (S. Karger, Basel 1998, co-edited with A. P. Hills). She is also the author of approximately 500 articles published in international and national scientific journals and proceedings, including international congresses. She has been an invited speaker at more than one hundred international congresses, conferences, etc. Dr. Pařízková was a chairperson and/or organizer of IUNS symposia and workshops in 1975, 1978, 1981, 1989, and 1997.

WHO appointed Dr. Pařízková visiting professor, International Course on Nutrition and Hygiene, Hyderabad, 1977 (in conjunction with SEARO); consultant in Geneva in 1978; member panel of experts on "Energy and Protein Requirements," Rome, 1981 (findings published in Geneva in 1985 as WHO

Technical Report Series, No. 24); and member of the consultation group on "Epidemiology of Obesity," Warsaw, 1987.

Among other rewards, Dr. Pařízková has received The Philip Noel Baker Prize, ICSPE by UNESCO in 1977, Memorial Medal from Charles University in 1978, Prize of the Rector of Charles University in 1996, and the International Memorial Medal of Ales Hrdlicka in 1996.

Dr. Pařízková is a member of the Czech Medical Association of J. E. Purkyne, (CzMA JEP), the Czech Society for the Study of Obesity, the Czech Association of Nutrition, and the Czech Anthropological Society. In addition, she is a member in the following organizations: the European Association for the Study of Obesity, International Association for the Study of Obesity, the International Commission for Anthropology of Food (ICAF) through the International Union of Anthropological and Ethnological Sciences (IUAES), the European Academy of Nutritional Sciences (EANS), International Society for the Advancement of Kinanthropometry (ISAK), and the European Anthropological Association. She has served previously as the Chairperson of the Nutrition and Physical Performance Committee through the International Union of Nutritional Sciences (IUNS), and as a member of the Scientific Committee of the International Council for Sport and Physical Education (ICSPE) through UNESCO. She was elected a member of the New York Academy of Sciences (1963) and was conferred an honorary appointment to the Research Board of Advisors of the American Biographic Institute.

**Dr. Andrew P. Hills** is a prominent exercise physiologist with a primary interest in pediatric obesity and exercise. He is currently Vice-President of the Australasian Society for the Study of Obesity and foundation member.

Dr. Hills trained initially as a physical educator before completing a Master of Science degree at the University of Oregon after having been awarded a Rotary Foundation Graduate Fellowship. His Ph.D. thesis, titled "Locomotor characteristics of obese pre-pubertal children" was undertaken at the University of Queensland in the Department of Anatomy. He is also a Fellow of Sports Medicine Australia and Secretary-Treasurer of the International Council for Physical Activity and Fitness Research.

His current appointment is Associate Professor and Clinic Director, School of Human Movement Studies at Queensland University of Technology. There he established a multi-disciplinary clinic with a special emphasis on weight management. Dr. Hills has published widely in the fields of physical growth and development and obesity, including 5 books, 11 book chapters, and over 100 papers and presentations. His most recent book is Body Composition Assessment in Children, T. Jurimae and A.P. Hills (Eds.) (Basel: Karger).

Current research emphases include adaptation to weight loss in the obese, the relationship between the energy cost of walking and adiposity, the relationship between body composition and body image in the obese, and submaximal markers of exercise intensity.

# Contents

# Part II    Treatment and Management Principles

**Chapter 13    Practical Programs for Weight Management during the Growing Years**

# Part I

# Main Characteristics of Childhood Obesity

# 1

## Introduction

During the recent past the prevalence of obesity has increased and the condition is developing in much earlier periods of life than was the case previously. This situation is a major concern, not only in the countries with a good food supply, predominantly the industrially developed countries, but also countries of the Third World,[3] where obesity is more commonly a problem of the upper socioeconomic classes.[4] Irrespective of the setting, increased attention must be paid to the problems of obesity during growth in the areas of prevention, treatment, and evaluation.[5,6]

Genetic factors and environmental conditions play central roles in the early development of obesity but the situation varies in different countries. This topic will be treated in greater detail in later chapters. The prevalence of obesity in all age groups varies significantly in different parts of the world, especially when comparing the populations in Asia with Western populations. For example, the prevalence of obesity, using the standard criteria of a body mass index (BMI) greater than 30, in a group of Japanese aged 15 to 84 years, and followed up from 1990 to 1994, was quite low compared with the data in Western populations.[7]

Some would argue that there are so many children in the world who are hungry and starving, why care so much about obesity, the health problem of affluence? One never sees a child from a poor Asian or African village who is obese! However, when the economic situation in such countries improves, the prevalence of obesity does increase. Thus, when problems such as malnutrition, decreased immuno-resistance, and other health outcomes are improved, new health problems appear. Childhood obesity has also been identified in lower social strata groups in the industrially developed countries, which suggests that obesity is due mainly to inadequate food preferences and reduced physical activity, in short, poor lifestyle behaviors. Given the widespread nature of obesity, particularly under conditions of an improving economic and social situation, the adequate management of obesity during growth is an urgent challenge for most countries of the world.

According to recent data from the United States, obesity affects approximately 25 to 30% of children, with estimates varying from study to study. Despite the variability, the prevalence appears to be increasing significantly.

To compound the situation, the status of the condition in the same country can vary considerably. For example, preschool children living in the north and central regions of Mexico have higher obesity prevalence rates than those living in the southeast. The risk of obesity in these regions was positively associated with the educational level of the head of the household and also with the social and economic situation.[8] This variability will be described and analyzed in detail in the following chapters.

An analysis of the variability of the prevalence of obesity, and the effect of the environmental conditions, both in the past and at present, is important. In addition, an understanding of the characteristic features of obesity in various parts of the world could help elucidate and define the most important mechanisms that promote the development of marked obesity during growth and, therefore, provide some assistance on how to treat and prevent the condition.

However, it must be acknowledged that an analysis of the available data on childhood obesity and comparisons of this work are far more difficult than comparable between-study analyses of adults. Differences exist in the aims, research design, criteria for assessment, terminology, protocols, and methodology, but there is an additional significant problem. It relates to comparisons confounded by differences in chronological age and maturational status. Further, the stage of development and maturation differs according to gender but may also be different in various countries, especially when comparing children from different economic and social situations. Differences in the age of onset and duration of obesity related to the critical periods of growth in subjects evaluated in various studies must also be considered.

The development of obesity in a growing organism is not the same as the obesity present in a fully mature adult or aging organism. The same diversity applies to approaches to prevention, treatment, and management with differences according to age, stage, character, and duration of obesity, and the type of treatment and its duration.

The relationships between various factors and variables in growing subjects are, therefore, largely peculiar to the specific study population. As such, it may not be surprising that the synthesis of findings and conclusions from the available publications is often controversial. However, despite a degree of pessimism surrounding the successful management of childhood obesity, a developing body of knowledge argues for a favorable outcome and solution to this major health problem.

In summary, despite some of the common features and characteristics of the condition, each child is an individual with a distinct personality, personal health, nutrition, and physical fitness background. As such, each individual should be evaluated and treated recognizing these inherent unique characteristics. A failure to recognize this uniqueness may contribute to an oversimplification and generalization of the situation of a particular child. This may be one of the main reasons for the lack of success to date in the treatment of childhood obesity.[2,9]

## 1.1 Evaluation of Obesity and Its Causal Factors during Growth

Obesity may be defined as a multifactor syndrome that consists of physiological, biochemical, metabolic, anatomical, psychological, and social alterations.[10] The condition is characterized by an increased level of adiposity and a corresponding increase in body weight, which must be evaluated according to the standard values for the individual age categories of girls and boys.

The precise level of fatness that defines obesity is somewhat arbitrary. Himes suggested that excessive fatness should be determined according to some health-related criteria.[11] At that time, he indicated that there was limited definitive knowledge regarding specific health implications of various levels of fatness and this void was particularly evident for the childhood population. Since the early 1980s there has been a progressive accumulation of health-related implications of higher levels of adiposity.

A useful start is to make a distinction between overweight and obesity. Overweight refers to an increase in body weight above an arbitrary standard, usually defined in relation to height.[12] Obesity, on the other hand, refers to an abnormally high proportion of the body composition as body fat,[13] or a surplus of adipose tissue.[14] A more precise definition of what constitutes problematic obesity in all individuals is a challenge as there is no universally accepted classification system or completely satisfactory numerical index of obesity, particularly for children and the immature adolescent.[15] The utilization of the BMI and measurements of skinfolds has contributed to an improvement in the evaluation of childhood obesity.

The criteria and methods used to evaluate obesity and the degree of the condition are serious problems. Similarly, the definition of factors contributing to the development of obesity is also a major challenge. Because the processes of growth, development, and maturation during childhood and adolescence do not proceed at the same pace in various countries, it is also not easy to evaluate the adequacy of changes in growth status, for example, in height, weight, and body composition.[9] This issue also complicates the definition of obesity in both industrially developed and developing countries where it is inappropriate to use the same growth and development standards.

However, considerable effort has been made to standardize measurement criteria with work undertaken by researchers and also by the World Health Organization (WHO),[16] the Food and Agricultural Organization (FAO), United Nations University (1985), and other institutions. From an anthropometric perspective, a number of groups are responsible for the progression of a standardized approach to measurement, for example, the International Society for the Advancement of Kinanthropometry (ISAK).

Obesity has commonly been defined in relation to certain limits of body fatness. For example, for prepubertal children, values for acceptable percent body fat levels are 17 to 18%, 15 to 18% for young adult males (aged 18 years), and 20 to 25% for young females of similar age.[17] However, the values for the individual age categories of girls and boys vary from year to year, and, in addition, are related to the level of sexual development.[18] There is also considerable merit in relating weight to weight for height values of the reference population being sampled and, as such, definitions of obesity in children have also taken the form of weight-for-height distributions (percentiles). Children above the 95th percentile for weight-for-height and age are often considered obese (yet in other studies this may be above the 97th percentile, or only the 90th percentile).

As is the case in other disciplines, publication bias appears to exist in the literature, particularly regarding the evaluation of obesity and the results of weight management. Therefore, it is necessary to evaluate the results of available studies with caution. Suggestions for the management of such bias once it has been identified, or reducing its likelihood, are also discussed in the literature.[19] This also applies to the results of various scientific meetings concerning obesity in children and adolescents, e.g., European Children's Obesity Group (ECOG), 1996, 1998.

A continuing theme is the paramount role of nutrition in the form of extra energy intake caused by a range of factors. In addition to an increased intake of food, a higher metabolic efficiency or energy utilization in certain subjects predisposed to obesity has been considered. The role of genetics manifested by family clustering has been the focus of extensive research more recently.[20] Composition of the diet has also received considerable attention, particularly high intake of fat. Energy output resulting from various levels and types of physical activity and exercise has also been considered, along with the interplay of all of these parameters.

A further problem is the reliability of methods and procedures used in the individual studies, up to the present day. For example, more recent studies using advanced techniques have revealed a clear discrepancy between self-reported and actual energy intake and self-reported and actual physical activity or energy expenditure in obese subjects. This is of particular concern for obese individuals who have had difficulties losing weight by dietary adjustment.[21] The same applies to food choice and habits, food aversions and preferences.

Limitations in the assessment of dietary energy intake by self-report have also been reported by other authors.[22] Two investigations of the validity of self-reported dietary records by measuring change of dietary intake indicated a considerable underestimation of the actual change. Therefore, self-reported data on dietary intake must be interpreted with caution unless independent methods of assessing their validity are included in the experimental design. In addition, intercorrelations between measures of body composition and adiposity are generally highly significant, but the data do not necessarily correspond.

Reasons for discrepancies have also been considered and analyzed according to the family situation. The obesity status of the mother, father, or other family members had no effect on the accuracy of the information recalled.

However, the results indicated that the lack of differences consistently observed in dietary intake between obese and normal-weight children could not be explained by differential accuracy of recalled information on food intake.[23] The same applies to reports on physical activity, as shown clearly by Mayer who followed obese and normal children during various physical activities.[24] Mayer found marked differences in self-reported and filmed levels of physical activity among normal-weight and obese children, despite the same findings in both groups.

Evaluation of the level of physical activity with the help of triaxial accelerometers (Tritrac) has yielded more reliable estimates of the level of physical activity in obese children aged 8 to 15 years than self-report questionnaire information.[25] This means that much of the information available on the level of physical activity in obese children may not be objective.

 There is evidence that energy intake, certainly in the United Kingdom, declined between the 1950s and 1970s; this was explained by the reduction of physical activity and increase in inactive behavior. Another explanation for some of the differences was that higher factors were used to calculate the energy derived from protein, fat, and carbohydrate in the 1930s and 1940s than were used later. If the later factors are applied to the results of earlier surveys, the values for energy are reduced by about 10%. This correction brings the results of the earlier surveys into line with those of the later ones for boys up to 14 years and girls up to 10 years.[26] However, older boys and girls as well as adults do appear to eat less than was the case in the past. This has also been confirmed by other comparisons.[27]

These issues are of concern for all periods of life, but they commence with the fetal period. Predisposition for the later development of obesity may start as early as during pregnancy. One of the key questions is whether women should increase their intake of food during pregnancy. It is postulated that metabolic economies enable women during pregnancy to produce an average of 4 kg of fat and a fetus weighing 3.5 kg without any increase in energy intake at all. However, a number of pregnant women "eat for two," which might be one of the main reasons for the development of obesity in both mother and child.[26]

Increased adiposity is also a serious risk for co-morbid conditions. The Framingham Study followed secular trends and risk factors for cardiovascular disease and showed that compared with 1957–1960, mean BMI and prevalence rates for overweight and hypertension were higher in 1984–1988, despite the higher levels of physical activity reported.[28] Closer cooperation between nutritionists and exercise physiologists, which is still insufficient, could also help provide a better solution for obesity, especially in children.

Risk factors for childhood obesity are similar in various parts of the world. In a group of Chinese children it was found that parents' weight (as evaluated by Kaup's index), birth weight, and breastfeeding were risk factors for childhood obesity (see Chapter 3). On the other hand, basal metabolic rate was not different in obese children compared to normal-weight individuals (Chapter 5). The earlier the appearance of overweight and obesity, particularly if earlier than 4 years of age, the more severe the condition was likely to be. Earlier onset of the condition may also be due to a different etiology. The earlier obesity was associated with prenatal factors while later onset obesity was related to the type of feeding in early life. Such results support the necessity of early interventions as recommended by a wide range of specialists in the field.[18,29–35] Generally, the earlier the commencement of treatment for obese children and adolescents, the higher the likelihood of long-term success.

Factors contributing to obesity may not always be the same in both genders. For example, in boys, physical inactivity, measured as both television viewing time and registrations of participation in sports activities, contributed independently to body fat mass. In girls, there was a weaker or no contribution of physical inactivity.[36]

## 1.2   Main Problems in the Treatment of Childhood Obesity

A number of ways to manage obesity have been defined, and these options provide a very useful guide to management of the obese child or youth. However, this is not the main problem. The most difficult challenge is for the individual to adhere to the principles of the treatment and permanently maintain a desirable weight and body composition. The treatment and management of obesity must ideally involve a range of health professionals in a team approach. Williams et al. have suggested that the process should involve pediatricians and other specialists who could play significant roles in addressing increased adiposity in children during the growing years.[37]

A more fundamental starting point is for all health professionals to be aware of the condition. Given the lack of understanding of the condition by many people this process must involve education regarding the actual and future risks of obesity, especially when the condition develops during the early phases of growth. Recent advances in the treatment of obesity during childhood have been presented at a number of scientific meetings,[38] for example, the ECOG meetings in 1997 and the European and International Congresses on Obesity in 1998.

Some suggest that the pediatrician's perception of the problem of childhood obesity is usually adequate and results in an appropriate approach to management.[39] However, some medical practitioners still underestimate the health risks of obesity and potential accompanying problems. Eating habits that are employed across the lifespan are established in infancy. During this period, pediatricians can have a significant impact on young mothers and their children by encouraging a diet low in saturated fat, cholesterol, and sodium. The diet should be adequate in energy and meet the recommended dietary allowances (RDAs) for all macro- and micronutrients corresponding to the needs of the growing child.[40]

In addition to counseling for dietary moderation, pediatricians should also encourage regular physical activity. Such an approach would not only assist in the prevention of obesity but also cardiovascular and metabolic diseases, especially coronary heart disease. Obesity is an essential predisposing factor for many of the common chronic diseases, especially when it is manifested during childhood. Regular physical activity and exercise provide the common essential elements in the prevention, treatment, and management of each condition.

As mentioned above, a poor child in a developing country never becomes obese. Similarly, a young track-and-field athlete or long-distance runner does not generally have excess body fat. Despite the potential contribution of genetic factors, the laws of the conservation of energy cannot be avoided or excluded. This provides some guidance on the management of obesity, and especially the prevention of obesity in many children. Common sense suggests that the employment of a highly restricted energy intake, or excessively hard physical training, as a means of managing childhood obesity is inappropriate.

Nevertheless, the illustrative example of a young adequately active youngster is an appropriate model to highlight the role of physical activity and exercise in the prevention of obesity. This approach has been repeatedly considered.[18,41] Unfortunately for too many people, an interest in physical activity and exercise does not extend beyond the exertion of being a spectator of sporting events either in person or watching on the television screen. Too few people of all ages do not have a personal commitment to physical activity and exercise and therefore do not actively participate.

A recent ILSI Europe Mini-Workshop on Overweight and Obesity in European children and adolescents concluded that a consensus on the definition of child obesity on the basis of BMI was not sufficient, especially for the monitoring of the secular increase in obesity prevalence. In most European countries there is significant variation in the prevalence of childhood obesity. Evidence presented at this meeting showed dietary patterns rather than simple energy intake may be responsible for children's obesity. In this respect more research is necessary. Regarding physical activity, more longitudinal studies are needed as changing demographic and social characteristics also play important roles in the changes to children's obesity.[42]

## 1.3   The Role of Lifestyle and the Mass Media in the Development and Prevention of Childhood Obesity

The lifestyle of most people in industrially developed countries is significantly influenced by the mass media. Due to the changing economic, social, and cultural situation in many countries of the Third World, the same factors may apply, especially for those in the higher social strata.

Paradoxically, the mass media, and particularly television, can play both positive and negative roles in the management of obesity during the growth period.[43] Many children and adolescents spend more time in front of the television and with computers and video games than in any other daily activity except sleep. A number of studies have confirmed that obesity is directly related to the number of hours spent watching television.[44-46] For many children, the world as displayed on television represents a greater reality than their wider "real world." For example, television stars are rarely obese; they generally represent the other end of the size and shape spectrum.

Further, the inactive behavior of television viewing is combined with frequent, very attractive commercials advertising food and drink.[47] Rather than promoting sound eating practices such advertisements more commonly promote foods that are not recommended for the optimal development of the health and fitness of children. Unfortunately, the power of advertising is such that young people are a captive audience and readily associate with the unfavorable practices that are presented, particularly involving highly processed and energy-dense foods.

Running in tandem with food advertisements is the portrayal and subsequent adoration of the ultra-slim, lean, and very tall "beautiful people" with bodily characteristics that approximate "Barbie" dolls.[48,49] Individuals with this shape represent an extremely small proportion of the normal population. Unfortunately, such images are powerful in the portrayal of an idealized shape. Those who attempt to make wholesale changes to size and shape to emulate a societal ideal may be at risk of serious nutritional problems such as anorexia nervosa, bulimia, bulirexia, and obesity. The extent of eating and weight disorders is poorly understood but the situation is clearly cause for concern in some places; for example, in the Czech population, about 5% of adolescents girls suffer from eating disorders.

Therefore, television reflects a cultural contradiction by promoting both food consumption and leanness.[31,50,51] However, there is an enormous reservoir of potential stimuli available for the wide spectrum of television viewers, both in the promotion of optimal nutrition for growing children as well as for the ecological sustainability of the food supply in the future.

The association between television viewing and obesity has been analyzed from the data collected during cycles II and III of the NHANES study. In all samples, significant associations between time spent watching television and the prevalence of obesity were revealed. The relationships were consistent even after controlling for a number of possible intervening factors studied simultaneously such as race, socioeconomic class, region, population density, family variables, season, and so on.[44] Television viewing was also positively associated with relative weight in Argentinian children and predicted the development of obesity 2 years later.[52]

Television commercials that encourage the consumption of poor quality but attractive foodstuffs may contribute to the development of obesity, particularly when the energy intake is not counterbalanced by an adequate energy output. It is well known that physically active people, particularly athletes, have more flexibility in terms of eating as a function of their large expenditure of energy. Such a lifestyle is certainly preferable as there is also a better chance of minimizing marginal or more serious vitamin and mineral deficiencies that could result if food intake were restricted.[53]

In fact, there is enormous potential for the media to portray attractive idols and their ways of life. For example, famous international movie stars and singers could be used to great effect to promote appropriate lifestyle practices such as optimal nutrition and exercise. Such individuals are able to perform at a high level and look attractive or glamorous, but at the same time, also achieve outstanding professional and social success including big earnings.

## 1.4 The Position of an Obese Child

The image of the obese child as "fat, friendless and unhealthy" is best prevented as early as possible. Societal perceptions of thinness and overweight echo the prejudices against the obese condition, even in very young children.[54] It is common for young girls to inappropriately judge their size and shape and have a greater than desirable perceived relevance of weight. Healthy eating is often confused with dieting, which is indicative of the need for better instruction on adequate eating and a more consistent presentation of the health implications of overweight in health promotion.

The conduct of research and the treatment of pediatric obesity have a long tradition in some countries.[24,55–57] Some new ideas and approaches have also appeared as the situation has worsened during the last decade. A large number of approaches to treatment and management have been developed to suit different contexts and psychosocial and economic costs.[58] New findings on selected factors such as insulin-like growth factor (IGF) and leptin may provide possibilities for future successes in the management of childhood obesity;[59] however, until now no positive results of leptin application have been found in the obese.

One of the main problems in obesity management is that no comprehensive explanations have been given for the significant increases in the condition during recent decades.[60] Therefore, there is no definite consensus on the main approaches to the treatment of obesity during growth. Major issues are the individuality of the particular obese child and the multi-factorial origin of the condition.

However, the best approach is the prevention of obesity by closely monitoring diet and physical activity levels from as early as possible in childhood, especially in children at risk;[2] for example, such individuals may include children with obese parents and a strong family history of obesity.[18,30,33,61]

---

## 1.5   Long-Term Consequences of Childhood Obesity

The association of long-term health risks with child and adolescent adiposity was reviewed by Power et al.[62] On the basis of large epidemiological studies, the child to adult adiposity relationship is now well documented, although methodological differences can hinder meaningful comparisons.[63] Fatter children are at a higher risk of becoming overweight or obese adults, despite the fact that correlations between, for example, BMI assessed at a younger age than 18 years and adult values are often only mild or moderate.

A study of Japanese youth showed that among obese subjects aged 17 years, most had tracked from the primary school or preschool. The earlier overweight or obesity commenced, the higher the BMI at the age of 17 years.[64]

The interference of many other factors along with increasing age may be responsible for this limited relationship. Therefore, more long-term studies are necessary to confirm the suggestion from some studies that adult disease risks are associated with a change in adiposity from normal weight in childhood to obesity in adulthood. However, population-based approaches to prevent and treat obesity are necessary for all age categories, as it is not only the obesity that starts during childhood that is problematic. Obesity that originates and develops at any period of life increases morbidity and mortality at any stage of the human ontogeny.

The prediction of adiposity in French adults from anthropometric measurements, including 4 skinfolds and BMI during childhood and adolescence was completed after 2 decades of follow-up. The best correlation between childhood and adulthood values in this population was found for BMI. Correlations between child and adult values of skinfolds were better in males than in females, especially for trunk skinfolds. In females, arm skinfold thickness, especially the biceps, showed a better predictive value than trunk skinfolds. Trunk skinfolds, which are more often associated with metabolic complications of obesity than limb skinfolds, are predictive from childhood measurements in males, but not in females.[65]

Assessment of BMI and skinfold thickness may facilitate the identification of children at greater risk of later obesity and the commencement of some preventive measures as early as possible. The utilization of natural approaches such as improvement of diet and physical activity is recommended in childhood and adolescence as they are far more preferable than the more drastic approaches for weight reduction when obesity is fully developed in later life. Epstein et al.[66] has suggested that targeting physical inactivity (such as television viewing and similar activities) along with an increase in vigorous activity is an important approach in the promotion of health and the prevention of obesity.

Contradictory opinions exist regarding whether obesity is preventable.[67] However, it is undisputed that it is possible to limit the deposition of excess fat by various procedures and therefore reduce additional health risks that may be even more dangerous. Finally, it must be stressed that starting a preventative approach as early as possible is always best.[18,30,33,51,61,68–70]

# 2

## Geographical, Historical, and Epidemiological Aspects

### 2.1 Changes in Obesity Prevalence and Accompanying Variables in Children during Recent Decades in Various Countries

The prevalence of childhood obesity varies in different populations. Some previously published results are difficult to interpret as different criteria and cut-off points were used for the definition of obesity. It is only recently that comparisons between studies and populations have become easier and this has corresponded with the utilization and widespread acceptance of the body mass index (BMI) as an indicator of body fatness.[16] Older studies did not use this criterion for the evaluation of obesity and its extent. Commonly, morphological characteristics of individuals' obesity have been used to categorize obesity.

The global prevalence of obesity has become the focus of attention for numerous countries and their respective professional and scientific bodies. Special attention of the World Health Organization (WHO) was given to this problem in some years but there has been a considerable worsening of the situation in the recent past.[16,71] An International Obesity Taskforce (IOTF) has been established and this initiative has the full support of the WHO. As a consequence of this interest, an increasing number of clinicians, general practitioners, nutritionists, dietitians, physiologists, and anthropologists are now working in the area of obesity prevention, treatment, and management. A major goal has been to define childhood obesity.

The confusion in the international literature has been substantially reduced since the acceptance in 1997 of the IOTF Childhood Obesity Working Group's decision to use BMI as an indicator of fatness in children and to develop a BMI-for-age reference chart.

The results of studies on the prevalence of obesity, physical activity, and preventive efforts have been recently compared between the United States and Europe.[72] As shown for MONICA (WHO monitoring of cardiovascular diseases project) populations, age-standardized proportions of BMI also vary for adults from country to country.

In adult males, the highest rates of obesity were found in Malta, in the region of Bas-Rhin in France, Kaunas (the former USSR, now Lithuania), the former Czechoslovakia (now the separate countries of the Czech Republic and Slovakia), and Germany. The lowest rates of obesity were found in China, Sweden, New Zealand, and Australia.

For adult females, the highest prevalence of obesity (BMI > 30) was also found in Kaunas, the Novosibirsk region, and Moscow (all former USSR), Poland, the former Czechoslovakia, and Italy. Lowest prevalence rates for females were also found in China. Otherwise, obesity prevalence was similar for both genders.[16] It should be remembered that these examples are for the years 1983–1986 and in China the situation has recently been in the process of change.[3,16]

Gurney and Gorstein evaluated the prevalence of obesity in preschool age children in selected countries and found the lowest prevalence in Papua New Guinea, Bangladesh, Philippines, Burkina Faso, and other developing countries.[71] The highest prevalence of obesity was found in Trinidad and Tobago, Iran, Mauritius, Canada, Jamaica, and Chile. However, not all countries included in MONICA studies were evaluated, which concerns especially the industrially developed countries.

More than 30% of the population in the Caribbean, the Middle East, Northern Africa, and Latin America is overweight. Inhabitats of Pacific and Indian Ocean islands are among those with the highest prevalence of obesity in the world. In Asia and black Africa, the overall prevalence of overweight is still low but the incidence is high in urban areas. In most of these countries, the increase in the number of overweight people has occurred within the last few years. Excess weight appears first among the affluent and then among lower income classes including young children and teenagers.

The main factors are a transition to a westernized diet with high lipids and reduced physical activity, particularly in the urban areas. Obesity and associated diseases could become even bigger problems in the future as malnutrition during the fetal period and early childhood is a predisposing factor for future obesity, often combined with stunting. The obesity problem and the economic costs of its management create an extra burden along with the existing malnutrition in these countries.[73]

## 2.1.1   North America

Obesity is most widespread in countries with the highest economic standards. For example, in the U.S. a significant increase (up to 30%) in the prevalence of obesity in children and adolescents has been evident in recent times. A comparison of the results of NHANES I and II showed an increase in the average values of BMI of the adult population and also an increase in the ratio of subjects with a BMI higher than 30. It has been shown that the problem is not limited to adults but is also an issue for young children. Most observations over time have not shown an increase in food intake, for example, comparisons between the 1970s and 1990s.[27,46,61,74]

Similar conclusions have been made on the basis of observations in other countries, such as Sweden.[75] An inadequate energy balance is due to both a reduction of energy output and restrictions in physical activity. This concerns the growing subjects of most socioeconomic levels in the industrially developed countries. The essential role of an inadequate macronutrient intake has also been defined.[76] The epidemiology of obesity is also related to nutrient intake.[77] An imbalance between the intake of protein, fat, and carbohydrate does not correspond to the RDAs of WHO, EU, and particular countries.

Secular changes in the trends for obesity prevalence were demonstrated by the Bogalusa Heart Study at the end of the 1980s. Height and weight were assessed in 5- to 14-year-old children, from 1973 to 1984. The age- and gender-specific 85th percentiles were used as the cut-off points for the ponderal index (weight/height$^3$). Secular trends for the increase of weight (2.5 kg), and ponderosity (0.5–0.7 kg/m$^3$) were revealed. Gains in ponderosity over the 11-year period were greater at the 75th percentile than at the 25th percentile. The prevalence of overweight increased from 15 to 24%.[78]

Further measurements have confirmed this trend. Data from national surveys in the United States indicate that the prevalence of obesity has increased during the last decades. As criteria for overweight and/or obesity, the 85th (obesity) and 95th percentiles (super-obesity) of triceps skinfold have been used. Compared with skinfold data from the 1963 to 1965 National Health Examination Survey (NHES), the 1976 to 1980 NHES indicates a 54% increase in the prevalence of obesity among children aged 6 to 11 and a 98% increase in the prevalence of super-obesity.

Compared with skinfold data from the 1966 to 1970 NHES, cycle 3 skinfold data from the second NHES indicate a 39% increase in the prevalence of obesity among children 12 to 17 years old and a 64% increase in the prevalence of super-obesity. The increase in the obesity prevalence was apparent in all age categories and both genders and was also the same for white and black subjects. Blood pressure data from the four surveys mentioned suggest that the share of pediatric hypertension associated with obesity in children has increased. According to the speed of changes in the prevalence of obesity, environmental causes are more likely to be responsible than changes in genetic and hereditary factors.[45]

The NHES were executed in five representative cross-sectional studies with an in-person interview and medical examination from 1963 to 1991. The periods were 1963 to 1965, 1966 to 1970, 1971 to 1974, 1976 to 1980, and 1988 to 1991. From 1988 to 1991, the prevalence of overweight according to the BMI was 10.9% based on the 95th percentile, and 22% based on the 85th percentile. Overweight prevalence increased during the examined period among all age and gender groups.

The increase was greatest between 1976 to 1980, similar to findings reported previously for U.S. adults. This increase of overweight among youth indicates the need for an increased focus on the prevention of the problem.[79,80] Associated negative phenomena in the growing population includes the decline of fitness in American children as discussed by other authors.[81]

Numerous observations have confirmed that overweight during childhood and adolescence is associated with overweight during adulthood. Previous reports have documented an increase in the prevalence of overweight among growing subjects and adults during the periods 1976 to 1980 and 1988 to 1991. The third National Health and Nutrition Examination Survey (NHANES III), which provided results of assessments from 1988 to 1994, is the more recent set of estimates of overweight among U.S. children aged 6 to 11 years, and adolescents aged 12 to 17 years. The results of this study indicate that the prevalence of overweight in the U.S. has continued to increase.

During the last 20 years, the prevalence of overweight has also increased in U.S. children aged 4 to 5 years of age. A comparable finding was not revealed in children aged 1 to 3 years. From 1971 through 1974, 5.8% of 4- to 5-year-old girls were obese, in contrast to 10% from 1988 through 1994. During the period 1988 to 1994, the prevalence of overweight among children from 2 months through to 5 years of age was consistently higher in girls than boys. Mexican-American children had a higher prevalence of overweight than non-Hispanic black and non-Hispanic white children.

These results parallel those reported for older children and adults in the U.S.[82] The prevalence of overweight among low-income U.S. preschool children in the follow-up studies of the Centers for Disease Control and Prevention Pediatric Nutrition Surveillance System increased from 18.6% in 1983 to 21.6% in 1995 (based on the 85th percentile cut-off point for weight-for-height, and from 8.5 to 10.2% for the same period based on the 95th percentile cut-off point).

Analyses by single age, sex, and race or ethnic group (non-Hispanic white, non-Hispanic black, and Hispanic) all showed increases in the prevalence of overweight although changes were greatest for older preschool children.[83] The level of economic and social class had no significant effect on the increasing prevalence of overweight in 4- to 5-year-old children in this study.

The results of the National Heart, Lung and Blood Institute's Growth and Health Study (NGHS) population at baseline, compared with the data of the two National Health and Nutrition Examination Surveys (NHANES I and II) in young black and white girls, revealed secular trends of obesity prevalence. Anthropometric measures, height, weight, and triceps and subscapular skinfolds were assessed, and body mass index (BMI) was calculated. Compared with age-similar girls in the 1970s, girls in the present study were taller and heavier and had thicker skinfolds. The differences in body size were most apparent in black girls who had a greater body mass than white girls as early as 9 to 10 years of age.

The prevalence of obesity also appears to be increasing among younger girls, especially black girls.[84] This situation is interpreted as an imminent health risk for these individuals in later life. In conjunction with these findings, poor childhood nutrition resulting in overweight and obesity and adult cardiovascular diseases are considered to be closely related.[85]

According to a 1995 National Center for Health Statistics study, 4.7 million American children aged 6 to 17 years were severely overweight. Another estimate from the New Jersey Department of Health and Senior Services indicated that one in four children weighs too much.[86] In addition to the increasing prevalence of obesity in adults, these results are a disturbing trend. If obesity commences in childhood, there are more serious health consequences than if obesity develops during adulthood.

Black and white 9- and 10-year-old U.S. females were followed longitudinally each year during a 5-year period. Parents were seen in year one and responded to a questionnaire in years three and five. Initial values for height, weight, BMI, and skinfold thickness were higher in black compared to white girls. On the basis of dietary history, black females consumed a greater amount of energy and a larger proportion was fat. White females were physically more active and spent less time watching television than black females. More black than white females expressed a desire to be "on the fat side," and body weight of black mothers was approximately 20 pounds higher than that of white mothers.[87] Findings from studies in the 1980s revealed that nearly half of the black American females were obese, and that adolescence is a critical period for the development of obesity.

The prevalence of obesity in American Indians is 13.7% for men and 16.5% for women. Obesity rates for Indian adolescents and preschool children are higher than the respective rates for all races combined.[88] In the native population of Navajo adolescents, 33% of the girls and 25% of the boys were obese according to the BMI criterion. Navajo youth tended to have larger skinfolds than their white (NHANES II) and Mexican American (Hispanic Health and Nutrition Examination Survey) counterparts.

A greater difference in the subscapular skinfold measurement is indicative of greater deposits of truncal vs. peripheral fat. In girls, BMI was positively related to systolic and diastolic blood pressure. In boys, systolic blood pressure was only higher in subjects with a higher BMI.[89] This study indicates the urgent need for interventions in Navajo children and youth as obesity is a significant health risk for blood pressure, as is the case in the white population. Similar conclusions have been drawn for other American Indian and Mexican-American children.[90,91]

The Hispanic Health and Nutritional Examination Survey (1982 to 1984) provided data on BMI, triceps and subscapular skinfolds and showed that in the U.S., Hispanics had a higher prevalence of overweight and obesity than whites. The prevalence in children was assumed to be similar to that in adults. In Mexican-American preschool children, obese subjects had a significantly higher birth weight and the mothers of obese children had a significantly greater BMI.

Analyses of responses to the ideal infant body habitus scale revealed that mothers of obese children selected a chubby baby as ideal significantly more often than mothers of non-obese children.[92] This could influence feeding habits and food intake of obese children early in their lives.

Attitudes and behavior related to nutrition vary significantly in white and black American adolescents and are also in contrast to the same characteristics in other countries. For example, Russian adolescents prefer a larger body size, are also less likely to diet, and are less concerned about being overweight. A study of Moscow students using questionnaires showed that the ideal weight was higher in black American boys and girls than in white American and Russian boys and girls. After controlling for BMI, black American girls were less than half as likely to report dieting compared with white American girls. There were significant differences between white American girls and Russian girls, and there was no ethnic difference among boys in the prevalence of dieting. White American girls and black American girls were much more likely to identify being overweight as an important nutritional concern than were Russian girls.[93]

The NHLBI Growth and Health study showed that at an early age black girls were more likely to engage in eating practices associated with weight gain. These included eating in front of the television, eating while doing homework, and skipping meals. Such practices may have implications for obesity development.[94] Along with the differences in the prevalence of obesity, for example, among Caucasian and African-American girls, it has also been shown that children who suffered neglect or abuse are also more likely to become overweight.[63]

The prevalence of obesity is higher in low-income and multi-ethnic Montreal school children. Diet and physical activity assessment in these children showed different patterns related to environmental conditions. Height, weight, dietary intake, physical activity record, lifestyle, and demographic characteristics were evaluated. 39.4% of children were overweight, higher than the 85th percentile of NHANES II.

Dietary fat intake was significantly higher in children from single-parent families and those with mothers born in Canada. Intake of vitamins was related to income level. Children who were more active had a higher intake of energy, calcium, iron, zinc, and fiber, but were not heavier. Overweight children systematically under-reported their food intakes and their reported intakes did not meet calculated energy needs. This situation makes it difficult to define the reason for energy imbalance and an enhanced deposition of fat.[95] It must be stressed that inadequate reporting is also possible in relation to the specific intensity, character, and duration of physical activity.

### 2.1.2 Latin America

Excessive fatness was found in 6.4% of the population of Argentinian children aged 6 to 12 years who were evaluated using local standards and Frisancho's norms for U.S. children. In this population the prevalence of obesity was generally below the expected values. However, the frequency of excessive fatness was significantly higher in the 8- to 11-year-old male group (8.9%) and in the girls (10.8%). The prevalence of fatness increased with age in girls and from the age of 8 years onward they exceeded the expected percentage.[96]

As a result of an anthropometric survey in Cuba the prevalence of overweight in preschool children from birth to 5 years of age was identified as the most frequent nutritional problem, with a prevalence of 5.2%. Of great importance, the prevalence of malnutrition, both chronic and acute, was reduced significantly (by 44.4%) in Cuba between the years 1972 and 1993.[97]

Obesity prevalence in Chile is also relatively high and increasing at a rapid rate. As reported by some observers, girls show higher rates than boys. First graders have a higher prevalence of obesity, a result that is probably due to their higher socioeconomic background.[98]

The nutritional status of children in an area of São Paolo (Brazil) was assessed by considering the distribution of z-scores of weight-for-age, height-for-age, and weight-for-height, in relation to growth charts of the NCHS reference population. Children were further sub-grouped according to socioeconomic status: 22% of children were stunted, 15% wasted, 22% underweight, and 5% overweight. Data were further analyzed by age, gender, ethnic group, and socioeconomic level; 32% of the very low socioeconomic group were both stunted and low weight-for-age. A total of 11.6% from the high socioeconomic strata were obese. These results emphasize the need for a range of programs to deal with nutritional problems in different groups of the population such as in Brazil.[99]

Nutrition transition can significantly influence the nutritional status in all age categories, including children. In Brazil, malnutrition is a major problem; however, obesity is the leading health issue among both adults and children in the urban areas of the south and southeast and in the rural south. Only in the rural northeast, the poorest region in the country, was malnutrition the main problem in children.[100] Similar to other countries, the economic situation has an important effect. However, this only applies within the framework of a certain range of nutrition and malnutrition.

### 2.1.3  Europe

The Belgian-Luxembourg Child Study was executed in an area with a cluster of obesity as well as other risk factors for cardiovascular diseases and non-insulin dependent diabetes (NIDDM). This study confirmed the important role of an increased BMI at a young age and later health development. In the initial phases of this study, children aged 6 to 12 years of age showed that the BMI of children was significantly related to birth weight in boys, but not in girls in the same age groups.

Blood pressure, fasting plasma triglycerides (TG), and insulin, but not blood glucose and total cholesterol (TC), increased significantly with higher BMI quintiles. These relationships were most pronounced for the fifth quintile of BMI. No significant relationship was found for BMI and breastfeeding, social or educational status of the parents, or estimated physical activity.[101]

The continuation of the above-mentioned study with children from 6 to 12 years of age revealed that BMI was strongly correlated between the children and both parents, and parents and grandparents.[102]

The Belgian-Luxembourg Child Study IV revealed a changed pattern of food intake and an increase in the prevalence of overweight.[103] Similar results were found in other industrially developed countries, for example, in Switzerland where there was a doubling in the proportion of obese children of both genders in the pre- and postpubertal periods.[104]

From 1975 to 1989 there was an increase in the prevalence of obese pupils in Hamburg, Germany, from 4 to 11%. Sequentially, the following age differentiation was reported. Overweight was diagnosed in 6.3% of preschool children, at approximately 10 years of age 17.2%, and in children aged approximately 14 years, 17.3%. The effect of social class was apparent both in the prevalence of obesity and in enrollment in regular exercise. In the low socioeconomic districts the reverse was noted; the rate of overweight and obese children was higher and enrollment in sports activity was lower. In high social class districts, the rate of overweight and obese children was lower and the rate of children involved in sports higher.[105]

In the eastern part of Germany (the former German Democratic Republic), there were significant changes in subcutaneous fat and BMI, especially between 1985 and 1995. Height increased less than body weight; BMI therefore increased significantly. The amount of subcutaneous fat increased, along with changes in its distribution. The ratio of trunk to extremity skinfolds decreased significantly between 1985 and 1996. Changes in nutritional habits and lifestyle, obviously related to the reunification of Germany in 1989, may be the reason for these changes.[106]

Marked increases in obesity prevalence have also occurred in the adult English population when values are compared between 1980 and 1991.[107] Lack of physical activity was considered one of the most important causes. On average, energy intake decreased during the same period. Trends in weight-for-height and triceps skinfold thickness were followed for English and Scottish children from 1972 to 1982 and from 1982 to 1990, in the framework of the National Study of Health and Growth. Data from 1972, 1982, and 1990 in children aged 4.5 and 11.99 years were compared. It was shown that all measurements increased from 1972 to 1990 except for weight-for-height in English boys, and that the increments were generally greater when comparing the measurements from 1982 to 1990 to those from 1972 to 1982.

Approximately one third of the increase in weight-for-height and triceps skinfold thickness from 1972 to 1990 was associated with increases in parental body mass indices and decreases in family size. No consistent differences in trends were found between social groups. More significant trends were found for girls and for Scottish children; Scottish boys are now heavier and fatter than their English counterparts.[108]

The values of height, weight, and body fat measured by bioimpedance analysis (BIA) in Scottish children were compared with the baseline values of Fomon et al.[109] after 12 months. All measures increased; the mean change in the percentage of body fat was +2.8% in girls and +1.8% in boys, although 21% of girls and 25% of boys decreased the percentage of depot fat over the 12 months of observation. No gender differences in height and weight were observed at either measurement. Compared with the values assessed by Fomon et al.,[109] children were taller and heavier, had a similar percentage of stored fat at the age of 7 years, but a greater percentage of fat at the age of 8 years.[110]

A study of the prevalence of obesity in French children showed an increase from 5.1 to 12.7% (Figure 2.1). In both adults and children, very severe obesity was about five times as frequent in 1996 than it was in 1980. The prevalence of obesity is still lower in France compared to other industrially developed countries. However, increase in prevalence and the overall trend in this respect is stimulating more and more of an interest in this health problem in France.[111]

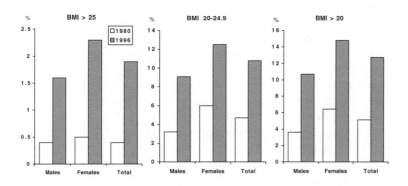

**FIGURE 2.1**
The changes in the prevalence of obesity (%) in French children during the period from 1980 to 1996. (Based on data from Ref. F1.)

An increase in pediatric obesity in French children from 1980 to 1990 (> 90th percentile of BMI) was 17%, and for super-obesity (> 97th percentile of BMI), 20%.[112] From 1976 to 1995, the prevalence of obesity in 10-year-old children increased from 6.3 to 14.4%. In addition, fatness and food intake and the composition of food have become more important issues.[113]

These increased trends in the prevalence of obesity[114] are consistent with those revealed in the U.S. and in Denmark. However, in France, severe obesity increased more than mild obesity. These changes are derived from an altered skewness of the distribution.[112] The prevalence of obesity in Danish recruits increased 50 times during the post-war period, from 0.1 to 5%.[115]

The prevalence of obesity also appears to have increased in other Eastern European countries.[116,117] In Russian adolescents, a different attitude about overweight and obesity was also evident.[93] Observations in 23,462 Bulgarian children and adolescents (BMI, skinfolds) showed several peaks in the prevalence of obesity at different ages. The first peak occurred between the ages of 3 to 6 years and reached 10%. The second peak occurred from 10 to 12 years, and reached 12 to 14% and coincided with the beginning of puberty. The third peak was between 15 and 17 years of age and was more obvious among boys. In more than 80% of cases, obesity started to develop at an early age, during the first 7 years of life.[118]

In the Czech Republic, BMI values increased from 1945 to 1952. From 1961 to 1991, and up to 1995, the prevalence of obesity based on average values of basic morphological parameters has not changed.[119] In girls, the continued trend of a reduction of overweight was observed. A recent comparison of BMI values of Czech and English children did not show any significant differences.[120]

In Austria, Elmadfa et al.[121] showed that the prevalence of obesity increased from 19% in the age range of 7 to 9 years to 29% in the range of 15 to 19 years in boys. In girls, the prevalence of obesity decreased from 16 to 13% in the same age intervals. Later it was revealed that the prevalence of obese children was approximately 5 to 8%.[122]

Overweight in children and adolescents accounted for about 8% of the entire population in the country. Furthermore, it is of great interest that there is no marked change in the percentage of subjects who can be classified as overweight or obese in the different age categories. Another estimate for Austrian children is 12 to 15% in 11- to 18-year-old youth.[122]

The prevalence of obesity also varies in different parts of countries where the environmental conditions are less homogeneous. For example, in a small rural community of Lazio (Italy), prevalence was 17.7%. Food intake of children 7 to 14 years old showed an imbalance of nutrients.[123] On the other hand, the prevalence of obesity in Roman adolescents was 6.9%. This was not particularly high compared to other localities in Italy and other industrially developed countries.[124] However, food composition was inadequate, with a high fat intake to the detriment of carbohydrates and starches. This might have a negative effect later in life.

A high prevalence of obesity was also found in the child population aged 9.6 years living in Naples, Italy.[125] The percentile values for triceps skinfold thickness were similar to those reported for other populations of children but BMI values were different. Children in Naples have the highest BMI values at the 50th, 75th, 90th, and 95th percentiles.

The prevalence of obesity among Neapolitan children was estimated using the BMI value at the 90th percentile as a cut-off. The comparisons revealed that the prevalence of obesity in Neapolitan girls was 5.2 times as high as in France, 3.3 times as high as in Holland, 1.7 times as high as in the U.S., and 2.5 times as high as in Milan, Italy. Among boys it was 4.3 times as high as in France, 4.0 times as high as in Holland, 2.1 times as high as in the U.S., and 2.5 times as high as in Milan.[125]

An update of obesity in childhood was also completed in one district of Rome.[126] The obese group was more represented in 8- to 9-year-old children. When overweight and obese children were evaluated together, these subjects represented more than 50% of all children followed in this study. These results indicate the alarming problem of pediatric obesity in the city.[126]

A cross-sectional epidemiological study that included anthropometric measurements and dietary surveys was undertaken with Spanish children aged 6 to 13 years. The prevalence of obesity in this community was 26%, which was considerably higher than the national average (6 to 15% in 1991 using the same criteria). The most important factors contributing to the development of obesity were low levels of physical activity, and genetic and environmental factors influenced by conditioned eating behavior.[127]

A study of Catalonian adolescents showed 15% were obese; 13.5% presented with Grade I obesity (BMI 25 to 29.9 kg.m2), and 1.3% presented with Grade II obesity (BMI 30 to 40 kg.m$^{-2}$). Obese subjects were more likely to show concern for their diet. The results of this study showed a lower prevalence of obesity in Spain than in the U.S. There was no linear relationship between the degree of excess weight and the restraint boundary in regard to eating behavior.[128] However, in some Spanish communities the prevalence of obesity in growing subjects can be higher, for example, 26%, which exceeds the national average mentioned above.

In Yugoslavia, overweight (that is, +1 to +2 SD) was registered in 19.4% of children in a sample of the national survey of children under 5 years of age;[129] 12.9% of children included in this study were above +2 SD relative to the reference weight for height value, and 5% were above +3 SD. The prevalence of obesity was highest in children aged 2 to 3 years (17.8%) while variations by gender were not significant. Regional distribution showed the highest prevalence of overweight (16.7%) and obese children (17.2%) in the Belgrade area where 8% of the whole sample had a weight-for-height +3 SD over the reference values.[129]

In representative samples of children aged 6 to 18 years from three cities in northern Yugoslavia, a relatively high prevalence of overweight and obesity was revealed when using different standards as criteria (WHO/NCHS standards and BMI NHANES using the software, CHILD). Using BMI criteria, the prevalence of overweight was 12.9% in boys and 12.0% in girls, and the prevalence of obesity was 8.76% in boys and 9% in girls.[130] Unbalanced nutrition had an effect on the nutritional status of these children, which was also reflected in an increased ratio of health risks (increased level of serum total cholesterol (TC) in 11.9%, low HDL-C in 16%, high LDL-C in 21.7%, and hypertriglyceridemia in 30% of subjects).[131]

A statistically significant difference between urban and rural children in the Skopje region of Macedonia was found with a greater prevalence of overweight in the urban area. In both groups, serum triglycerides were higher in obese children. The same trend was identified in the observed association between the nutritional status and HDL-C levels, where a greater percentage of the obese urban children had lower values of HDL-C.[132]

Environmental conditions in the Arctic region of Finland may be the cause of early maturation associated with higher BMI and a body fat distribution with a higher amount of trunk fat during adolescence, leading to overweight and obesity. However, it is not clear whether early maturation is a causal factor or the result of the conditions in this region.[133]

In Denmark, the prevalence of obesity defined by the 99.9 or 99.0 percentile of BMI has increased in boys born in the 1940s and since the mid-1960s. This occurred without corresponding changes in the central part of the BMI distribution. When the obesity cut-off was the 95th percentile, there was a sharp, distinct age-dependent increase in the late 1940s.[134] These results indicate that the obesity epidemic is a heterogeneous phenomenon resulting from environmental effects starting with preschool age individuals, and influencing various sets of population in different ways. This is due to varying sensitivities and predispositions of particular individuals, as well as different exposures to the effects of the environment including nutrition and physical activity level (PAL).

## 2.1.4   Asia

Childhood obesity is also a fast emerging problem in Asia.[135] Results gleaned from studies of Chinese children in 1985–1986 were compared with those of the present day. The prevalence of obesity was 5% in 1998 compared with 2.1% in Beijing in 1986, and 0.9% in all cities studied in 1985. Significant relationships among infantile obesity, consumption of junk food, and physical inactivity ($p < 0.05$, $p < 0.01$) were noted. In China, television viewing was not yet associated with obesity.[136]

The patterns and correlates of obesity in China were also considered in the framework of a national longitudinal survey (the China Health and Nutrition Survey) conducted in 1989 and 1991. In adults, BMI was positively correlated with energy and fat intakes. Household income and physical activity were also significantly associated with BMI. Those living in an urban environment with a higher income displayed lower energy intake, higher fat intake, and lower physical activity levels compared to those in rural settings and other income categories.[137,138]

In countries where food insecurity and malnutrition have had detrimental effects on child growth and metabolic processes, increased accessibility and choice of various foodstuffs including those with high fat and energy, along with sedentary lifestyles introduced during recent periods, may promote obesity development.[138] This also applies to the stunted children suffering from malnutrition during earlier periods of growth.

Elementary school children in Tokyo were examined for nutritional status and obesity prevalence. The intake of lipids exceeded the recommended levels. Mean BMI and Rohrer's Index scores were slightly higher than Japanese standards. With these parameters for obesity, triglycerides (TG) and the atherogenic index were positively correlated, and HDL-C and HDL-C/TC were negatively correlated with obesity.[139]

Comparisons of the prevalence of overweight (BMI over 21) in Japanese and Korean junior high school pupils showed a higher prevalence in Korean girls. No differences were found in boys. Body fat measured by BIA in Japanese children was significantly higher than that of Korean children due to a greater lean body mass in Korean subjects, especially in girls. Further observation in younger age categories showed a lack of difference in certain food habits (such as intake of snacks and sweet drinks), but Korean pre-schoolers spent more time playing outdoors than their Japanese peers.[140]

A cross-sectional growth survey in Hong Kong from birth to 18 years enabled the refinement of weight-for-age and weight-for-height percentile charts for boys and girls. There was an average increase of 8.5 kg and 5.1 kg in the 18-year-old boys and girls, respectively, compared to those surveyed 30 years ago. The percentile curves between 6 and 18 years were similar to those of Singapore. Weight-for-height percentile curves were also similar to those of American children in the prepubertal years.[141] Health risks of obesity were also comparable to those revealed in other parts of the world.[142]

According to an island-wide survey in Taiwan, the prevalence of obesity varied from 4.3 to 17.4% in children aged 3 to 19 years. The weight-for-height index was used for assessment as local BMI standards were not available. Obese children had a high prevalence of hypertension, hyperlipidemia, and abnormal glucose metabolism. Colored striae located predominantly on the thighs, arms, and abdomen were also often found.[143]

Malaysian preschool children aged 3 to 6 years showed significantly more severe grades of obesity compared to Chinese and Japanese children of the same age in Singapore.[144] In Asian countries such as Thailand, with rapidly growing economies and changing lifestyles, obesity has become a serious problem. A study was executed in 6- to 12-year-old children and the preva-lence of obesity (as diagnosed by weight-for-height greater than 120% of the Bangkok reference) rose from 12.2% in 1991 to 13.5% in 1992 and to 15.6% in 1993.

However, obese children who attended a weight control program showed body weight and triceps skinfold thickness increases that were significantly less in the first year than in children of the non-attendees, and also during the second year when the differences were less apparent.[145] The effect of changes in nutrition due to transition and acculturation to a different lifestyle has been noted, as is the case in other similar countries.

The prevalence of obesity in Bombay was analyzed and related to age group, income, diet type, family history, and occupation. The usual criteria of BMI underestimated, and that of body fat content overestimated the preva-lence of obesity. This result indicates the variable character of morphological development in different parts of the world, and can also lead to a misinter-pretation of the values in India.

Students had the lowest (10.7%) and medical doctors the highest (53.1%) prevalence of obesity. Prevalence was positively associated with financial income and family history. This study shows the extent of the obesity prob-lem in Bombay and provides direction for nutritional planning in the future.[146] Some comparisons show that the prevalence of obesity in Asian countries in the higher socioeconomic groups is very similar to those found in the U.S. and other industrialized countries.

## 2.1.5   Middle East, Africa, and Oceania

Measurements in Israeli high school girls showed 17% were obese. A much larger percentage expressed dissatisfaction with their body weights and shapes. Comparisons with earlier studies in Israel indicate a large increase in concern for weight and dieting behaviors, with prevalence rates similar to those reported in other Western countries.[147]

The assessment of BMI in Lebanese adolescent girls showed that the mean BMI value in each age range was situated between the corresponding 90th and 97th percentile of the French reference population. The mean percentage of adolescent girls with severe obesity was 11%.[148] Obesity among secondary school students in Bahrain, aged 15 to 21 years, revealed a prevalence of 15.6% of boys and 17.4% of girls who were either overweight or obese, according to BMI. Family size, parents' education, and family history of obesity were significantly associated with obesity among boys, while family history was the only socioeconomic factor significantly related to obesity among girls. Patterns such as eating between meals, number of meals per day, and the method of eating were not associated with obesity in Bahraini subjects, but boys who ate alone were three times more likely to be obese than those who ate with family members.[149]

School children in Cairo aged 11 to 16 years were evaluated for nutritional status using measurements of weight, height, and skinfold thickness. A triceps skinfold greater than 18 mm in boys and 35 mm in girls was considered as a lower level of obesity. Age at menarche, birth order, social class, obesity in other members of the family, food habits, and dietary intakes were also followed up. The results showed that the prevalence of obesity in Egyptian children in the capital was comparable to that in the U.S. The study also emphasized the importance of social and cultural factors in the development of childhood obesity in Egypt, however, the situation may be different in rural areas.[150]

In Cameroon, the level of urbanization is one of the highest in sub-Saharan Africa. Dramatic demographic changes facilitate modifications in lifestyle, notably in nutritional patterns. Rapid shifts in the composition of diet and activity patterns plus subsequent changes in body composition may contribute to the increased prevalence of obesity and related adverse health effects.

In a Youandee population, 18.2% of girls and 1.7% of boys aged 12 to 19 years were obese. In children aged 9 to 11 years, 3.3% of boys and girls were overweight, lower than in France and the U.S. Menarche in this population appears to be linked to the increased prevalence of overweight with a dramatic increase from premenarcheal to postmenarcheal status.[151]

A survey of anthropometric profiles, expressed in terms of the National Centre for Health Statistics (NCHS) standards conducted in the Cape Town metropolitan area in 1990, revealed evidence of growth retardation and wasting in this population. These features coexisted with an emergent obesity among 3- to 6-year-old children.[152]

A dramatic increase in the prevalence of obesity was also seen in Western Samoa during the period 1978–1991. Great differences in the prevalence of obesity (BMI > 30) were found between urban and rural populations in 1978. In 1991, the prevalence of obesity was greater in urban than in rural areas. By contrast, waist-to-hip ratio (WHR) varied little between each area. Even in subjects aged 25 to 34 years, more than 50% of women from each location and 45% of urban men were obese. Increased physical activity in men, but not in women, was associated with lower values of BMI. Increased levels of education and professional work were associated with increasing BMI, but only significant in men. Multi-variate analysis showed age, location (urban), occupation (high status, women), and in men, physical inactivity, to be independently associated with increased risk of obesity. It can be speculated that a comparable increase in obesity prevalence for children and adolescents may also be a concern in this country.[153]

Similar changes were described in coastal and highland Papua New Guinea.[154] The association between obesity and individual degree of modernization was investigated. A modernity score was gained based on the area of origin, father's employment, type and duration of individual's employment, education, years spent in an urban center, housing type, and spouse score. More "modern" subjects had higher mean BMIs and lower levels of physical activity. Mean WHR also varied with modernity in men, but not in women. In a linear regression analysis, total modernity score was significantly associated with both BMI and WHR in men and women.[154] When components of modernity were examined, younger age, more sophisticated housing, and increasing number of years in an urban center were independently associated with BMI in both genders, while education level and reduced physical activity were also significant predictors in men. Associations with WHR were weaker.

A sub-study of dietary intake suggested that the lowest intake occurred in the least modern subjects of both genders. Children and adolescents were not included in this study but a similar situation regarding the effect of modernity may be assumed during growth period. The adoption of Western ways, which are associated with physical inactivity and increased availability of energy-dense Western food, has already promoted obesity in this rapidly developing Pacific region.[154]

### 2.1.6  Australia

There is evidence that the prevalence of obesity in Australian children is increasing. Trend data support substantial increases in BMI between 1985 and 1997 consistent with the situation in other parts of the world. The work of an Australian research group has made a significant contribution to decision making regarding the measurement of childhood obesity.[155,156]

A very recent study (the New South Wales Schools Fitness and Physical Activity Survey) showed no difference between anthropometric measures when comparing urban and rural boys and girls. Only the WHR ratio was higher in urban girls. Among boys, there were no differences between the socioeconomic status (SES) tertiles in any of the parameters measured (height, weight, waist and hip girths, skinfolds). In girls, each of the anthropometric measures except skinfolds was negatively related to SES. Girls from the highest SES group tended to be less fat than those from the lowest tertile of SES.[157]

## 2.2   Problems of Obesity in Third World Countries

### 2.2.1   Prevalence

Obesity among smaller children has appeared more frequently in Third World countries. These findings have commonly been seen in children from families in higher socioeconomic categories, for example, children in Cairo and elsewhere.[143,150] The lifestyle characterizing these individuals is very similar to the situation in the industrially developed countries.[158]

Generally, children in developing countries have very different problems than those in developed countries as they are subjected to poor nutrition and health care. Traditionally, such children have exhibited a relatively low prevalence of obesity irrespective of the criteria used. According to WHO and NCHS 50th percentile, 20 to 30% of children are stunted at the age of 2 to 3 years. While childhood obesity is not usually associated with such growth patterns, a high prevalence of female adolescent obesity has been reported.

### 2.2.2   Obesity and Stunting

Excess deposition of fat can occur in subjects whose height was delayed by early malnutrition and who became stunted. If the availability of food improved and children resumed a more consistent energy intake, they could become quite obese because of a shorter stature that usually did not catch up. This phenomenon has been seen in growing subjects in China, Brazil, Cameroon, etc.[159–161] An increased risk of obesity in stunted children was also reported in Hispanic, Jamaican, and Andean populations.

A study by Popkin et al.[138,159] analyzed the relationship between stunting and the overweight status of children aged 3 to 6 and 7 to 9 years in nationally representative surveys in Russia, Brazil, and the Republic of Southern Africa, and a nationwide survey in China. Identical cut-off criteria for BMI were used for each of the populations mentioned. The prevalence of overweight in these countries ranged from 10.5 to 25.0% (based on the 85th percentile). Recent NHANES III results indicate that the prevalence is around 22% in the U.S.

Stunting was common in the surveyed countries and affected 9.2 to 30.6% of all children. A significant association between stunting and overweight was observed. The income-adjusted risk ratios for overweight for a stunted child ranged from 1.7 to 7.8. When sufficient food is available, an important association between stunting and increased weight-for-height can appear and applies to the populations of various ethnic, environmental, and social backgrounds. This association can have serious public health implications, especially for lower income countries that have recently experienced significant changes in dietary and activity patterns.[159]

The underlying mechanisms have not been fully explored. Results of experiments in pigs malnourished *in utero* and/or over 1, 2, or 3 years indicate the pigs were retarded in growth and became smaller adults. The longer the period of undernutrition, the greater the impact on the length of the body. Limbs were progressively smaller the fatter the animals became. The standard measurements of the thickness of the subcutaneous fat layer in these animals did not provide a true picture of how fat the animals became. The muscles in the animals rehabilitated after 2 and 3 years of undernutrition were so infiltrated with fat that the muscle fibers were completely embedded within it.[162]

This raises an important question regarding the development of fat cells. It has been suggested that overfeeding in infancy causes rapid multiplication of cells in the adipose tissue which in turn leads to an excessive number of fat cells resulting in adult obesity.[163–166] The finding in pigs suggests that the opposite can also be true. The animals studied had cells full of fat at 10 days of age when undernutrition began, but these cells became completely empty and remained so for the entire period of undernutrition, whether it lasted 1, 2, or 3 years. The pigs began to deposit fat rapidly in their bodies as soon as plentiful food was supplied and the longer the period of deprivation the fatter they tended to become.

Marasmic children may also become fat when they are rehabilitated but there is little information on the number of adipose tissue cells before and after rehabilitation. Brook's hypothesis on the sensitive period for fat cell multiplication during the first year of life in man could lead to the conclusion that children who are severely malnourished during the first year of life develop less than the average final number of fat cells.[166] Alternatively, this may occur, but like pigs they may lay down fat rapidly when rehabilitated. Deposition of fat during such a situation is more rapid after the period of severe malnutrition than the rehabilitation of other tissues of the body as shown in adults.[167]

Problems concerning the effects of early nutrition on the deposition of fat in the body, and the number of cells in the adipose tissue produced to accommodate this fat, have yet to be resolved and deserve some primary attention by scientists. Delayed effects of early nutritional factors can explain some of the contradictions concerning, for example, obesity prevalence under comparable conditions, which was impossible to interpret until recently.

Studies on the population of children in a shantytown in São Paolo showed that nutritional stunting may increase the risk of obesity. To elucidate the mechanism of the relationship between stunting and obesity, a 22-month longitudinal study was executed in two groups of girls aged 7 to 11 years, one with mild stunting but normal weight-for-height, and a control group with normal weight and height. The energy and macro-component intake and energy output were comparable in both groups. The same applied to their insulin-like growth factor (IGF-1) levels that were below the normal range. A significant positive relationship between baseline IGF-1 and the change in height-for-age during the study was found in all subjects combined.

Another significant association was found during the follow-up between the baseline percentage of dietary energy supplied by fat and the gain in weight-for-height in girls with mild stunting but not in the normal control girls. The slope of these relationships was not significantly different. These results raise the question of whether the mildly stunted children may increase their susceptibility to excess fat deposition due to a diet with high fat. The etiological role of low levels of IGF-1 should also be considered in this respect.[168]

In the industrially developed countries similar associations are revealed. For example, the high prevalence of overweight and short stature among children involved in the Head Start program in Massachusetts.[169] Prevalence varied by race and ethnicity with a statistically significant upward trend in overweight among Hispanic children in this study. Children 4 years of age or older were more likely than younger children to become overweight. The prevalence of short stature did not vary significantly by year, gender, or age.[169]

## 2.3   The Effect of Acculturation on Obesity in Children

The trend of obesity development due to acculturation seems to be changing in some developing countries. However, obesity accompanying stunting has also been revealed in the countries that previously demonstrated a low prevalence of childhood obesity. Although there is still unsatisfactory data for a comprehensive investigation, it would appear that the documented increases in obesity are associated with both dietary change and altered physical activity patterns. In turn, these changes occur as a result of social, cultural, and psychological processes related to economic and nutritional transitions.

Increasing fat consumption due to the availability of cheap vegetable oils and fats in low-income nations and social classes may easily result in an increased childhood obesity as well as in stunted children in the developing countries.[160]

The effect of acculturation is significant in the obesity patterns of ethnic sub-populations living in the U.S. Changes in second and third generations were analyzed in the framework of the National Longitudinal Study of Adolescent Health. Height and weight data collected in the second wave of the survey in a national representative sample of 13,783 adolescents were used. Multi-variate logit techniques were used to analyze the interactions between age, gender, and inter-generational patterns of adolescent obesity. The results were compared with those of NHANES III. The smoothed version of the NHANES I, 85th percentile cut-off was used for the measure of obesity in this study. For the whole sample, 26.5% of adolescents were obese.

The rates in the individual ethnic groups were as follows: white non-Hispanics, 24.2%; black non-Hispanics, 10.9%; all Hispanics, 30.4%; and all Asian-Americans, 20.6%. Chinese (15.3%) and Filipino (18%) samples showed markedly lower obesity rates than non-Hispanic whites. All groups showed more obesity among males than among females, except for blacks (27.4% for males and 34.0% for females). Asian-American and Hispanic adolescents born in the U.S. are more than twice as likely to be obese as are the first generation residents of all 50 states.[170]

There has been an upward shift in both weight-for-height and height-for-age distributions since 1968, indicating that Mescalero children today are, on average, heavier and taller. However, no secular trends in obesity (weight-for-height above the 95th percentile) were found in Mescalero Apache Indian preschool children from 1968 and 1988. The prevalence throughout the 21-year period was as much as two to four times higher than expected when compared with the Centers for Disease Control (CDC)/WHO reference.[171]

Similar changes have also been found in populations transferred to developed countries and undergoing significant modifications in their lifestyle, especially in regard to nutrition and physical activity regimes. However, this also concerns tribal populations living permanently in their territories, where the conditions of life have changed markedly. For example, the Canadian Inuits, during the 1970s and 1980s showed significant changes in dietary intake and daily workload. As a result, an increase in BMI and percentage of stored fat along with a significant decrease in functional capacity measured as max $VO_2$ (aerobic power) occurred. Diabetes and other health problems have appeared simultaneously in the whole population.[172,173]

Children of immigrants from countries of the Third World who move to better social conditions may become overweight or obese. Nutritional status and obesity prevalence were followed in resettled refugee children from Chile and the Middle East. Obesity was common in Chilean children on arrival in Sweden and increased further after resettlement.[174] Obesity does not necessarily result from significant overeating under these new conditions. Rather, the increased availability of food in subjects adapted to a restricted energy intake and diet with a different composition of macro-components (especially saturated fats) early in life could be one of the reasons for the increased prevalence of obesity.

In children born to Maghrebian immigrants in the Parisian area in France in the 1970s and 1990s, an increase in body mass was found.[175] Compared to non-immigrant children, the prevalence of obesity in children of Maghrebian origin was 11% of the boys and 19% of the girls at the age of 3 years. Obesity was more frequent in girls. Between 1970 and 1990 the frequency of obesity increased from 9.5 to 29.5% in girls at the age of 3 years. Nutrition and the method of feeding during the first weeks of life did not influence the BMI values after 1 year of age.

Adiposity rebound (AR, or the subsequent increase in BMI in young children) was precocious, with 27% of the obese children experiencing AR between 36 and 48 months. It can be concluded that two types of adiposity appear in the measured subjects. The first occurs among very young children before 1 year of age, and is transitional in relation to hyperphagia of the newborn. The second obesity begins after 1 year and continues in relation to biological factors (such as parent to children correlation), and to diet and nutritional habits resulting from migration. The migrants adapt their traditional diet to the new food patterns.[175]

## 2.4   Concluding Remarks

The prevalence of childhood obesity has been a major concern in many parts of the world in recent years. As mentioned earlier in the chapter, the assessment of childhood obesity has been complicated by the lack of consensus on the criteria and cut-off points for the evaluation of obesity. The IOTF and ECOG are working toward a unified approach to a definition based on BMI. There has been a suggestion to draw the line from the point of the 85th percentile of an individual's BMI at the age of 18 years to younger age categories and use it as a criterion.

BMI alone may not be sufficient to monitor the rising prevalence of the condition, as increasing body fat seems to be matched by the fall of lean, fat-free body mass as a result of physical inactivity.[176] Therefore, skinfold thickness measurements and circumferences may supplement the evaluation of the adequacy of development of body size and composition during growth.[177]

Obesity has become a global health problem and is no longer limited to the industrially developed countries but is also present in countries of the Third World. This is particularly the case in the social strata where the economic and social situation has changed significantly during the recent past.

The implantation of the Western way of life, especially the intake of attractive energy-dense food of undesirable composition, along with a lack of physical activity has resulted in an increased prevalence of obesity. The management of childhood obesity has become a central issue in many countries, although the trends of obesity development are not identical in each country. Increases in obesity have continued, for example, in the U.S. and U.K., but in other countries prevalence appears to have plateaued since the 1960s (for example, in the Czech Republic and other countries of Eastern Europe).

Differences in BMI between the U.K. and Czech children have disappeared, mainly due to an increase in the average BMI in the U.K.[120]

Despite the lack of homogeneity of results it can be concluded that obesity in children has increased. However, exact international comparisons are only possible if based on studies with the same or comparable methods, sampling techniques, protocols, choice of parameters and criteria, apparatus, statistical treatment, and evaluation.

# 3

## Main Factors Associated with Obesity in Various Periods of Growth

### 3.1 Attitudes toward Obesity during Different Periods of Life

The different views on obesity at various periods of growth and development are an interesting phenomenon; for example, in young children a degree of fatness is commonly viewed as acceptable, even desirable, a sign of healthiness. Such an attitude may stem from the long-held belief that a degree of fatness helps guarantee an enhanced survival rate due to better resistance to disease, most commonly from respiratory and gastrointestinal infections. During previous centuries the ideal child was depicted as the chubby little angel in paintings of the great masters.

Today, with advances in medical knowledge, antibiotics, and other treatment modalities, additional fat is no longer essential to the survival of a young child. Quite the contrary, in the developed nations of the world, there may be a greater danger if a young person carries a higher level of body fat. Excess fat may jeopardize the individual's health status by increasing the risk of developing the 'diseases of modern living' later in life. In sharp contrast, some of the people living in Third World countries could benefit from greater fat deposits, particularly those in the lower social strata.

Most people, but particularly the families of obese children, do not start to perceive excess weight and fatness as serious problems in youngsters until puberty. At this time, a growing child starts to feel his/her position among the peer group, and commonly reports concerns in relation to fatness, lack of friends, and a belief that one is unhealthy ("fat, friendless and unhealthy"). Parents of obese children often believe that such children will outgrow their childhood body fatness and will be 'normal' later in life. Too often, this does not happen. Even after a temporary reduction of weight and fatness and an overall amelioration of the status of the child during sexual maturation, excessive fatness is often a continuing problem. The problem may become more pronounced following the cessation of growth, or after some other major life-changing event during adulthood; for example, pregnancy (or repeated pregnancies) in women, change in employment, or marriage may all be catalysts for people at different times.

A consistent message throughout this volume is that fat children more easily become obese adults, especially when overweight and obesity commenced early in life. Even though it is always possible to improve body composition status and lose excess fat later during growth or young adulthood, the achievement of such a change is progressively more difficult. Commonly, despite great effort, a sustained reduction of weight and fat is difficult to maintain and in many cases weight is regained (often surpassing the starting weight).

The prevalence of obesity varies markedly according to age. In preschoolers it is relatively low compared to the other age groups; prevalence increases along with chronological age.[61] In a population study of children and youth aged 3 to 18 years in Milan, Italy, the prevalence of obesity was highest in older students (aged 11 to 18 years). This corresponded to 17.9% compared with 4.7% of nursery school pupils.[178] Similar results have been reported for Czech children.[61]

Compared with other chronic diseases, including cardiovascular disease, diabetes, and related metabolic problems, the prevention, treatment, and management of obesity is different. Many of the diseases mentioned are now recognized as having their genesis in childhood. Therefore, appropriate and targeted interventions have been very successful, for example, in preventing and treating atherosclerosis. However, it has taken an extended period of time for such changes to materialize; atherosclerosis has been considered a pediatric problem since the 1960s.

Interestingly, obesity is a significant risk factor for cardiovascular problems and is also the common denominator in most of society's chronic health problems. The same is true of the modalities of regular physical activity and appropriate nutritional practices. For many years, definitions of health have stressed the importance of an adequate nutritional status that excludes overeating from the earliest periods of life.[179]

The dramatic increase in childhood obesity, over 30% in the past decade in some countries, has focused attention on various factors and their interactions during growth that may result in the deposition of excess fat. Some studies have tracked the effects of individual factors; however, most studies have considered a range of factors and their interplay over time in relation to the development of obesity. The variability in studies on children and adolescents makes comparative analyses of all data much more difficult than in adults.

## 3.2 The Role of Nutrition in Early Periods of Life

Numerous factors influence and interact with the nutrition of children. These factors include the family environment and status, heredity, nutritional knowledge, and feeding behavior (including food choice and preferences). Additionally, demographic, geographic, climatic, social, economic, and cultural parameters may play a role at different times in the development of the child. The perception of obesity as a positive or negative characteristic during growth also plays an important role in the growth and later development of the child in his/her family and school environment.[61]

During the first 2 to 3 years of life humans acquire basic knowledge of what foods are safe to eat.[180] A willingness to eat a wide variety of foods is greatest between the ages of 1 and 2 years, and this declines to lower levels at 4 years of age. Infants introduced to solid food unusually late have a narrower dietary choice throughout childhood. These data indicate that various factors can change food preferences and aversions to food during this early period of growth, which may result in an early predisposition to the development of obesity at a young age or later.

A considerable amount of experimental data on obesity has been accumulated in relation to growth and development. The greatest attention has focused on the critical periods of the preschool and prepubertal years. Adolescence is also a period during which the effect of certain factors could result in more marked and significant physical changes.[181]

Studies of obese children or adolescents who became obese adults have suggested that obesity that begins in childhood is more severe than obesity that begins in adulthood. The primary reason cited for this increased severity is the longer timeframe in which the individual carries additional body fat and the consequent increased risk of co-morbidities and enhanced mortality.[16,61]

Increased weight in the early years of life (as opposed to increased adiposity) appears to have little effect on adult obesity, but parental obesity represents an essential risk factor for the young person to develop adult obesity. At the time of the adiposity rebound, parental and child obesity carry a comparable risk for the subsequent development (or maintenance) of adult obesity.[182] By the time of adolescence, parental obesity has a more powerful influence on the risk of adult obesity in comparison to the adolescent's body weight.

The variable effects of parental and childhood obesity during the growing years on the risk of adult obesity suggest an interaction and, potentially, changing relative influences of heredity and environmental factors.[183] However, not enough is known about the interrelationships between genetic and environmental factors. Nevertheless, results from longitudinal projects such as the Fels Longitudinal Study indicate that those who were overweight early in life (up to 5 years of age) represented the majority of obese adults later in life.[184]

### 3.2.1 Fetal Period, Birth Weight, and Maternal Practices

The intra-uterine environment plays a critical role in the growth and development of the child. Malnutrition during early stages of pregnancy may be a likely cause of obesity later in life. Also, children exposed to hyperglycemia *in utero* are more likely to develop insulin intolerance and obesity during childhood.[185,186] To date, the mechanisms underlying these changes have not been fully explained.

Animal experiments suggest that stimuli such as a markedly increased or decreased food intake during pregnancy may affect hypothalamic development or pancreatic β-cell development.[187] Apart from the immediate intra-uterine environment, the health status of the prospective mother, maternal practices during her pregnancy, and subsequent breastfeeding (or lack of breastfeeding) can significantly influence the nutritional status of the child. The potential influences may have an immediate impact on the functional status and growth characteristics of the child, or be major mediators in the likelihood of the presence of delayed effects of body fatness.[51,61]

As independent factors, increased birth weight, massive weight gain in the first months after birth, and the level of overweight of the mother or both parents appear to be the major risk factors likely to promote the development of childhood obesity.

During recent years, the psychosocial domain has also received considerably more attention. Physiological or metabolic consequences should not be considered in isolation but rather, a broader perspective needs to be taken. Nutrition in early childhood and fat-cell hyperplasia and hypertrophy induced by nutritional factors probably do not imply persistence of obesity but may promote obesity and worsen the prognosis of therapeutic interventions.[188] Certainly, experiences in the treatment of adolescent obesity are such that many individuals show poor results and potentially, a predisposition to the yo-yo effect of weight cycling.[18,189] Such results provide more concrete evidence for the importance of early interventions.

An observational twin study, independent of genetic factors, that tracked the size and shape of individuals from birth to adulthood had the following results. The correlation of birth weight with adult body height was $r = 0.236$, and with adult weight, $r = 0.188$ (all p values $< 0.0005$). Further analyses of these data indicated that intra-uterine influences on birth weight have an enduring impact on adult height but not on adult relative weight. These results suggest that the intra-uterine period may be considered critical for height, but not for weight and adiposity.[190]

The role of birth weight and body habitus during the early periods of life was also followed in a longitudinal study in Japanese children. Changes in weight and height at birth, 3, 6, 11, 14, and 17 years of age were evaluated using the body mass index (BMI) which was calculated at birth, 3, and 17 years, and the Rohrer index (weight/height$^{-3}$) which was used at 6, 11, and 14 years of age. In girls, obesity at the age of 17 years was related to habitus at birth, and in boys it was related to body habitus at the age of 3 years. According to these results, the recommendation for the prevention of obesity is that interventions be commenced as early as possible.[191]

Nutrition is a key factor at any stage in life but at a critical or sensitive period in early life it influences future metabolism, performance, and morbidity in experimental models with laboratory animals. It also relates to the development of adipose tissue that can significantly influence the animal's later development.[163]

Similar data have been collected in humans but the methodologies of these studies may be questioned. Preliminary results from a prospective multi-center, randomized longitudinal study suggest that the way a pre-term infant is fed in the early weeks postpartum may have a major impact on later growth and development, including predisposition to overweight.[192,193]

A study of infants showed that the time of doubling and tripling of birth weight occurs later today compared to 2 to 3 decades ago. The group of children who tripled their weight had a higher percentage of fatter children but the type of feeding was not significant.[194]

Parents who use food to satisfy their children's emotional needs or to promote good behavior in the children may promote obesity by interfering with their children's ability to regulate their own food intake.[195] Interventions in child-feeding practices should not only include parents, but also grandparents and/or any care providers of children. Observations in a Brazilian population has also suggested a positive relationship between maternal and child obesity.[196]

In the early 1970s, the prevalence of obesity in British infants was attributed to early weaning and feeding practices such as overfeeding. However, this cannot provide a complete explanation as fat deposition in early infancy is succeeded by lean body mass development, and then again, a further acceleration of fat accretion.[197]

Studies on the relationship between infant milk feeding and adiposity have provided inconsistent results. Children aged 3 to 4 years from 3 ethnic groups who experienced different infant feeding practices were assessed using anthropometric parameters. Although a weak relationship was detected between the duration of breastfeeding and body weight, none of the measures of infant feeding were related to the 3 indicators of obesity, namely, body weight, BMI, and the sum of 7 skinfolds. Black American girls had smaller skinfolds than Anglo- and Mexican-American girls, with no ethnic group differences evident among boys. Concerns about adiposity due to methods of infant feeding can be allayed, at least for young children.[198]

### 3.2.2 Effects of the Relative Composition of the Diet

#### 3.2.2.1 The Intake of Protein and Adiposity Rebound (AR)

The relative composition of the diet early in life is important. Longitudinal studies (from 0.8 to 10 years of age) in children born in 1955 and 1985 revealed that the upper arm muscle/fat area estimates (calculated from arm circumference, C and triceps skinfold, TS; UFE = C × [TS/2]) increased during this period.[199] This result indicates a significant change in body composition. As energy intake has decreased in many places and the percentage of protein in the diet of children has increased, an excessive intake of energy has not been considered as the main cause of increased adiposity. Rather, decreased physical activity is considered responsible.[113,114]

One of the most important simple markers of the predisposition to later obesity is the adiposity rebound (AR) in children. Individual adiposity curves, assessed by BMI scores were drawn for a group of children from the age of 1 month to 16 years. Changes in BMI indicate that adiposity increases during the first year of life and then decreases. Another increase occurs at about 6 years of age.

In a longitudinal follow-up of French children, it was shown that the individual BMI curves differed regarding their percentile range level and age at AR. Results of this study also showed that there is a significant relationship between the age of AR and adiposity later in life. An early AR, that is, before 5.5 years of age was followed by a significantly higher adiposity level than when AR occurred after 7 years of age. This phenomenon was observed independent of the individual's adiposity at 1 year of age.[200]

Food intake data, along with anthropometric measures, were gathered from 10 months to 8 years of age in French children.[114,201] The BMI at the age of 8 years is positively correlated with energy intake at the age of 2 years, but this correlation becomes insignificant after an adjustment for BMI at 2 years. Protein, as a percentage of energy at the age of 2 years, is positively correlated with BMI and subscapular skinfold at 8 years, after adjustment for energy intake at 2 years and parental BMI. The percentage of protein at 2 years is negatively associated with age at adiposity rebound (AR), that is, the higher the protein intake at 2 years, the earlier the adiposity rebound and the higher the subsequent BMI level. Protein intake at 2 years was the only nutrient intake related to fatness development during later growth. A high protein intake enhances body fatness at 8 years of age, via the early AR, and a higher BMI is also found later in life.

The association between protein intake and obesity is consistent with the increased body height and accelerated growth in obese children. A high-fat, low-protein diet such as human milk corresponds to the needs for growth during the early growth period.[201] Bottle-fed children exposed to various milk formulae that contain a higher amount of protein can be at increased risk of obesity and other pathologies later in life.

As shown by assessments of 10-year-old French children, along with an increased prevalence of obesity, increased intake of proteins, especially animal protein, and lower intake of carbohydrates, sucrose, vegetable proteins, and saturated fatty acids were found. The intake of mono-unsaturated (MUFA) and polyunsaturated fatty acids (PUFA) remained the same while the P/S ratio increased (Figure 3.1).[113,114]

The increased proportion of protein in children's diets during recent decades may have also affected hormonal status. Nutrient imbalances are

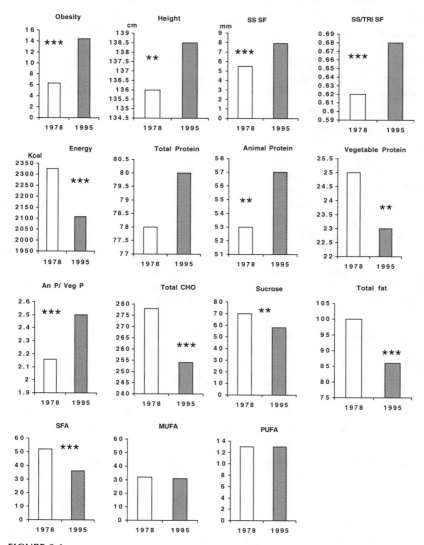

**FIGURE 3.1**

Comparison of obesity prevalence (% of obesity), average stature (cm), subscapular skinfold (mm) and centrality index (the ratio between subscapular/triceps), and intake of energy, protein (animal and vegetable, g) and their ratio, total carbohydrates (CHO), sucrose, total fat, saturated (SFA), monounsaturated (MUFA) and polyunsaturated fatty acids (PUFA, g), and the ratio between PUFA and SFA in French children evaluated in 1978 and 1995. **(p<0.01), ***(p<0.001). (Based on data from Refs. F2, F3.)

particularly apparent in early childhood when a low-fat, high-protein diet is not justified because of high energy needs for growth and because it is the period of a high rate of myelination of the nervous system.[202]

At older ages, the proportion of fat exceeds the recommended level with protein intake remaining high.[203] An increased ratio of proteins can have an effect on insulin-like growth factor-1 (IGF-1) which results in an increased cellularity of all tissues, including adipose tissue. Generally, obese children become taller at an earlier age, but normal-weight children catch up later. Therefore, a diet including more vegetable products is recommended in order to decrease metabolic risks during growth. Adiposity rebound in the early school years is thus an essential developmental marker. In summary, the earlier AR occurs, the greater the chance that obesity will be experienced later in life.[202]

In another study of Czech children, it was shown that the intake of protein during the first month of life in pre-term girls (born at 32 weeks) was significantly associated with later somatic development. A tendency for higher weight, BMI, sum of skinfolds, waist circumference, and sagittal diameter at the L 4/5 level was revealed at the age of 7 years in girls who consumed more protein during the first month of life. Serum leptin levels, assessed at the age of 7 years, reflected fat stores.

A significant correlation of protein intake during the first postnatal month with body weight ($r = 0.430$, $p < 0.05$), and fat-free mass ($r = 0.480$, $p < 0.05$) at the age of 7 years was observed. Birth length and height at the age of 7 years correlated significantly. It was concluded that the first postnatal month in pre-term infants represented a critical nutritional period that affects body weight and body composition at the age of 7 years.[193]

Retrospective analyses of the data of Dutch children treated for obesity showed that the mean age at which obesity begins is 5.5 years, but the mean age at which medical help is sought is 9.5 years. Seventy-eight percent of these children had one or both obese parents. The average energy intake of these children in pre-treatment feeding was 924 kJ less than the recommended dietary allowances for children of the same age category.[204]

As confirmed by other studies, parental obesity, high levels of body weight at the age of 1 year, and time of the BMI rebound are the main risk factors for obesity. The severity of obesity was negatively correlated with the age at the time of BMI rebound, and was not related to spontaneous intake of energy.[205]

A careful and routine monitoring of growth status, particularly of height and weight, enables one to notice undesirable changes in the accumulation of fat that may be indicative of a trend toward obesity. Such a strategy may be the most productive in terms of prevention of obesity at the individual level, particularly with those identified as at risk.

Family members represent the main avenues of support for all children. They should serve (where possible) as role models to reinforce and support the acquisition and maintenance of appropriate food habits and sound eating behaviors. Equally, family members provide the best opportunity for direct support in the establishment of appropriate physical activity and exercise practices. In short, the family environment in early life has the greatest potential for significant impact on the development of obesity in children.

In the area of development of food preferences children can be strongly influenced by the family environment, particularly very early in life, recognizing that food habits are established at the age of 2 to 3 years.[180,206,207] The impact of the family environment can have a decisive positive or negative impact, that is, by introducing and reinforcing good or poor food and physical activity habits.

One might suggest, therefore, that the strict distinction between genetic influence as opposed to environmental impact is a difficult one to make. Where does one factor begin and end? Does genetics encompass both the inherited biological features that are undisputed, plus a characteristic way of life? Certainly, the impact of the family's "way of life" has a profound impact on all facets of growth and development.[61]

For example, factors associated with obesity in preschool age children have been analyzed simultaneously with their parents. Familial aggregation of obesity, socioeconomic status, and parents' attitude toward the use of food for non-nutritive purposes were followed up using questionnaires and compared with the children's health status, specifically through height, weight, and skinfold thickness measurements. NHANES percentile rankings were used for the evaluation.

Mother–child anthropometric correlations were significant as were relationships between infant feeding practices and childhood obesity. Further, the educational level of the mother was inversely related to the children's weight for height.[208]

### 3.2.2.2  Fats and Carbohydrates

Since the beginning of this century, trends in fat consumption have changed markedly in the U.K. (from 1900 to 1985).[209] Most of the studies used to generate these comparative data involved 7-day weighed intakes as the method of dietary assessment. Quadratic regression equations were applied to the fat intakes from all of the available studies across this period, with each study weighted by the number of individuals examined.

Fat intakes were subsequently calculated for individual decades. Results indicate that fat represented 30% or less of dietary energy in the U.K. until the 1930s, when it began to increase. This rise was curtailed by rationing during World War II, but afterward fat intake continued to increase, reaching a plateau of about 40% of energy in the late 1950s. There was little subsequent change until the late 1970s.

Trends were similar in all age groups, including children, which might be one of the reasons for the increasing adiposity during growth. Interestingly, these results of fat intake change differ from those in the U.S., where the individual intake has fallen steadily since the mid-1960s. However, during the corresponding period, the prevalence of obesity has also increased dramatically in the U.S., and a high ratio of fats in children's diets has been assumed to be one of the reasons for increasing obesity in that country.

Composition of the diet and frequency and energy distribution in individual meals during the day also play an important role in the development of obesity. When the percentage of daily energy intake contributed by carbohydrates (ECH) equaled or was greater than 51.5%, this was associated with a greater leanness in French prepubescent children aged 5 to 11 years. This result was reflected in skinfold thickness measurements, waist-to-hip ratio, and relative weight differences between children whose ECH was less than 51.5%.

When the frequency of meals increased from three to six per day, relative weight increased from 94.3 to 101.3%. This relationship was not seen in children whose ECH was equal to or greater than 51.5%. In addition, children who had a ratio of energy intake ascribed to the two main meals, that is, lunch and dinner, of a value equal to or greater than 55%, were leaner than those who had a higher ratio. These results indicate the importance of an increased ratio of carbohydrates in children's diets and the relevance of reducing the energy intake during each of the main meals to prevent obesity.[210]

## 3.3 The Role of Physical Activity

Children in the U.S. were recently evaluated as fatter, slower, and also weaker than counterparts from other industrially developed countries. This finding may be the result of the adoption of a sedentary lifestyle earlier in life than was commonplace in previous decades.

Nutrient intake data of the past decade show that the energy and fat intakes of children in the U.S. may have reduced slightly but have been fairly constant. However, data also indicate that the level of physical activity has declined. Such data strongly suggest that the apparent prevalence of pediatric overweight and obesity may not be as much a function of nutrition as a reduction of physical activity and exercise from the levels that existed in the past.[211]

In spite of the recent trend toward decreased fat consumption in the diet, the increased prevalence of obesity might reasonably be considered to have increased due to the lack of health and dietary instruction, including inadequate exposure to and opportunity for physical activity and exercise.[2,10] There is still a limited understanding of physical activity levels and energy expenditure in children, but particularly obese children.[212–215]

The effect of physical activity level in the early periods of life has also been studied but somewhat intermittently. A study of 4- to 6-month-old infants considered body size, rate of growth, energy intake, subcutaneous fat (triceps skinfold), and physical activity (measured by actometer). The energy intakes of these infants were more closely related to the degree of activity than to their body sizes and were not at all related to growth.

Obese children tended to be hypoactive and consumed correspondingly less energy. The reverse was found in thin infants. Significant negative correlations were found between activity and the triceps skinfold ($r = -0.80$).[216] It was recommended that energy intake be adjusted to suit the individual child's needs, his/her body build, degree of activity, and inclination for food.

The influence of the mass media on children and youth has already been mentioned. The impact of television viewing on nutrition, physical activity (inactivity), and subsequent body size and shape has been considered an important issue for some time.[217,218] Generally, the time spent television viewing has increased markedly since the 1960s (Figure 3.2). In Germany, of children aged 5 to 6 years, 34% of boys and 44% of girls spent between 1 and 3 hours daily watching television.[219]

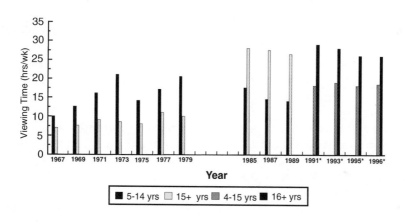

**FIGURE 3.2**

Changing trends in television viewing time (hrs.week$^{-1}$) of children aged 5 to 14 years and 15+ years. *Base changed to 4- to 15-year-olds and 16+ years in 1991. (Data from Social Trends, 1998. With permission.)

Competition between attractive television programs and exercise is too difficult a choice for many children and youth because many are not adapted to any form of increased physical activity or workload. In this respect, children throughout the industrially developed world are similar, with comparable risks of obesity.[220]

A longitudinal study was undertaken to examine the relationships between hours of television viewing, adiposity, and physical activity in female Californian multi-ethnic adolescents in the sixth and seventh grades.[221] After-school television viewing was not significantly associated with either baseline or longitudinal change in BMI or triceps skinfold thickness. Baseline hours of after-school television viewing were weakly, but negatively associated with level of physical activity in cross-sectional analyses, but not significantly associated with change in level of physical activity over time. Adjustment for age, race, parent education, and parent fatness had no significant effect on the results of this study. Only limited associations with the present level of adiposity, physical activity, or change in either variable over time were revealed.[221]

Another study showed a weak negative association between television watching and physical activity levels. Physical activity was lower during television watching than during non-television watching time.[222] Viewing behavior was not associated with body composition status. However, as the range of physical activity of youth, especially girls, is generally low in the industrially developed countries, it is possible to speculate that more marked relationships might appear when more extreme differences in all parameters of physical activity measured are present.

The observations of Klesges et al.[223] considered the effects of television viewing on resting energy expenditure (metabolic rate) in normal weight and obese children. Measurements were executed in a laboratory setting with children aged 8 to 12 years. In all subjects, the metabolic rate was measured twice under resting conditions and once during television viewing. The results revealed that during television viewing, the metabolic rate was significantly lower (with a mean decrease of 211 kcal extrapolated to a day) than usual resting conditions.

Obese children tended to have a larger decrease, but this was not statistically significant compared to normal weight children, 262 $kcal.day^{-2}$ vs. 167 $kcal.day^{-2}$, respectively). Television viewing has a marked and profound effect on the reduction of metabolic rate, and this might have additional implications for the development of obesity during childhood. In adults, energy expenditure during television viewing is higher compared to resting energy expenditure and is similar to other sedentary activities. Similarly, obese adults spend more time viewing television than non-obese individuals.[224]

What is the relationship between the nature of television programming and metabolic rate or energy expenditure? Inactivity represents a wide spectrum of "activities," a so-called "continuum of inactivity." At one end of the spectrum, gross inactivity or immobility may be combined with the over-consumption of snack foods. At the other end, television may be combined with low levels of activity, including fidgeting, but be significantly different than the former example in terms of energy expended.

Time spent viewing television at the age of 9 years can predict, along with the low levels of physical activity, the development of adolescent obesity. The measurement of body composition using BIA and physical activity questionnaires at baseline and 8 years later in Pima Indians as compared to Caucasian peers showed greater body dimensions, increased fatness, less time spent participating in sport activities, and more time viewing television.[136]

After 8 years, subjects who spent a longer time viewing television and less time with more vigorous sporting activities at baseline (hours per week engaged over the past year) had a higher increase in BMI.[225] These longitudinal observations also confirmed the role of inactivity in the development of adolescent obesity. However, in other countries like China, television viewing is not yet associated with obesity.[136]

With respect to the effect of television viewing on food choice and food intake, weekly viewing hours in a group of children correlated positively with reported requests by children for purchases by parents of foods influenced by television, and also the energy intake of children. However, the requests of children for sport items and physical activities did not significantly correlate with the number of hours of television viewing.[226] One must not necessarily assume that all television viewing is counterproductive.

The role of lack of physical activity in the development of obesity was also examined in a group of obese and non-obese African-American girls. Participation in vigorous (greater than or equal to 6 multiples of the basal metabolic rate (METs)) or moderate physical activity (greater than or equal to 4 METs) was inversely associated with BMI and triceps skinfold thickness. $PWC_{170}$ (physical working capacity at a heart rate of 170 per min$^{-1}$) and isometric strength tests gave similar or better results in both obese and non-obese girls. This did not apply when these parameters were related to body weight. In this case, obese girls demonstrated significantly lower values. These results support the hypothesis that lack of physical activity and low levels of physical fitness are important contributing factors in both the development and maintenance of obesity.[227]

The use of doubly labelled water for the determination of free-living energy expenditure has shown that obese children under-report intake significantly more than lean children. When measurements are appropriately adjusted for differences in body size, there are generally no major differences in energy expenditure between lean and obese groups. However, in some cross-sectional studies, a low level of physical activity has been related to current body fatness. Also, some longitudinal studies have shown that a low level of energy expenditure, particularly the energy spent in physical activity and exercise, is associated with both increasing body weight and fatness.[18,55,56,228,229]

Other potential contributors to the development of pediatric obesity have been considered. For example, the possible association between low levels of exercise and exposure to high-fat foods was analyzed in a group of Texan children aged 8 to 10 years. The prevalence of obesity in these children was 100% higher relative to national normative standards. Neither a high-fat food intake nor reported levels of physical activity were independent risk factors for this condition. However, it was speculated that high fat and inactivity might exert a synergistic effect when both are present in the same child.[230]

## 3.4  Familial Clustering of Obesity and the Effect of Genetic Factors

As indicated by some of the above-mentioned studies, the importance of genetic factors cannot be underestimated.[20] However, the differentiation between environmental and genetic factors is extremely difficult and where suggestions have been made they are still speculative.

In the context of the family, it is far more common for a child to be obese if one or both parents are obese than in families with normal weight and/or lean parents. It has been suggested that heredity doesn't concern only the genes, but also the inheritance of dietary habits, food intake, and lifestyle including physical activity level and spontaneous interest in exercise. Where there is a family risk of obesity, it is even more critical to pay close attention to the development of the child.

Incorporation of dietary and physical activity habits to limit, or even better, eliminate the deposition of excess fat should be the goal. Routine measurements of height and weight (plus calculation of BMI) can track the growth and development of the child. Obesity prevention strategies must commence early, particularly in families with a history of obesity. A study of obese adult female monozygotic twins during long-term reduction treatment showed greater similarity in the reaction of morphological, hormonal, biochemical, and clinical variables than in unrelated subjects.[231]

Similar studies in growing twins have not been reported. As mentioned above, familial predisposition may also influence how subjects react to particular life events, such as special diets (especially with a high fat content), or a sedentary lifestyle. However, there is still considerable uncertainty about the role of the interactions between specific genotypes and exposure to various environmental stimuli in both the short-term and long-term development of obesity.

In all instances, obesity cannot develop without sufficient energy being available, a consistently high level that exceeds the base needs of the growing organism. The fact that genetic influence contributes to the inter-individual differences in the population where energy is available may in itself be considered a gene/environment interaction. Also, the rare cases of obesity based on identified mutations in single major genes, for example, the leptin gene and the leptin gene receptor, may be considered as examples of specific genotype/environment interactions.[232]

Substantial advances in the genetic underpinning of obesity have emerged during recent years, but behavioral genetic methods are used rarely. Obesity is largely determined by environmental factors directly related to human behavior. Therefore, eating and physical activity habits in the family have become the special focus of attention in recent research.

There are important reasons why this aspect of the development of obesity should be studied in more detail, since behavior resulting in an enhanced deposition of fat is also genetically conditioned.[20,233] For example, the volume and character of physical activity during certain periods of time are more similar in mono- than in dizygotic twins.[234,235]

Genetic factors, or more specifically, polygenic factors, may be the most important for the development of obesity; recessive monogenic inheritance may be involved. The aggregation of additional environmental factors at the family level may be very decisive, particularly when the family lives together.[236] Similarly, delayed effects of the factors influencing the growing organism in the early stages of development may not be manifested until later periods of life. The situation is further complicated by additional factors outside the family environment. Such factors may be equally important in the establishment and maintenance of later onset obesity.

Familial behavior indicators such as parental physical activity may also be predictors of the activity levels of prepubertal children.[237] Respiratory quotient (RQ) and energy expenditure (EE)[237] correlated significantly in mothers and a cohort of children, and then also in mothers and girls in terms of percentage of moderate physical activity. In contrast, the only variable that correlated significantly in fathers and children was time spent in low level activity. The strong relationship between activity habits of parents was also evidenced by results in this study. Boys in the highest tertile for EE were 2.4 times more likely to have parents in the top tertile for EE. A similar trend for RQ was not significant.

Mother and child correlations in anthropometric parameters are significant in preschool children. Also, statistically significant relationships have been found between infant feeding practices and obesity in preschool children. The educational level of the mother varied inversely with the children's weight for height. The parents' child feeding attitudes had no obvious relationship with the anthropometric parameters of children in preschool age.[208]

A longitudinal study in 504 obese Norwegian children over a 40-year period showed that the degree of overweight in the family and at puberty were the determinants of adult weight level. The mean level of persistent overweight in the adults was 35% (20 to 60%). Body weight was increased even when food intake was within the recommended range. Additionally, excessive overweight in puberty was associated with greater adult morbidity and mortality.[238]

The Belgian-Luxembourg Child Study evaluated children from 6 to 12 years of age, and showed that BMI is strongly correlated between children and both parents.[101] The familial link extended beyond one generation as the obesity problems of grandparents were related to the BMI of parents, and also to obesity in the children. In addition, the correlation between birth weight and current BMI of the children was confirmed in the youngest age group in girls and birth weight also correlated with mother's BMI. The energy intake was high in these children, and energy output low due to low levels of physical activity.

These results indicate that obesity can be traced through three generations in familial clustering in this area, and is already evident at birth. Statistical analyses suggest that familial factors have a more significant effect on obesity in children than other broader environmental factors.[102]

The results of a study by Locard et al.[239] showed that parental overweight and birth overweight are closely related to the degree of the child's obesity at the age of 5 years. In this study, the environmental factors that contributed to childhood obesity were southern European origin of the mother, snacks, excessive television viewing and, more interestingly, short sleep duration. A logistic regression model, after taking parental obesity into account, showed that the relationship between obesity and short sleep duration persisted independent of television viewing.[239]

A number of factors that can predispose an individual to obesity were assessed in preadolescent girls at varying risk of obesity. The girls were obese or non-obese children of parents with or without obesity. Total energy expenditure (TEE) was measured by doubly labelled water (DLW) and resting metabolic rate (RMR) by indirect calorimetry. After adjusting for age, body composition, and degree of pubertal development, there were significant differences in RMR between the groups. The lowest RMR values were revealed in obese girls born to two overweight parents.

However, the largest differences in adjusted RMR were found between the normal weight and obese girls with two obese parents each. Neither TEE, nor non-basal energy expenditure (TEE − RMR) as an indicator of energy spent on physical activity, differed between the groups. Height and weight development up to the age of 1 year did not differ. However, at the age of 2 and 4 years, obese girls with both parents obese had significantly higher values of BMI. As shown by this study, preadolescent girls at risk of obesity are not generally predisposed to overweight and obesity because of a reduced RMR. Furthermore, obese girls seem to spend less time engaged in exercise and physical activity.[240]

A 4-year longitudinal study of Italian children who were 8.6 ± 1.0 years at the beginning of the study confirmed that the main risk factor for obesity was parental obesity. Sedentary behavior, such as television viewing, was independently associated with overweight at the age of 8 years. Physical activity, plus energy and nutrient intakes, did not significantly affect the change in BMI over the 4-year period of observation when the parent's obesity was taken into account.[241]

A study of risk factors in a transitional society in Thailand found that the prevalence of obesity among school children was 14.1%. Statistically significant associations with obesity were found for the family history of obesity, a low exercise level and obesity in both parents. Increased risk was associated with higher family income and smaller family size. Specifically, the highest population attributable fraction was for family history of obesity, followed by a low level of physical activity and exercise, and an obese or overweight mother.[242]

To elucidate the role of genetic factors, measurements of BMI and percentage of body fat by BIA and skinfolds in mono- and dizygotic twins (MZ, DZ) were conducted. Standard statistical procedure revealed a stronger association among MZ than DZ twins for BMI and also for percentage of stored fat, suggestive of a consistent genetic influence. Considering the percentage of body fat, the model of best fit included additive genetic and unique environmental influences. Using a more precise measure of adiposity than BMI confirmed a substantial genetic influence. As was the case for adults, the mix of environmental determinants of pediatric adiposity were "unique" rather than "common" in nature.[243]

The findings of the Stanislas Family Study emphasized that weight is a composite phenotype reflecting different components that evolve in distinct ways during the whole life span. In research related to susceptibility genes in obesity, the evaluation of fat mass should be the preference over weight or BMI.[244]

In another study of Italian children, the association between obesity and parental and perinatal factors was evaluated. After an adjustment for age, significant relationships between the risk of obesity and body weight at birth, and the mother or father's BMI were found both in boys and girls.

When parental and perinatal variables were included as independent variables in a multiple logistic regression model controlling for the effect of age, parental BMI and children's birth weight remained independently associated with childhood obesity. In females, an interaction between birth weight and the mother's BMI was found. Thus, parental obesity and birth weight were the most important risk factors for obesity among children in northeast Italy.[245] It is important to acknowledge the mixture of contributing factors that result in variability in size and shape.

Metabolic rate and somatic development were evaluated in a longitudinal study of children, of obese (group O) and normal weight (group N) parents, who participated in a study of metabolic rate and food intake when 3 to 5 years old. When the final measurements were conducted 12 years later, a marked gender difference was revealed. In boys, parental obesity predicted a more rapid growth, but not adiposity, along with an earlier decline in resting metabolic rate (RMR/kg weight). Childhood energy intake/kg body weight was not predictive. In girls, the reverse was found; that is, childhood energy intake/kg body weight (BW) predicted both body size and adiposity, while parental obesity had limited predictive value. These gender differences are consistent with the earlier sexual maturation of girls. Growth differences are consistent with the hypothesis that a low BMR/kg body weight is associated with a precocious pattern of growth and development in children and youth with a predisposition for obesity.[246]

The familial risk of obesity was examined in another study of children 4.4 to 5 ± 0.5 years old. Children were subdivided according to parental weight status; the high-risk group had one or both parents overweight, the low-risk group had both parents of a normal weight. The initial body weights of the children were the same, but after 1 year the high-risk group gained marginally more weight. The total energy intake was similar, but the high-risk group consumed a larger percentage of energy from fat, and a smaller percentage from carbohydrate. Only slight differences were observed in the level of physical activity of both groups. In summary, a distinctive pattern that may lead to increased weight gain may be present in the high-risk group.[247]

Obese children in Taiwan were about five times as likely to have an obese parent than were control children. There was also a significantly greater chance that members of the obese group had an obese sibling compared to the control group.[143]

In Scandinavia, a 40-year longitudinal follow-up of children treated for obesity between 1921 and 1947 was executed in Sweden. Questionnaires at 10-year intervals showed that 47% of patients were still obese in adulthood. A large proportion (84.6%) of these individuals were two standard deviation scores (SDS) above the norm for BMI than in childhood. Family history of obesity (in grandparents and parents) and the degree of obesity during puberty were the most important markers for obesity in adulthood. Food intake in the study population corresponded to RDAs, but this was not sufficient to prevent the development of obesity in adulthood. Excess overweight in puberty (SDS greater than +3) was associated with higher than expected morbidity and mortality in adulthood.[248]

Measurement of energy expenditure in parents and children did not support the hypothesis that the obesity of children of obese parents is caused by major defects in energy expenditure. Total energy expenditure (TEE) was measured over 14 days in children aged 5 ± 0.9 years and in their parents using the DLW technique. Physical activity energy expenditure (AEE) was derived by subtracting resting energy expenditure (REE) under post-prandial conditions. Fat and fat-free mass (FFM) was measured by bio-electrical impedance (BIA). There were no significant relationships between TEE and AEE in children after adjustment for FFM and body fat content in children or body fat in mothers or fathers. A three-way analysis of co-variance, with FFM as the co-variate, showed a significant effect of gender in children, obesity in mothers, or obesity in fathers on TEE or AEE in children.

There was a significant effect of gender and a significant interaction between obesity in mothers and obesity in fathers on REE. Relative to children with two non-obese or two obese parents, REE was approximately 6% lower in children when mothers only, or fathers only, were obese. Results of this study did not show any effect of parent's obesity on energy expenditure of children.[249]

Allison et al.[250] studied the heritability of BMI in pairs of adolescent black and white male and female twins. BMIs were adjusted for age and transformed to approximate normality. Hierarchically nested structural equation models were tested. These analyses showed that both the genotype and the environment exerted greater influence on the BMI of black than white adolescents. Variance in BMI was greater for blacks, but the heritability was the same for both black and white adolescents.

The challenge of obesity along with insulin-dependent diabetes mellitus (IDDM) is also paramount in Native Americans. The specific reasons for this have not yet been elucidated, but it has been hypothesized that Native Americans have a genetic predisposition to overweight under conditions of a "westernized" environment of abundant food and decreased levels of energy expenditure. Most studies show a high prevalence of overweight in this population in all age categories. Historical comparisons have shown that this is a relatively recent phenomenon. Preliminary evidence for two formative school-based programs in the southwest U.S. suggests that Native American communities are receptive to school-based interventions. Such programs, which should be diversified according to the particular Native culture, may slow the rate of excess weight gain and lead to improved fitness in school children.[251]

A 3-year longitudinal study to investigate the dietary, physical activity, family history, and demographic predictors of relative weight change was conducted in a group of preschool children.[252–254] Results showed that boys of normal-weight parents, or those who had only one parent overweight, showed the usual reduction in BMI values while those with both parents overweight showed increases of BMI. Girls with an overweight father showed BMI increases while others experienced the usual decreases of BMI during this period of growth.

As shown by Rolland-Cachera, the earlier than normal rebound of BMI predisposes the later development of obesity.[255–257] In addition, baseline intakes of energy from fat as well as decreases in fat were related to decreases in BMI. At higher levels of baseline aerobic activity, subsequent changes of BMI decreased. There was also a trend toward changes in leisure activity in that increases in children's leisure activity were associated with decreases in subsequent weight gain.

Modifiable variables, namely, diet and physical activity, accounted for more variance in child BMI change than non-modifiable variables, for example, the number of obese parents.[23] This result indicates that at an early age, the role of genetic factors might be weaker than that of environmental factors, including energy output from exercise. However, this might not be true during later periods of development; therefore, an early intervention in lifestyle, especially in children of overweight parents, is plausible.

Klesges et al. followed up parent–child interaction correlates of physical activity in preschool children.[253] Activity levels were evaluated with a system that directly quantified physical activity in the natural environment. Significant relationships were revealed using regression-modeling procedures between the child's relative weight, parental weight status, and percentage of time spent outdoors, and children's activity levels. Parental obesity was associated with lower levels of physical activity in children.

Children's relative weight was associated with slightly higher levels of physical activity and more outdoor activity was associated with higher activity levels. The participation of parents in the activities of children also significantly interacted with levels of parental obesity in predicting activity levels. Those children with a 50% risk of obesity (as defined by both, one, or neither parent being overweight) had small changes in activity across levels of parent–child interaction, whereas those at high risk for obesity responded with increased activity as parent–child interactions increased.[253]

A review of the existing literature on the role of the genetic determinants in daily physical activity, sports participation, and resting metabolic rate (RMR) indicated variability from low to moderately high. Transmission and heritability coefficients were calculated from twin and family data. Heritability coefficients for sports participation varied between 0.35 and 0.83, and for daily physical activity between 0.29 and 0.62. If one of the parents or co-twins is active in sports, it is more likely that the child or co-twin is also active in sports. Twin and parent–child correlations for RMR also indicate a moderate genetic effect. At present, only a linkage between RMR and uncoupling protein-2 markers has been reported.[258]

## 3.5 The Effect of Social Class

The effect of social conditions is apparent, especially in Third World countries. Under conditions of significant change in the economic, social, and cultural situation, obesity may manifest even more markedly than in other countries. Some of the studies in industrially developed countries focused on this topic.

Social and economic conditions have a significant relationship to nutrition and dietary intake; therefore, the relationships between social class and obesity have also been analyzed. The influence of social class on the development of obesity was examined in a 1958 longitudinal study. In childhood, the social class differences in the prevalence of obesity were negligible, but were quite marked in early adulthood, with a greater percentage of overweight and obesity in lower social classes (provided a certain level of economics usual in industrially developed countries existed). This difference was threefold among obese men and twofold in obese women when respondents were classified on the basis of their own occupation.[259]

A lower social class position, a lower level of social support, and if the primary care-giver is unmarried are all associated with a high food intake and a higher weight-for-height score of children.[260] A long-term effect of early class background was also manifested. Children from families with fathers involved in manual professions were more likely to become overweight and obese young adults compared with peers having fathers in non-manual professions. These subjects were also more likely to remain overweight or obese through early adulthood.[259]

Another study showed that children from low-income families, who were exposed to less cognitive stimulation, and who had obese mothers, showed an increased risk of obesity independent of other demographic factors. In contrast, the increased rates of obesity in black children, and those with a low family education and non-professional parents may be mediated through the confounding effects of low income and lower level of cognitive stimulation.[207]

Measurements of children in New York State showed that those who tended to be fatter were from two-parent households of low socioeconomic status rather than those with few or no siblings and those who ate school lunch or skipped breakfast. Overweight was revealed as a problem among many elementary school children in this locality.[261] The identification of socio-demographic characteristics may be particularly useful in targeting preventive efforts against later obesity development.

## 3.6 The Role of Sudden Changes in Lifestyle

Commonly, childhood obesity has its genesis during recovery from illness or accident (for example, fracture or major sprain) when anxious parents or care givers allow increased food intake (including delicacies) while the child is still limited by a reduced regime of physical activity. Sometimes the child succeeds in reducing his/her body weight and fatness after recovery, but too often this is the beginning of a long-lasting increase of weight.

Under such circumstances it is very difficult to follow an optimal regime because a high quality diet with sufficient energy, along with a degree of rest, is necessary. However, the maintenance of an optimal energy balance is possible but depends on the child's environment. Medical, exercise, and/or dietetic support is highly desirable under such circumstances in order to limit unnecessary health risks resulting from the previous pathological situation and also to reduce the risk of obesity.[18,61]

There was a rapid increase in the prevalence of obesity in children in the former East Germany after the reunification of the country.[106] Between 1975 and 1995 the prevalence of overweight (BMI over 90th percentile) of Jena children increased from 4.7 to 8.1% in boys, and from 7.0 to 10.9% in girls. The prevalence of obesity (BMI over 97th percentile) increased from 5.3 to 8.2% in boys, and from 4.7 to 9.9% in girls. Changes in the nutritional situation resulting from social, economic, market, and living conditions after reunification are considered the main factors in the changing prevalence of obesity in German children.[262] This result was something of a special contrast with growth characteristics from 1880 when secular changes began to be studied.[263]

Obesity is also a risk in growing subjects who have adapted to a high level of energy output, for example, young athletes, who, for whatever reason, stop their sports training. Some would contend that after an interruption in training fat is deposited excessively. A number of practical examples exist to portray the sudden effect of a decrease in workload and exercise causing a reduced level of energy expenditure.[18,264]

## 3.7  Recommended Dietary Allowances during Growth

Recent observations of Prentice et al. showed that the RDAs for energy for infants and young children were too high, and that normal growth has been demonstrated in children who had an energy intake of approximately 10% lower than RDAs.[265] Measurements of total energy expenditure (TEE, using DLW) in healthy normal babies has also shown that the current RDAs for energy were considerably higher than the estimates calculated from the direct measurements of TEE.[266] This excess of energy might play a significant role in predisposing one to obesity later in childhood.

New estimates for energy requirements of young children have been derived by combining the energy deposited during growth with measurements of total energy expenditure obtained using the DLW ($^2H_2\,^{18}O$) method in healthy infants aged 0 to 3 years. The resultant values of energy from 1 to 36 months (Figure 3.3) are substantially lower than current Department of Health and Social Security and FAO/WHO/UNU RDAs. Therefore, it is recommended that dietary guidelines be revised to avoid overfeeding of infants.

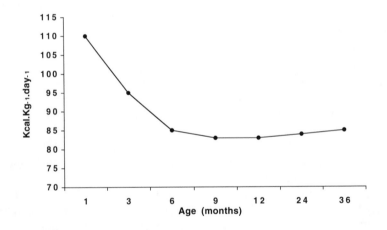

**FIGURE 3.3**
Estimates for the energy requirements of young children obtained by using doubly labelled water ($^2H_2\,^{18}O$). Values are lower than the present RDAs. (Based on data from Ref. F4.)

A modification of the estimations for the energy requirements of infants and children was then proposed as the basis of new FAO/WHO information. The requirements were also validated by measurements of energy intake in both breast- and bottle-fed infants. In addition, assessments were made of 1- to 3-year-old children in the Dortmund Nutritional and Anthropometric Longitudinal Designed Study, the results of which showed considerably lower values of energy intake compared to the energy allowances recommended by FAO/WHO/UNU in 1985. Height and weight development of children measured corresponded to suitable standard values (The Netherlands' third nationwide survey). To avoid early overfeeding and predisposition to childhood obesity, new estimations should be mentioned and would be preferable with regard to health promotion.[267]

# 4

---

## Physical Characteristics of the Obese Child and Adolescent

---

### 4.1 Basic Morphological Characteristics, Criteria, and Methods

Anthropometric methods for the evaluation of overweight and obesity have enjoyed widespread acceptability in all countries,[268] but, comparisons of the occurrence of obesity in various parts of the world to date have been very difficult, because the criteria for classification have not been homogeneous and reference values have varied.[16,29] What is deemed to be overweight in one country may be normal-weight in another country or continent. Substantive efforts have resulted in the ability to define more exactly levels of development and nutritional status during growth.[269,270]

Tables of standard reference values for body weight and height in individual age categories have been widely used as criteria for the evaluation of overweight and obesity in different populations. Growth grids that enable a quick orientation to the degree of overweight of an individual during growth have also been used. Some of the more common growth grids used extensively in the past include Wetzel,[271] Tanner et al.,[272] Kapalin,[273] and others.

During recent decades, growth charts for height and weight prepared for individual children have also been in widespread use. However, there has been considerable discussion as to whether percentiles and/or standard deviation (SD) values should be used for evaluating populations during their growing years. The World Health Organization (WHO) uses cut-offs based on SD scores rather than percentiles, which are more suitable for the extremes of growth status in the developing world.[274] However, this approach is not compatible with charts based on percentiles. A proposition for a unified growth chart was advanced, with 9 rather than 7 percentiles spaced two thirds of a SD score apart, rather than the more usual unit spacing. This gives a set of curves very much like the conventional 3rd and 97th percentiles, but with additional curves at 2.67 standard deviation (SD) below and above the mean (roughly the

0.4th and 99.6 percentiles). The 0.4th percentile is a more practical cut-off for screening purposes than the 3rd or 5th percentile.[275]

Weight-for-age, height-for-age, weight-for-height, and their standard values have also been frequently used in the evaluation of children and youth.[16,274,276] This approach provides a better approximation of the evaluation of children's growth and nutritional status. Retardation of growth in height and weight, stunting (shorter stature related to age), and wasting (reduced weight related to height) can be differentiated. This approach is considered the most important for evaluating children's development in the countries of the Third World, especially where malnutrition exists and most commonly affects the child population. This approach has enabled comparison of different growing populations living under conditions of various levels of nutrition and malnutrition.[274] The same procedure is also suitable for the evaluation of childhood obesity.

Obese children commonly have higher values of height-for-age and higher values of weight-for-age than normal-weight children. Falorni et al.[277] showed that more information on the growth of obese subjects may be obtained when evaluating height and height velocity according to specific reference standards from the same population of origin. When adopting this modality, no significant variations in height during reduction therapy are apparent. Slower growth during weight loss in obese children appears only when standards for normal-weight children are used.

---

## 4.2   Body Mass Index (BMI)

The most widely used method for defining obesity in adults, particularly in population studies, is the Body Mass Index (BMI = $kg/m^2$). Some believe that the index is more suited to adults than children and adolescents unless alternative values for p are used at different ages ($Wt/Ht_p$). The major limitation cited is the BMI's inability to distinguish weight from adiposity. Nevertheless, support for the use of the index with children is extensive. BMI tends to misclassify individuals at the extreme ends of the height spectrum, with very short and very tall individuals often incorrectly categorized as obese.[176]

Variability in the timing of the pubertal growth spurt, increase in height velocity in the year prior to menarche, and earlier menarche in taller and heavier children may contribute to distortions in weight-for-height measurements around puberty.[278]

BMI or Quetelet's index has been frequently used for the evaluation of children's growth and development.[279] A certain lack of precision is unavoidable using this technique because of the different stages of growth observed at a given age. Therefore, in children, the evaluation of size and shape is not easy since proportionality of the growing organism changes significantly during various periods of growth.[176]

Greater linearity is a natural phenomenon during preschool, and/or prepuberty and puberty. On the other hand, greater bulkiness and predisposition to adiposity appear in infants, toddlers, and those in the earlier years of schooling. This is also reflected in the changes of BMI.[112,279]

The utilization of the BMI to categorize under- or overweight is no problem for adults as the criterion is the same for all age periods, that is, 25. A BMI value of 25 to 30 defines overweight or pre-obese status, 30 to 35 moderate obesity (obesity class I), 35 to 40 severe obesity (obesity class II), and higher than 40, a very severe or morbid obesity (obesity class III).[16] Nevertheless, the cut-off point for any category or grade of overweight or obesity can vary according to different authors. For example, an adequate BMI for some may be extended to 26, while for others it would be only 24.

The first developmental BMI grids for children and youth were prepared by Rolland-Cachera et al.[255,279] and were based on data from a longitudinal study of French children.[65] Other developmental curves for BMI have been produced in many countries.[278,280–282] Some are based on older data, or cover only certain age ranges. Newer BMI grids have been derived for the United Kingdom,[283] Sweden,[284] and Italy,[285] among others. In preparing these grids, the least mean square (LMS) method elaborated by Cole was used.[275] This enables the adjustment of the BMI distribution for skewness and allows the BMI expression of an individual to be an exact percentile or standard deviation score.

Elaboration of approaches has been continuing to try to make comparative evaluation of childhood obesity on an international basis possible. This has also been the aim of several ECOG (European Childhood Obesity Group) meetings. It has only been possible thus far to compare conclusions on the prevalence of childhood obesity, which is most commonly evaluated by different procedures (reference values based on the measurements of different populations, using ± SD for the definition of growth percentiles).

### 4.2.1 Grids for the Evaluation of BMI and Its Rebound in Children

Developmental grids of BMI by Rolland-Cachera et al.[255,279,286] are presented (Figures 4.1 and 4.2). BMI increases significantly during the first year of life, then decreases until approximately 6 to 7 years of age when it increases again. This return and the further increase of BMI are defined as the adiposity rebound (AR) of BMI. Standardized percentile curves of BMI for children and adolescents have also been used for U.S. children and Czech children.[281,282,287]

As mentioned previously, AR that occurs earlier than 6 years of age is a marker of later adiposity. That is, subjects who increase their BMI at an earlier age are more prone to becoming fatter and potentially obese later in life.[256] This has also been confirmed by the results of the Fels Longitudinal Growth Study.[288] Therefore, the age of adiposity rebound (AR) and the BMI at that age are significantly associated with BMI in early adulthood. Correlations between BMI at the age of 7 years and BMI at ages 18 and 21 were similar in magnitude. This indicates the possibility of predicting BMI in early adulthood from BMI values at the age of 7 years.[289]

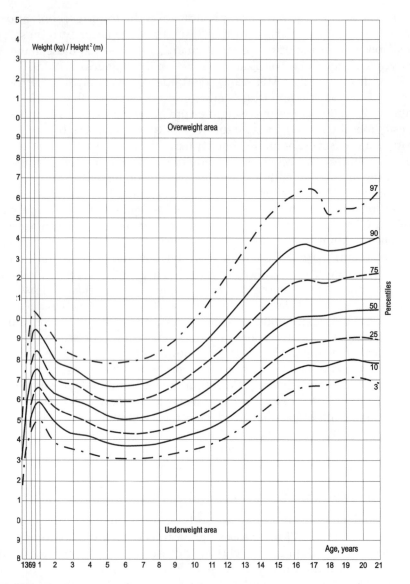

**FIGURE 4.1**
Growth grid with percentiles for body mass index (BMI, kg.m⁻²) for girls. (Based on data from Refs. F2, F3.)

### 4.2.2 Dissimilarities of BMI in Various Countries

The development of BMI varies in different populations. For example, in the former Czechoslovakia, a cohort of children was followed longitudinally from birth, with measurements taken at the ages of 3, 6, 9, and 12 months, and twice a year from 1 to 20 years of age. The inverse relationship between age at AR and the BMI was confirmed. In the leanest adults AR had occurred by

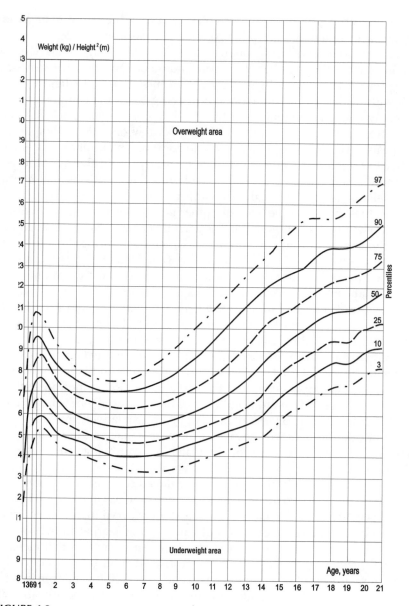

**FIGURE 4.2**
Growth grid with percentiles for body mass index (BMI, kg.m⁻²) for boys. (Based on data from Refs. F2, F3.)

7.6 years and in the heaviest adults, age at AR was approximately 5 years. Many lean (44%) and fat (58%) infants developed into average-size adults. The risk of becoming obese as an adult, as compared to non-fat infants, was 31/22 or 1.8.[290,291] Individual growth curves of children with very high or very low adult BMI values demonstrated convincingly the relationship between BMI at 12 months, age at AR, and adult BMI.

In the Czech population, in which obesity later in life seems to be a more frequent phenomenon than in the countries of Western Europe, the prevalence and morbidity of cardiovascular diseases are also significantly higher than in Western Europe, the U.S., Japan, and other countries. The genesis of these problems may occur in early childhood and is related to dietary intake, both with respect to the total amount of energy, and the composition and ratio of the macro-components of the diet.[292] For example, Czech RDAs for children aged 4 to 6 years are higher (65 g per day of protein) compared to European or U.S. RDAs of 24 g per day. In addition, intake of protein is often higher in Czech children.[61] This is in agreement with the hypothesis of Rolland-Cachera that an increased ratio of protein in the diet is an important factor relating to greater weight and earlier AR.[114]

The values of BMI at the 50th and other percentiles vary not only during growth when they express the developmental changes from relative bulkiness-adiposity with linearity and leanness, but also during the adult years until the ninth decade.[293] BMI changes between 20 and 65 years cannot be explained by an increase of energy intake; on the contrary, a reduction of energy intake was observed during the age range of 30 to 35 years. Sex and age variations in energy intake were similar to variations in lean, fat-free body mass, and opposite to fat mass of the body.[278] This may be related to the reduction of physical activity observed in most aging subjects.

A comparison of BMI curves from countries with different nutritional environments shows that the U.S.,[294] Swedish,[295] Czech,[282] and French curves are very similar. Data from Senegal,[296] Burundi,[297] and India[298] indicate that BMI values are not very different from those of the industrially developed countries for children up to 6 years of age. Adiposity is relatively low during this period of development irrespective of the nutritional conditions in a given country. Differences are more apparent later in the growing years.

In the more affluent countries, BMI values usually increase after the age of 6 years, but in Burundi, this increase is delayed to 7 years. In Senegal, an increase occurs at approximately 8 years of age whereas in India, no increase in BMI is evidenced. The individual age at which BMI increases correlates with bone age.[255] The increase in BMI values occurs earlier in the obese, at 3 years of age.[299] Differences in BMI trends reflect the notion that increased dietary intake accelerates growth but restricted food intake retards it.[300] When comparisons of the individual percentiles of BMI for children in different industrially developed countries are made, they show considerable similarity that is not found for percentiles of children from the countries of the Third World (Figure 4.3).

Therefore, the choice of an adequate developmental grid for BMI evaluation is a critical issue. At present, it is recommended that national standards suited to the particular situation of the country be used, especially in the developing countries. It is preferable to use those that were derived on the basis of the measurements of the healthy and normal local children, rather than of those living under quite different environmental (especially more favorable nutritional) conditions.

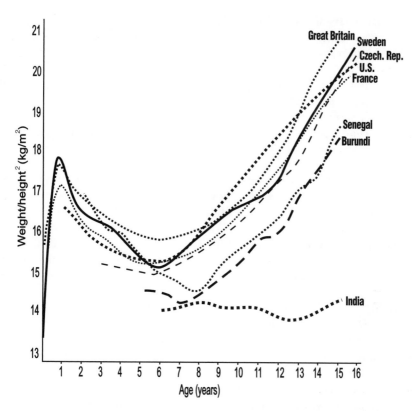

**FIGURE 4.3**
Development of BMI in different countries. (Based on data from Refs. F2, F3.)

### 4.2.3 Validation of BMI

BMI has been validated as a measure of size and shape through significant correlations with percent body fat (measured by densitometry) and/or by skinfolds in children and adolescents ($r = 0.86$, $p < 0.001$) and similarly in adults (women $r = 0.934$, $p < 0.001$, men $r = 0.85$, $p < 0.001$).[18,158,189,301–303] This also indicates the possibility of estimating the percentage of body fat from the BMI value. However, it can only give an approximate characteristic of body adiposity.[176] The BMI of obese prepubertal boys is also significantly correlated with the percentage of total extracellular and intracellular body water, calculated from the data gained from the multi-frequency bioimpedance method, and using special equations.[301]

Further validations of BMI were conducted by simultaneous measurements with the following methods. A significant relationship between body composition measurements by TOBEC and BMI was demonstrated in obese children and adolescents aged 6 to 17 years.[302] The screening performance of BMI with respect to adiposity was tested using dual energy X-ray absorptiometry (DXA) in Australian subjects aged 4 to 20 years. Receiver-operating characteristic (ROC) curves were prepared for detecting total body fat percentage at or beyond the 85th percentile. Screening performance was slightly but not significantly better for girls than for boys. The analysis showed that screening for excess adiposity using an appropriate percentile cut-off for BMI gives acceptable performance. ROC curves facilitate the design of screening programs by allowing an explicit trade-off between true-positive and false-positive rates. Although large sample sizes are necessary for precise estimates, the recommended cut-off points appear to offer a reasonable compromise between true- and false-positive rates.[156]

High correlations may be reported for BMI and body fat; however, further analyses have revealed that BMI is not an appropriate exact evaluation of body composition, especially in obese youth.[303,304] This is in spite of high correlations of BMI and absolute (TBF) and relative amounts of stored fat measured by DXA (PBF %) (girls PBF r = 0.84, boys r = 0.56, p < 0.0001; TBF girls r = 0.93, boys r = 0.85, p < 0.0001). Correlations between BMI and skinfold thickness measurements have been reported as follows: girls r = 0.84, boys r = 0.58).[305]

Widhalm and Schonegger measured body fat in obese children using total body conductivity measurements (TOBEC), which correlates highly and significantly with the results of DXA measurements (r = 0.948, p < 0.0001).[176] The relationships were similar for girls (r = 0.65) and boys (r = 63, p < 0.0001). However, when the obese children were divided into groups with different values of BMI, the groups with the lowest and/or highest values of BMI had poor correlation, while in the group with medium values of BMI, no correlation was revealed. The curvilinear relationship, which starts inclining at a BMI of approximately 25 to 27, demonstrates that an increasing BMI is not necessarily linked to a higher relative amount of fat. When the same children were divided according to age, the highest correlation for BMI and percent body fat was found for subjects aged 6 to 9 years (r = 0.79, p < 0.0001). The correlation decreased in the older age groups despite remaining significant.

Therefore, interpretation of BMI results for obese children across different age groups should be treated cautiously. Direct measurements of fat and lean body mass are preferable for the evaluation of obesity whenever possible.

A significant relationship between body composition measurements by TOBEC and BMI in obese children and adolescents aged 6 to 17 years has also been reported. However, there was also a curvilinear relationship between BMI and fat content (r = 0.609, p < 0.0001) indicating that with increasing BMI, between 25 and 27, the correlation becomes weaker. These results indicate that BMI can be a useful standard for defining obesity in children and adolescents, but only to a moderate degree in terms of adiposity. In cases of severe or morbid obesity in this age group, BMI does not reflect the real degree of fatness.[302]

## 4.2.4  Critical BMI Values as Cut-Off Points for Obesity

Until recently there has not been a general consensus regarding the cut-off points for overweight and obesity in children and adolescents. The 85th percentile has often been used to operationally define obesity, and the 95th percentile as gross, or severe, obesity. Race-specific and population-based 85th and 95th percentiles of BMI and also of triceps skinfold for humans aged 6 to 74 years were derived from the anthropometric data gathered in the National Health and Nutrition Examination Survey 1 (NHANES I). Racial differences in the extremes of the distribution do not emerge until adulthood. It is possible to choose population-based, race-specific, or age-specific criteria for obesity on the basis of assumptions underlying their specific research and clinical aims.[280]

More cut-off points were used, for example, the 95th for overweight, 97th for obesity, and/or 99th percentile for gross obesity. The cut-off points used in different countries to define obesity range from the 85th (Australia) to 90th (Finland, France, Greece, Hungary, Japan, U.K.) or the 95th (U.S., Canada, Saudi Arabia) and 97th percentile (Belgium, Netherlands).[306]

Some studies have confirmed that the cut-off points for evaluating obesity should be derived from measurements of the local growing population. For example, smoothed Australian cut-offs for BMI were similar to those derived from the first U.S. National Health and Nutrition Examination Survey (NHANES I) values for whites. However, the NHANES I cut-offs would result in systematic misclassification, for example, among 7-year-olds. The NHANES I 85th percentile cut-off would wrongly classify 4.6% of normal males and 9.1% of normal females as at risk of overweight. At the age of 14 years, the NHANES I 95th percentile cut-off would misclassify 3.5% of children as "overweight" instead of "at risk of overweight."[155]

These results indicate some variability in the cut-off points that might appear among various populations. The differences may be even greater among growing populations that vary more markedly in regard to environment, way of life, and cultural conditions. The elaboration of BMI grids for individual parts of the world should be one of the important issues for pediatric research in future years.

A study of the predictive value of BMI during growth for overweight in adulthood (defined as BMI > 28 in males and > 26 in females) was conducted during a 35-year longitudinal study. Analyses of data in white children indicated that overweight at the age of 35 years could be predicted from BMI at younger ages. The prediction is excellent at age 18 years, good at 13 years, but only moderate at ages younger than 13 years.[307]

In summary, the BMI is most often used as a guide to levels of adiposity in population studies and also for monitoring change in the obese as a function of treatment for overweight.[308] The index has proved to be most useful in these respects, and particularly in studies executed under field conditions where more accurate measurements are not possible.

## 4.3 Body Composition and Stored Fat

An essential characteristic of obesity is the excess deposition of fat relative to the body mass. Therefore, the most important criterion of obesity is a measurement of the amount of the adipose tissue represented in either absolute (kg) or relative (%) values. A number of methods exist for the evaluation of body composition. For clinical research purposes, for example, a five-component model may be preferred as this allows one to follow the changes of body composition in greater detail with regard to pathological processes in the organism.[309–311]

Body composition studies vary greatly with respect to aims and methodologies. Numerous reviews describing the approaches, methods, and opportunities for the measurement of body composition have been published during recent decades. The development of new methodologies has enabled more sophisticated measurements in healthy, as well as pathological subjects, including infants and young children.[300,309,312–315]

Evaluation of the total amount of fat and other components in a two-compartment model may be sufficient for the evaluation of simple obesity without the complication of other co-morbidities. Lean body mass (LBM), or fat-free mass (more exactly, adipose tissue-free body mass, FFM) is often used as a reference standard for evaluating the level of various variables. Measurements in obese children have showed that along with increased weight, BMI, and stored fat, they often have a significantly larger LBM when compared to normal-weight children.[18,68,158,316]

There has also been considerable discussion regarding the usefulness of more definitive body composition data as a range of benefits may be derived from this information. For example, it has been suggested that medication doses should be related to body composition status such as lean FFM.

Lean FFM, along with total body weight, is also used as a reference characteristic to which various functional parameters are related.[18,264] It applies mainly to aerobic power, other functional characteristics, and also to food intake and the individual macro-components of food. Developments in methodology have made it possible to complete a number of studies that were not possible previously, especially in diseased subjects.[314,315]

However, with respect to children and adolescents during various periods of growth, the selection of exact methods is more limited, and/or gives less reliable results.[317] Generally, direct validation of available procedures by anatomical or biochemical methods is still lacking. Some "reference methods," such as densitometry, are difficult to use in young children, or recently developed techniques such as DXA have a small yet documented health risk.

Changes in body composition follow a certain pattern during growth from childhood until adulthood (Figure 4.4).[18] Similar gender differences in body composition are already evident at the age of 6 years (Figure 4.5).[318] In children 5 to 7 years old, body weight and BMI were higher in boys, independent of the percentage of body fat (BIA, skinfolds). This was apparent until the 90th percentile of values, but not above it; that is, in fatter children no gender difference in the amount and distribution of fat was noticeable.[18,319] Growth changes have been demonstrated in a range of studies such as The Fels Longitudinal Study of children aged 8 to 20 years. The conclusions of this study revealed that there are gender-associated differences in the patterns of change of percentage of body fat and lean FFM, but not for total body fat. The percentage of fat and FFM increased in size with increased rates of maturation.[320] These findings may also apply to early tracking of obesity development during growth. Figure 4.6 shows differences in height, weight, BMI, and percentage of fat (measured by hydrodensitometry) in normal and obese children aged 11, 12, and 16 years.[18]

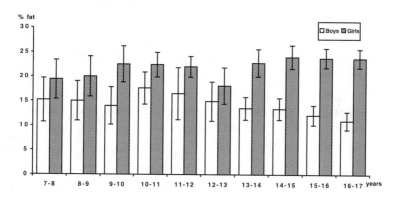

**FIGURE 4.4**
Body composition changes in normal boys and girls aged 7 to 17 years (hydrodensitometry with simultaneous measurements of the air in the lungs and respiratory passage). Age and gender differences are statistically significant except for ages 10 to 12 years. (Based on data from Ref. F6.)

Regarding the cellularity of adipose tissue, there is poor proliferation in non-obese children until 10 to 12 years. In contrast, in the obese there is a constant proliferation from the age of 1 year. As a result, the number of fat cells at the end of growth is significantly higher in obese individuals.[321] Both early, high-fat adipocyte content and hyperplasia in these children could account for the early adiposity rebound (AR) which appears with respect to a BMI increase in the obese before the age of 5.5 years.[255] This is significantly associated with increased weight at the end of the growth period. Wabitsch et al.[322] demonstrated that *in vitro* fat cells cultures, IGF-1, stimulated fat filling of the pre-adipocytes and proliferation of mature adipocytes. An excessively voluminous "fat storehouse" could be formed early in life and then later be filled by an inadequate food intake as related to energy needs. However, a positive excessive fat balance, more than a chronic positive energy balance, has been considered recently as a major factor contributing to the increase of fat deposits.[323] The results of the measurements using different methods correlate significantly, but usually do not give identical results.

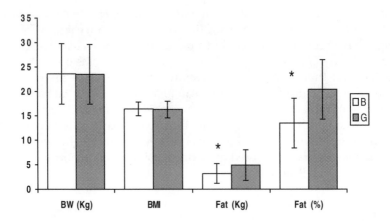

**FIGURE 4.5**
Body composition characteristics in boys and girls aged 6.4 ± 1.7 years. (Based on data from Ref. F7.) * indicates ($p < 0.05$).

### 4.3.1   Methods

There are numerous advanced methods recommended for the measurement of body composition in children. These include DXA (dual energy X-ray absorptiometry), bioelectrical impedance (BIA), $D_2O$, TOBEC (total body conductivity), densitometry, MRI (magnetic resonance imaging), and others. However, the equipment needed is expensive and generally exists mostly in a limited number of laboratories, hospitals, and other institutions. This type of equipment is also used more for diagnostic and clinical purposes, and is less accessible for physiological measurements.

For measurements of large experimental groups, or for checking the effects of different weight management approaches, more accessible and cheaper methods include bioimpedance analysis (BIA), $D_2O$, and anthropometric methods. The application of these techniques has been described in a number of studies following both normal and obese children.

There are other methods that measure body composition using, for example, voluminometry. In addition to water and air displacement, the anthropometric estimation of body volume can also be used.[324] Further, use of inert gas absorption or dilution methods to assess the content of body water using various items (antipyrine, urea, isotopes, $D_2O$, or tritiated water, $T_2O$) is available. Lean body mass can be estimated using creatinine excretion, 3-methyl-histidine, or $^{40}K$ measurement.

Many methods are too demanding to expect the cooperation of young subjects, or may be considered too risky for small children even though only slight doses of radiation are provided, for example, with DXA. However, technological advances are such that risk reduction has been maximized in many areas and an increasing number of these methods are now available for use with children and adolescents.

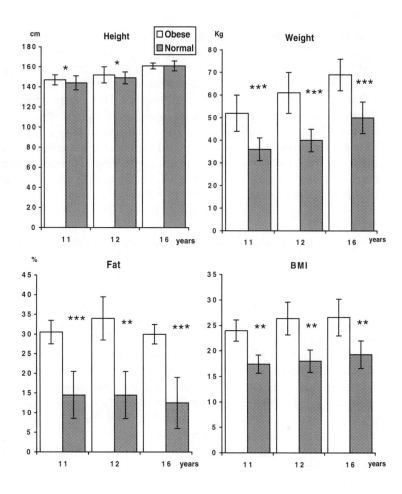

**FIGURE 4.6**
Differences in height, weight, fat percentage (assessed by hydrodensitometry), and body mass index (BMI) in obese and normal boys. * (p < 0.05); ** (p < 0.01); *** (p < 0.001). (Based on data from Ref. F8.)

In the recent past, the following methods have been used. Some are considered reference methods, for example, densitometry using hydrostatic weighing with the simultaneous measurement of air in the lungs and respiratory passages. This method has a very long tradition and for many years was recognized as the gold standard measure.[18,55,56,325–328] The technique is still widely used in laboratories throughout the world. However, because it is often very difficult for younger children to cope with being underwater, the procedure has been more commonly used with school-age children and older subjects.[18,56,330]

### 4.3.1.1 Anthropometric Methods

Anthropometric measurements have been considered too simplistic by some researchers. Nevertheless, anthropometry still represents a good opportunity for evaluating the nutritional status and degree of obesity in children.[331] This is especially the case when evaluations are conducted under field conditions, or in more modest clinical conditions. The common measurements, circumferences, breadths, lengths, skinfolds, and ratios between individual measures have been correlated with results from numerous "reference methods" such as densitometry and DXA, and showed high correlations and sound predictive ability. Other advantages relative to ease of use are the price of the equipment such as anthropometers, pelvimeters, and various calipers, and their portability for use in field settings. However, despite the apparent simplicity of anthropometric techniques, researchers need to be well trained.[8,18]

Commonly, skinfold thickness measurements are used as a more direct index of body fat. While the technique is not difficult to perform, considerable attention to detail is imperative to avoid inter- and intra-observer errors.[10,18,56,329] The amount of subcutaneous fat measured by skinfolds correlates significantly with the amount of total body fat assessed by other methods. Thus, the total amount of fat can be calculated from the results of various sets of skinfold measurements, for example, 2, 4, 5, or 10.[18,55,56,328,335]

The most common skinfolds used are the triceps and subscapular sites, the suprailiac, calf, and biceps.[332-335] Measurement of a larger number of sites, for example, 10 skinfolds, can give more reliable results as the measurements are more representative of a wider cross-section of the body surface, over which the subcutaneous fat layer can vary substantially.[18,330,335] The maximum number of skinfolds measured as reported in the literature is 93.[167]

For the evaluation of body composition from various anthropometric parameters including skinfolds, regression equations derived by Matiegka have been used.[18,331] The results of the estimated values of body composition in adults using these equations correlate well with the results from densitometric measurements ($r = 0.75 - 0.97$).[18] Age, gender, and other factors have a significant effect on the character of these relationships; therefore, regression equations and any nomograms developed vary in different age groups of males and females. This also applies to growing subjects, with marked variances between prepubertal and pubertal subjects and different regressions available for boys and girls before and after 12 to 13 years of age.[335]

However, the relationships can vary during shorter time periods of growth and development. This has been shown by the comparison of regression lines between the sum of 10 skinfolds and/or abdominal skinfold on the one hand and the total amount of fat measured by densitometry in a longitudinal study of boys from 11 to 15 years of age.[333,334]

Regression equations are only available for growing individuals and then for adults of both genders, not for individual categories year by year. For more specific evaluations, additional factors such as the degree of sexual maturation, nutritional status, and adaptation to various workloads and exercise can influence the character of the relationships between total and subcutaneous fat. In this respect it may be preferable to characterize fatness on the basis of individual skinfolds and/or the sum of various skinfold measurements. If required, a number of regression equations exist that enable evaluation of body fat percentage from skinfolds in children.[18,335,336]

Individual skinfold measurements are also often used to evaluate the development of adiposity. The triceps and subscapular skinfolds are the most commonly selected sites. For example, the triceps skinfold was used for the evaluation of fatness in Indian children aged 11 to 18 years. In this population, the trends for this age, gender differences, and the relationship to socioeconomic status were similar to the results found in other child populations. As a single site, the triceps skinfold also correlated significantly with weight and BMI.[337]

Under field conditions, there is generally a preference to measure the smallest number of representative sites, particularly those that are readily accessible. Recently, the submandibular skinfold measurement was recommended for children aged 3.0 to 15.1 years given the high correlation of this measure with other fat indices, especially BMI and circumferences.[338] This skinfold was previously included in the above-mentioned sum of 10 skinfolds.[18]

The morphological characteristics of obese and normal-weight prepubertal children have been assessed by both authors in a number of studies.[18,55-57,158,189,316,325,339-342] The obese possess greater overall height and weight and higher values on all anthropometric parameters, indicative of greater physical maturity.[18] As found by Hills, the sum of 4 skinfolds in each group reflects the differences in subcutaneous fat. The mean value for the obese group was 92.26 mm, significantly greater ($p < 0.001$) than the normal-weight group's 27.87 mm. Differences were also pronounced in percent body fat values with means of 32 and 17.37%, respectively.

Correlation coefficients between body composition measures are characteristically high, particularly in the obese group. The sum of 4 skinfolds in each group was significantly related ($p < 0.001$) to percent body fat and individual skinfold measures showed varying degrees of association. Subscapular skinfold ($p < 0.001$) for the obese and triceps plus subscapular for the normal-weight group ($p < 0.001$) showed the best relationship with percent body fat. Triceps and suprailiac for the obese were significant at the .005 level while the latter skinfold was insignificant for normal-weight subjects. For both groups, the biceps skinfold provided the lowest levels of association.

A similar trend was found when relating individual skinfold sites to the sum of skinfolds. The biceps skinfold in the obese group was not significantly associated with other skinfold sites. The triceps site ($p < 0.001$) followed closely by the suprailiac and subscapular represented the strongest associations in the obese while suprailiac, subscapular, biceps, and triceps were the most useful in that order for the normal-weight subjects. Biceps for the obese and biceps plus suprailiac for the other group were poorly correlated with the BMI score. Lean body mass (LBM) was significantly related to the sum of 4 skinfolds and percent body fat in the normal-weight group only.

Significant correlations were found between lean body mass and all anthropometric variables ($p < 0.001$). Each correlation coefficient was greater than 0.748 with the strongest association being lean body mass and body weight ($r = 0.981$). A similar result was found with normal-weight comparisons, all anthropometric variables bearing a direct relationship to lean body mass. In this group, coefficients ranged from 0.686 (chest circumference) to 0.993 (weight). Each of height, weight, sitting height, and bi-acromial diameter exceeded 0.918.

For the obese group, two skinfold sites (triceps and biceps) plus the sum of four skinfolds were significantly related to anteroposterior diameter ($p < 0.001$). Similarly, the triceps and biceps skinfold measures were associated with body weight ($p < 0.005$). Interestingly, the skinfold measure of note in the normal-weight group was the suprailiac measure which was associated with all anthropometric measures except anteroposterior diameter and bicristal width. Strongest associations were between weight (0.831) and hip circumference (0.822). BMI for the same group was significantly associated ($p < 0.001$) with weight, each circumference measure, and each diameter except anteroposterior chest. The only other associations of significance were between some of the body circumferences and skinfold measures in the obese group.[340]

Somatotyping has also been used for the estimation of body composition. Somatotype is expressed by a three-digit evaluation comprising three consecutive numbers (1 to 7, that is, from lowest to highest) and always listed in the same order. Each number represents the evaluation of one of the three basic components: endomorphy (relates to the relative adiposity), mesomorphy (relates to skeletal muscle development) and ectomorphy (relates to the relative linearity of the body).[343,344]

### 4.3.1.2　Methods for the Measurement of the Individual Body Components

Body composition can be evaluated from the broader perspective of gross components such as fat and fat-free mass, lean body mass, or the sub-components of fat-free tissue, such as water, mineral and protein. Other methods can evaluate the mass of the individual tissues, organs, or body segments. The choice of specific method(s) for a particular study depends on various considerations including the aim of the study, required accuracy and precision, availability of apparatus, subject acceptability, convenience, cost, the need for trained personnel, and health issues such as radiation exposure.[9]

As mentioned above, reference methods such as densitometry, isotope dilution methods ($D_2O$), dual energy X-ray absorptiometry (DXA), computerized tomographic scanning (CT), magnetic resonance imaging (MRI), and *in vivo* neutron activation analysis (IVNAA) are in use. In the category of bedside or field methods, anthropometry including skinfold thickness, impedance/resistance (bioimpedance analysis or BIA), near-infrared interactance (NIRI), and 24-hr creatinine excretion can be used.[315] Various methods have been described and analyzed in extensive reviews by a number of authors.[167,172,300,312,313,345,346]

The suitability of these techniques for the evaluation of body composition in children varies greatly; therefore, only some have been used for measurement during growth. In most recent studies the trend has been to use simultaneously a range of methods for the evaluation of body composition. Some of these methods are briefly described in the remainder of this chapter with examples of the results provided.

### 4.3.1.3 Densitometry

Body density is assessed by hydrostatic weighing based on the Archimedean principle, ideally with the simultaneous estimation of the volume of air in the lungs and respiratory passages.[18,167,326,330] For the assessment of the air in the respiratory passages, a nitrogen or helium dilution method can be used.[18] Body density is then calculated using the formula of Brozek et al.:[326]

Body Density = Weight in air × 0.996/ weight – weight under the water – volume of the air LRP × 0.996 (LRP = respiratory passages and the lungs; 0.996 = density of the water during weighing, that is, 37°C).

Percent fat is calculated using the following formula:[167]

Percent fat (% fat) = (4.201/density – 3.813) × 100

Brožek et al.[326] later used another constant in this formula, that is,

% fat = (4.950/density – 4.50) × 100.

A number of other equations are in use.[172] Lean body mass (FFM) can be calculated:

% LBM (FFM) = 100 – % fat, kg fat = % fat × body weight/100.[18]

During repeated measurements the results varied by 0.5% and during the day variations in body density were minimal.[18]

Some researchers measure the volume of the air separately in the normal atmosphere under similar conditions after a maximal expiration; however, this may cause some imprecision. Also, a certain proportion of the vital capacity (24% of VC) can be subtracted from the value of the volume ascertained by underwater weighing (volume of the body = weight in the air – weight under the water).

This method requires a great deal of cooperation by the subject and lack of fear when submerging the whole head during the underwater weighing. The method has been used mainly for school children and adolescents[330,335] but it has not always been easy for obese youth, and the measurements require longer preparation and training time.[18] Therefore, air displacement plethysmography or body line scanners employing the principles of three-dimensional photography were suggested as they are also potentially able to measure body surface and body volume (total, segments) which can be used for the derivation of body density.[324]

### 4.3.1.4   Dual Energy X-ray Absorptiometry (DXA)

Dual energy X-ray absorptiometry (DXA) is a relatively new scanning technique that measures the differential attenuation of two X-rays as they pass through the body. It differentiates bone mineral from soft tissue and subsequently divides the latter into fat and lean FFM. The method provides information on total body composition, and that of individual body segments, which is an advantage over densitometry, [40]K measurements, or water dilution. The method has excellent reproducibility as shown in adults; however, the machine is very expensive.

Comparisons of boys and girls aged 3 to 8 years of age with the same age, height, weight, BMI, or bone mineral content showed that boys had a lower percentage of fat, lower fat mass (kg), and higher bone-free lean tissue mass than girls. These measurements revealed that girls had approximately 50% more fat than boys.[318] The measurement also confirmed that gender differences in body composition are present a long time prior to the onset of puberty.[318]

The accuracy of body composition measurements (DXA) was assessed experimentally by comparing the method with total carcass chemical analysis in 16 pigs, with a weight range of 5 to 35 kg. All estimates of body composition were highly correlated with the results of direct chemical analysis. For the absolute mass of body fat, one DXA analysis underestimated by 9.5% the reference chemical method, whereas an alternate software package resulted in overestimates averaging 15.5%. Conversely, the average fat-free compartment was initially overestimated by 968g, then underestimated by 892 g. The impact of these differences in the body composition measurements using DXA was also examined in a group of 18 young boys aged 4 to 12 years.[347] When using this method, results need to be interpreted with caution.

Another study using DXA followed both genders from 4 to 26 years and showed that lean body mass (LBM) and bone mineral content (BMC) increased with age in females until 13.4 and 15.7 years, respectively, and in males until 16.6 and 17.4 years. Significant correlations between LBM and BMC were found for both genders ($r = 0.98$, $p < 0.0001$ for females, and $r = 0.98$, $p < 0.0001$ for males). The body fat percentage according to DXA measurements (%BF DXA) increased with age in females ($r = 0.52$, $p < 0.001$), but not in males, and was higher in females than in males at all ages.

The trunk-to-leg fat ratio (TLFR) has also been calculated as trunk fat/leg fat measured by DXA. After puberty, TLFR was higher in males than in females, which was not the case during younger ages when no gender differences in TLFR were found. The trunk-to-leg fat ratio, as measured by DXA in

Brazilian children, was almost twice that in obese as in normal children.[348] DXA underestimated the body weight measured by scales by a mean of 0.83 kg. The %BF DXA correlated with %BF derived from skinfold thickness measurements. The results corresponded well in males, but overestimated the %BF by skinfold thickness in females. Therefore, the measurements of body composition using DXA confirmed the findings on age changes and gender differences gained by densitometry and other methods.[18,288,330]

### 4.3.1.5 Bioelectrical Impedance (BIA)

Tetrapolar bioelectrical impedance analysis is widely used in clinical practice and also in experimental growth studies of both normal and obese children. The tetrapolar BIA method applies a small (800 mA) alternating (50 kHz) current which is mainly conducted by the body's water and its dissolved electrolytes. The resistance of the current is in theory inversely proportional to the amount of conductive material, that is, to total body water (TBW) and its dissolved electrolytes. The specific resistivities of intracellular (ICW) and extracellular water (ECW) vary according to differences in the type and amount of dissolved electrolytes in the intra- and extracellular spaces. Therefore, the relationship between body impedance and total body water will be theoretically different between individuals who differ in the proportion of extra- and intracellular water.[317,349,350]

The BIA method was validated against reference methods such as densitometry, deuterium oxide dilution ($D_2O$), or $^{40}K$ in adults and later also for children and adolescents.[351–354] Total body water was measured using the stable isotope $^2H_2^{18}O$, and body resistance was measured using a tetrapolar technique with a constant 50 kHz, 800 mA alternating current. Total body water was highly correlated with height$^2$/body resistance (r = 0.97, p < 0.001). This method may be suitable as it is non-invasive, rapid, and acceptable for children.[355] However, further cross-validation studies are needed, especially with regard to markedly changed body composition in obese children and adolescents.

When bioelectrical resistance was used for the assessment of body composition in children and adolescents, there were doubts about which age-specific equation should be used during growth. The relationship between height$^2$/resistance and total body water (TBW) is fairly reliable across a wide age range, but for preschool children some validation is necessary. TBW was assessed from $^2H_2^{18}O$ dilution in groups of children aged 4 to 6 years, and bioelectrical resistance and reactance were measured in two independent laboratories; no significant differences in the results of TBW measurements were found. Using Kushner's equation, TBW can be transformed into an equation for fat-free mass (FFM) by using published gender- and age-specific constants for the hydration of FFM. The intra-class reliability for estimates of fat mass and FFM using bioelectrical resistance in another independent group of children was > 0.99 for duplicate observations performed 2 weeks apart.[354,356]

The results of measurements using tetrapolar whole-body bioelectrical impedance analysis (BIA) were compared with the measurements of total body potassium (TBK) using [40]K spectrometry, and skinfold thickness measurements in subjects aged 3.9 to 19.3 years. A best-fitting equation to predict TBK-derived FFM from BIA and other potential independent predictors was developed and cross-validated in two randomly selected subgroups of growing subjects using stepwise multiple regression analysis.

The technical error associated with BIA measurements was much smaller than that of skinfold measurements; however, the reproducibility of BIA-derived FFM estimates was only slightly better than that of FFM estimates obtained using weight and 2 skinfold measurements. Best-fitting regression equations for FFM using BIA measurements have been derived.[357] In this study, conventional anthropometry, using published equations for the evaluation of FFM from skinfolds, slightly overestimated TBK-derived FFM, but predicted FFM with a precision similar to the best-fitting equations involving BIA.

Bioelectrical impedance analysis (BIA) has also been used to study the effect of dietary supplementation in malnourished children. A positive effect was found with a high-protein diet contributing to the acceleration of growth and restoration of body composition.[358] BIA has also been used for evaluating body composition in obese children to assess the effect of reduction treatment.[301]

### 4.3.1.6    [40]K Measurement

[40]K measurements using whole-body counters evaluate body potassium as related to its natural gamma-activity in the human organism. This method was also used, e.g., for the estimation of body composition in a group of adolescents using hydrostatic weighing, BIA, and whole-body counting of [40]K. Estimates of body fat percentage by total body potassium were significantly greater than by either hydrostatic weighing or BIA. When current estimates for the fat-free mass (FFM) density in children were employed to derive the [40]K/FFM, the value for boys was 58.9 mEq, and for girls 54.2 mEq. These data indicate that the FFM can be underestimated in growing subjects when using adult-derived values for [40]K/FFM.[359]

### 4.3.1.7    Total Body Water by Deuterium or Tritium Oxide

Total body water may be measured by isotope dilution by administering a tracer which dilutes equally throughout body water and which can then be measured. Stable, non-radioactive isotopes of water containing deuterium or [18]O are used; deuterium is used more often because it is cheaper, and can be analyzed by mass spectrometry. Gas chromatography or infra-red absorption can be used, but requires the use of a greater amount of deuterium. Tritium can also be used as the analysis is cheap and rapid, but it is radioactive and so is not suitable, especially for younger subjects.

At present, deuterium oxide ($^2H_2O$) is used for measurements of body water and body composition. Most often it is used as DLW ($^2H_2^{18}O$) which enables the simultaneous assessment of TEE.[360]

### 4.3.1.8 Total Body Electrical Conductivity (TOBEC)

Measurements of body composition by total body electrical conductivity (TOBEC) are used mainly for the evaluation of hospitalized infants and children for whom permanent monitoring of nutritional status is indispensable. This approach is considered more suitable for infants and young children because methods using density assume a constant relationship between water and the fat-free component of the body and "adult" composition of lean FFM.[1,361] The anthropometric assessment of body composition using skinfolds has not been satisfactory in very young children. Methods such as total body potassium, neutron activation, hydro-densitometry, and body volume measurements also require a relatively long confinement within special devices. This is difficult for younger children and unthinkable for those who are sick or any children who are shy and afraid of laboratory and clinical procedures.

TOBEC is one of the most promising methodologies available for the evaluation of body composition, especially for those in the youngest age categories. The technique is safe, quick, totally non-invasive, and more accurate than the majority of other methods.[362] The method is based on the principle that a living organism placed in an electromagnetic field perturbs that field. This perturbation is caused by the electrolyte mass within the organism. Since electrolytes are included in fat-free body mass exclusively, it is possible to accurately separate this tissue from body fat, which is enabled by adequate calibration. One measurement requires one second, and is usually repeated three times to achieve a desirable level of accuracy.[1] The pediatric instruments usually give more exact results because they can be calibrated using animal carcasses such as miniature pigs or mature rabbits.

All TOBEC instruments are constructed around a large electromagnetic coil to which sensors are attached. As electromagnetic energy dissipates when an individual enters the coil, more current needs to be fed into the coil to maintain a constant electromagnetic field strength. The amount of current needed for this measurement is directly proportional to the perturbation of the electromagnetic field, that is, to the electrolyte mass of the measured subject. Thus the "TOBEC number" is derived.

For older children and adults, larger TOBEC devices have been developed with motorized carriages in contrast to those for infants. The subject is passed through the instrument at a constant rate and a total of 64 readings are obtained in a sequential fashion. These readings result in a computer-generated curve that is then de-convoluted by Fourier transform.

The Fourier-derived constants are used in the calibration equation to assess fat-free body mass.[1]

TOBEC was used for the assessment of body composition in obese children as compared to children with Prader-Willi syndrome who also have a high fat content; their ages were $11.5 \pm 3.6$ years and $10.1 \pm 3.5$ years. The percentage of fat was higher, but the development of lean body mass was significantly lower in children with Prader-Willi syndrome as expressed by a special index relating FFM to body height. This latter index improved in some of the patients when treated with growth hormone, which was possible to evaluate properly by TOBEC measurement in a longitudinal observation.[1]

### 4.3.1.9    Magnetic Resonance Imaging (MRI)

The principle behind this method is that certain nuclei with intrinsic magnetic properties range in a certain direction of the magnetic field during the transmission of the radiofrequency wave. After interruption of the wave's transmission the nuclei return to their original position, and transmit the absorbed energy that it is now possible to measure and evaluate from the explored tissue image. There is no irradiation in this method, and it does not require any cooperation of subjects but the measurements take a long time. MRI is used for the measurement of visceral fat.[363]

In children, this method has been used to assess the muscle and fat tissue of the thighs in subjects who were treated with growth hormone (GH), children with Turner's syndrome, and those with intra-uterine growth retardation (IUGR). Children administered GH were examined before GH treatment and then at regular intervals. MRI revealed an increase in muscle tissue and a reduction of adipose tissue in the thighs, and also a dramatic change in muscle/adipose tissue cross-sectional area ratio in each period of the treatment. BMI correlated with the muscle and adipose tissue cross-sectional area at each time point ($p < 0.0001$). The muscle cross-sectional area increment also correlated with height velocity.[364] MRI could be used in studies of children treated for various purposes, including obesity, but no such observations have been reported.

### 4.3.1.10    Computed Tomography (CT)

Whole-body scans provide information on the size of individual tissues. However, the organism is subjected to some irradiation; therefore, this method is not recommended for younger children. The measurements are also time consuming and costly. Intra-abdominal fat was measured using CT in some studies.[365]

### 4.3.1.11    Ultrasound

High-frequency sound waves pass freely through homogeneous tissues and part of the emitted energy is reflected at any interface between different tissues, for example, fascia separating muscle and adipose tissue. This reflection is then converted to an electrical signal. Correlations with carcass fat measurements are statistically significant, but are not sufficiently high. The results of this method correlate significantly in adults with measurements of the distance between the tip of the abdomen and L4-5 using a pelvimeter.[366]

### 4.3.1.12 Comparison of Several Methods: Measuring Children Using BIA, TOBEC, and DXA

Ellis used several methods simultaneously for the evaluation of body composition in children and young adults.[367] Estimates of the relative and absolute amounts of body fat were highly correlated among several methods: bioelectrical impedance analysis (BIA), total body conductivity, and DXA (r = 0.72 to 0.97, p < 0.001). However, use of a Bland and Altman comparison among the estimates revealed significant differences between methods. The mean differences between methods for measuring body fat ranged from 0.30 ± 6.7 kg to 4.2 ± 2.7 kg while the difference for the percentage of fat ranged from 0.8 ± 3.5% to 9.9 ± 5.2%. Therefore, classification of fatness into simple categories such as normal, overweight, and obese with regard to the % of fat was significantly method dependent. This important study led to the conclusion that the lack of interchangeability for fatness classification makes it difficult to ensure that similar groups of subjects, homogeneous with regard to fatness, can be accurately selected when different methods are used. This limitation can also restrict possible comparisons with the results of various studies, both cross-sectional and longitudinal, that also relate to treatment follow-ups of obese subjects.[367]

### 4.3.1.13 Creatinine Excretion

This final product of nitrogen metabolism gives information on the amount of muscle tissue in the body. To obtain sufficiently precise results it is necessary to collect urine over several days (at least three) and adhere to a certain diet. This is difficult when subjects are not measured in a metabolic unit or in a hospital.[276] This method has been used in the past with children.

## 4.4 Fat Distribution

Another important morphological characteristic of obesity is subcutaneous fat distribution or fat patterning. Gender differences in the amount and distribution of fat appear at birth.[18] The measurement of 10 skinfold thicknesses during the first 48 hr after delivery revealed significant gender differences, especially in the suprailiac skinfold.[55] Generally, there was a trend for higher deposition of fat in all 10 skinfolds measured in girls in whom the suprailiac skinfold was significantly greater immediately after birth.[55,335] This gender difference increased during further periods of growth and was largest during puberty.[18]

Fat patterning is evaluated via ratios, for example, between subscapular and triceps skinfold (centrality index), or the sum of skinfolds on the trunk and on the extremities. In later periods of adulthood, when the amount of subcutaneous fat increases even when BMI remains the same, there is less of a gender difference in fat due to an increasing amount in males.[18] Similar differences were also found in the total amount of fat as measured by densitometry.

As one gets older an increasing amount of fat is deposited in body cavities, especially in the abdomen. An increased amount of visceral fat is considered the most important health risk with regard to cardiovascular diseases, diabetes, and other metabolic problems. Various methods are used to measure internal fat, most commonly CT. The importance of central adiposity was revealed several decades ago when it was shown that individuals who have a larger deposition of fat on the trunk as compared to the extremities have a higher risk of pathological features including increased blood pressure, diabetes, and dyslipoproteinemia.[368,369] More recently a similar situation was described in children. This means that not only the total amount of excess fat, but also its distribution on the body surface and body cavities, can be a risk and must be evaluated in growing individuals.

### 4.4.1   Skinfold Thickness Ratios (Indices)

Figure 4.7 outlines the distribution of subcutaneous fat in normal and obese children at the age of 12 to 13 years. A comparison of the thickness of the individual skinfolds shows not only markedly higher values but their mutual relationship is different. The distribution of fat is similarly increased both in obese boys and girls; the usual gender difference in the amount of total fat and its patterning is lacking. Both obese boys and girls resemble older women as shown by comparing the results of measurements in various age groups using the same method.[56] Also, the relationships between individual skinfolds (for example, using the centrality index of the subscapular/triceps skinfold ratio), and those between the sums of skinfolds on the trunk and on the extremities were different as compared to normal-weight children.[18,56] In another study in severely obese children aged $10.15 \pm 2.01$ years, the centrality index was positively correlated with TC, LDL-C, TG, and negatively correlated with HDL-C.[370]

### 4.4.2   Waist-to-Hip Ratio

Fat distribution has also been evaluated using ratios of various circumference measurements, most often the waist-to-hip ratio (WHR) or waist-to-thigh ratio. Gender differences in normal children aged 4.0 to 14.5 years living in the central part of Spain were described. These values may serve as standard values of fat distribution for clinical practice.[371] This index, along with the

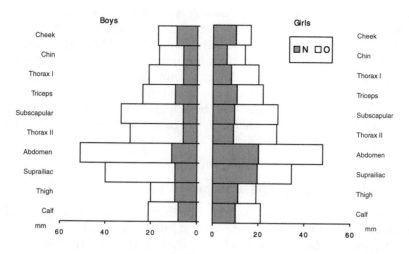

**FIGURE 4.7**

Comparison of skinfold thickness (mm) distributions in obese (O) and normal-weight (N) boys and girls (12 to 14 years old); centrality index (subscapular/triceps ratio) in obese boys (1.2), in obese girls (1.4); in normal-weight boys (0.8), in normal-weight girls (0.7). (Based on data from Refs. F6, F8, F9.)

percentage of overweight and percentage of stored fat was validated by significant correlations with triglycerides (TG), alanine aminotransferase (ALT), and insulin in boys, whereas only WHR/Ht showed a close relationship with TG and insulin in girls. Moreover, this index differentiated subjects with abnormal values of TG, insulin, and ALT, especially in girls.[372] WHR was negatively associated with HDL-C and positively associated with TC/HDL-C ratio in pre- and postpubertal girls independent of age and BMI.[306]

Marelli et al.[370] found a significant correlation of WHR and TG level. These results confirm that even during childhood, severe obesity is related to blood lipid alterations and at this early stage of life the truncal distribution of adipose tissue is associated with an adverse serum lipid spectrum. WHR/height standard deviation score (SDS) can serve as an index predicting occurrence of biochemical complications, that is, abnormal values of TG, ALT, and insulin in obese children ages 6 to 15 years.[373]

To validate the above-mentioned indices of fat distribution, interrelationships were examined between BMI, the WHR, and serum concentration of immuno-reactive insulin (IRI), C-peptide, and sex hormone-binding globulin (SHBG). In central and gluteal obesity, differentiated by WHRs, IRI, C-peptide and SHBG differed significantly. WHR did not correlate with IRI, C-peptide, and SHBG. These results suggest that using WHR for the differentiation of central and gluteal obesity does not help in adolescence, which may be due to morphological changes during puberty.[374]

In a 2-decade longitudinal study the relationships between adiposity on the trunk and on the extremities were followed up in French males and females from the age of 1 month to 21 years. The relationship between adult and childhood skinfold ratio measurements is weak in boys and slightly better in girls. From this study and also previous follow-ups, adiposity measurements in children that are associated with metabolic and health problems that have the best correlations with the adult values could be selected: BMI in both genders, trunk skinfolds in boys, and subscapular/arm skinfold thickness ratio in girls. Consequently, a boy with both high BMI and trunk skinfold thickness values, or a girl with both high BMI and subscapular/arm ratio skinfold values are at a greater risk of centralized obesity and accompanying comorbidities later in life.[201,257]

### 4.4.3   Subcutaneous and Intra-Abdominal Fat

Body fat distribution was assessed and quantified using MRI in girls in late puberty. The amounts of subcutaneous and intra-abdominal fat were derived from transverse slices at the levels of the waist, hip, and trochanter using magnetic resonance imaging (MRI). The results were compared with simple anthropometric measurements. Waist, hip, and trochanter circumferences were highly correlated to the respective related MRI total fat surface area both in early and late pubertal girls ($r = 0.79 - 0.97$), while waist circumference, and waist-hip, waist-thigh, or skinfold ratios were not significantly correlated to intra-abdominal fat areas.

Further measurements showed that in late puberty the MRI derived amount of subcutaneous fat was significantly larger at the trochanter level compared to that in girls in the early stages of puberty. This was due to greater deposition of fat in the gluteal area. It could be concluded that while circumferences at the trunk are good measures for the related amounts of fat in pubertal girls, this is not true for various ratios of circumferences and/or skinfold ratios.[375]

Possible prediction of visceral adiposity from measurements of waist circumference was further validated by MRI assessments at a level of L4 in subjects with simple obesity aged 8.6 to 15.5 years. Best correlations were found for MRI and waist circumference. In addition, waist-arm, and waist-thigh ratios correlated with visceral fat measured by MRI.[376]

Internal fat was measured in children and adolescents using computed tomography imaging along with anthropometric methods for the evaluation of intra-abdominal adipose tissue (IAAT) in children aged $6.4 \pm 1.2$ years, weighing $24.8 \pm 5.4$ kg.[365] Body composition was assessed using BIA, and fat distribution was evaluated from individual measurements of 8 skinfolds. The ratio of IAAT to subcutaneous adipose tissue (SCAT) was $0.15 \pm 0.08$, and the ratio of IAAT to total body fat mass was $1.44 \pm 0.84$ cm$^2$/kg. IAAT was significantly correlated with body weight ($0.54$, $p < 0.03$), all skinfold measures ($r = 0.60 \pm 0.78$, $p < 0.02$ to $0.0003$) except at the calf, fat mass ($r = 0.69$, $p < 0.003$), and trunk-to-extremity skinfold ratio ($r = 0.78$, $p < 0.0003$). No significant relationship between IAAT and WHR was found in obese children of this age. These preliminary results show the existence of IAAT in young children and also reveal that individual skinfold thicknesses on the trunk and the trunk/extremity skinfold ratio provide a better marker of IAAT than WHR.[365]

For evaluating IAAT it is also possible to use another anthropometric approach, the measurement of the distance between L4 and the tip of the abdominal wall. The correlation between these two measurements and the results of ultrasonography in adult obese subjects was significant in adults.[366]

Rolland-Cachera and Deheeger examined the relationships between waist circumference, WHR, and waist-to-stature ratio in children. WHR was not correlated with either fatness index but the absolute values of waist circumference as well as waist-to-stature ratio correlated significantly with fatness indices (BMI, triceps, and subscapular skinfolds).[377]

The findings from the Bogalusa Heart Study also emphasized the importance of body fat distribution in children, in particular as waist circumference. This parameter may help to identify children likely to have adverse concentrations of insulin and lipids. Compared with a child at the 10th percentile of waist circumference a child at the 90th percentile was estimated to have, on average, higher concentrations of LDL-C, TG, and lower concentrations of HDL-C. These highly significant differences were independent of weight and height, and consistent across race–gender groups.[378]

### 4.4.4 Arm Muscle and Fat Circumferences

Upper arm fat area (UFE = arm circumference × triceps skinfold/2) was used for the definition of malnutrition and also for the identification of obesity in Brazilian children aged 1 to 5 years. The prevalence of obesity was analyzed in various regions of the country.[379] Rolland-Cachera et al.[377] used this parameter to evaluate obesity in children as mentioned previously.[113,380]

### 4.5 Striae in Obese Children

Excess fatness can also cause striae in obese children and adolescents. In a group of 3- to 19-year-olds assessed in a pediatric nutrition clinic, striae were identified in approximately 40% of patients. Generally, striae were symmetrical on both sides of the body and were most prominent on the thighs, arms, and abdomen. Less frequently they appeared on the back, buttocks, and over the knees. There was no gender difference in the prevalence of striae but they were more marked in older subjects and after longer periods of obesity.[381] Colored striae were also observed in Taiwanese children, most commonly appearing on the thighs, arms, and abdomen.[143]

Measurements of type III procollagen propeptide and adrenal function suggest that striae in obese children are associated with lower collagen synthesis. As adrenal function was similar in all groups of obese children, those with and without striae, it was supposed that the higher estrogen levels in the obese with striae are due to aromatase activity of fat tissue.[382]

## 4.6   Growth, Skeletal Age, and Bone Development

As mentioned above, obese children are frequently taller than their normal-weight or lean peers. In a group of Italian obese children aged 3 to 16 years percentile distribution of height for age showed that stature was higher in obese children than in normal-weight control children by about 5 to 6 centimeters. This was the case in both genders until about 11 years in girls and 12 years in boys, which indicates accelerated growth in obese subjects. After this age, percentile distribution was similar in both obese and normal-weight children. With respect to controls, skeletal age tended to be advanced by about 0.75 year in obese girls at all ages, and about 0.75 to 1.0 year in boys up to 11 years. After this age, skeletal age of boys was similar to controls and relative to age. Maturation according to skeletal age tended to be earlier as BMI increased and early maturers had higher values of BMI.[383] Similar differences in height were also found in obese Czech children (Figure 4.6).[18]

Child weight and level of maturity accounted for 54% of the variance in predicting baseline height percentile. Initial values of height and parental height accounted for only 9% of the variance in height percentile changes, both adjusted for parental height. Weight change did not correlate with growth when adjusted for parental height.

In obese children bone development is usually advanced, as shown, e.g., in studies of South American children.[28,384] Development of body frame is also different in growing subjects with a longer history of obesity with some larger measurements in obese adolescents, for example, bi-iliocristal diameter, greater lean body mass, (Table 4.1) and others.[18,316] Obese Bulgarian children displayed accelerated growth and bone maturation varying about ± 1SD over the norm. This was more prominent in girls.[118]

Another study of Italian obese subjects showed that growth charts (97th, 50th, and 3rd percentile) were superior to those of the normal-weight population up to the age of 13 and 12.5 years for males and females, respectively. Later, growth decreases in both genders. The obese subjects did not differ in height compared to their normal-weight peers at the age of 18 years.

Bone age estimated by radiograph of the left hand and wrist using the Tanner-Whitehouse II system was more advanced over chronological age in both genders. Increase of bone age over calendar age did not show substantial difference during pubertal maturation in boys, whereas in girls this difference decreased with advancing sexual maturation.[385]

**TABLE 4.1**

Morphological Characteristics in Normal and Obese Boys and Girls
Aged 13 to 14 Years

| | BMI | Fat % | FFM (kg) | Bi-Iliocristal (cm) | Chest Circumference (cm) | Arm Circumference (cm) |
|---|---|---|---|---|---|---|
| *Boys* | | | | | | |
| Normal x̄ | 19.3 | 12.5 | 43.9 | 22.8 | 78.6 | 23.1 |
| SD | 2.1 | 5.9 | 5.1 | 1.8 | 3.3 | 1.2 |
| Obese x̄ | 26.6[a] | 29.5[a] | 48.6[a] | 27.7[a] | 88.3[a] | 27.0[a] |
| SD | 2.9 | 3.2 | 5.0 | 1.0 | 5.5 | 2.3 |
| *Girls* | | | | | | |
| Normal x̄ | 20.4 | 18.1 | 40.7 | 26.8 | 79.2 | 24.3 |
| SD | 3.1 | 6.0 | 4.9 | 2.3 | 4.2 | 2.5 |
| Obese x̄ | 27.8[a] | 31.9[a] | 46.7[a] | 27.4 | 95.18[a] | 29.6[a] |
| SD | 4.0 | 3.7 | 6.4 | 1.1 | 3.8 | 3.3 |

[a] Statistically significant differences between groups; Bi-iliocristal breadth significantly larger after reduction of suprailiac skinfold thickness.
Based on data from Ref. T1.

Obese subjects in this study had significantly higher plasma insulin levels compared to lean controls. A significant positive correlation between plasma insulin levels and height standard deviation score was also found. The study revealed that the growth increase in an obese child starts in the first years of life. This stature advantage is maintained until the beginning of puberty with growth velocity equal to that of lean individuals.

Skeletal maturation is markedly increased and accelerated in both genders. Bone age in this follow-up remained advanced during the period of pubertal development and obese subjects showed a less notable growth spurt than normal-weight subjects. The growth advantage gradually decreases and final adult height of obese and normal-weight subjects is not different.[385]

The excess load from increased deposition of fat might be one of the reasons for the changes in the bone mineral density in obese children. In a study of obese children aged 11.8 ± 2.7 years, determinations were made at the level of the lumbar spine (L2-4) by a commercial dual photon absorptiometer. Bone mineral density was similar in obese and normal children and was highly correlated with age (r = 0.70), body height (r = 0.65), and body weight (r = 0.55). The highest values for bone mineral density were found in obese adolescents with the most advanced pubertal status. No gender differences were observed in obese children when pubertal stage was taken into account. Lumbar spine bone mineral density corrected for age was not related to the degree or duration of obesity. No effect of physical activity could be demonstrated in spine mineralization in the obese group.[386]

## 4.7   Lean Body Mass in Obese Children

Increased fat deposition is accompanied by greater development of lean, fat-free body mass (LBM) as shown by hydro-densitometric measurements and increased bone mineral content (BMC).[18,386] These variables were followed up in children aged 7.3 to 16.5 years with mild, moderate, and severe obesity, using DXA and measuring BMC in various parts of the body. No significant differences were revealed in the upper or lower body or trunk, and total BMC and LBM of these three groups of obese growing subjects.

Upper and lower fat mass was significantly greater in the severely and moderately obese than in mildly obese or in normal groups. No differences between moderate and severely obese subjects were observed. Similar differences were found for trunk and total fat mass. In this study, more marked levels of obesity were thus associated with increased fat mass but not increased BMC and LBM.[387]

In contrast, a DXA study in obese Brazilian children (aged 94.67 ± 10.89 months) showed a significantly greater amount of LBM, higher bone mineral content, higher bone mineral density, and higher total body calcium in the obese compared to normal-weight children of a similar age.[348]

The reported differences of LBM in obese growing subjects in other studies can be explained by variations in the duration, time of the onset, and degree of obesity, plus different methodologies.[18,348]

## 4.8   Muscle Fiber and Obesity

The relationship between muscle fiber type and body adiposity has been studied using skeletal muscle biopsies. Such studies have mainly been conducted with adult subjects; however, some information can apply to younger age categories. Findings need to be verified in the future when additional methods suitable for children may be available.

The presence of slow fibers in muscle biopsies of the vastus lateralis was inversely related to body fatness in adult subjects. Metabolic evidence evaluated using the respiratory exchange ratio (RER) indicated that fatter men with a lower proportion of slow muscle fibers used less fat during exercise on a bicycle ergometer at a work load of 100W than lean men (those with a higher proportion of slow fibers).[388] This evidence supports the hypothesis that muscle fiber type is an etiological factor in the development of obesity and that the processes concerning the metabolism of lipids during work load are related to the proportion of various types of fibers in skeletal muscles. These mechanisms can apply at earlier periods of life since a ratio of slow to fast twitch muscle fibers is present at birth.[389]

Decreased activity of fat-oxidizing enzymes in biopsies from the vastus lateralis muscle was shown in obesity-prone adult subjects but a similar study was not executed in children for obvious reasons. No differences in fiber type composition were found, but a smaller area of type I and 2B fibers was discovered in post-obese women compared to controls. Significantly lower values for hydroxyacyl-coenzyme-A-dehydrogenase (HADH), a key enzyme in β-oxidation of fatty acids, and of citrate-synthetase, a rate-limiting enzyme in the Krebs cycle, were revealed in the post-obese women. These findings matched a trend for lower aerobic power (VO$_2$ max) and lower food and fat intake. As shown in other studies, a high level of aerobic power facilitates the utilization of lipid metabolites and contributes to a reduction and/or maintenance of a low amount of stored fat.[18] RMR and RER did not differ but tended to be lower in the post-obese women. This could explain the lower fat oxidation previously found in post-obese subjects; however, when adjusting data for age and VO$_2$ max, the differences in enzyme activities were no longer significant among post-obese and control subjects.[390] As mentioned earlier, a high level of aerobic power is a condition under which higher utilization of lipid metabolites occurs.

# 5

## Energy Expenditure and Physical Activity

Energy expenditure as related to energy intake, and the resulting energy balance and turnover, play an essential role in the deposition of fat in the human organism and in the development of obesity. Physical activity is the main variable that can change the energy expenditure at all ages. A reduction of physical activity due to sedentary activities during leisure time can have a negative effect on energy balance.

There are still numerous gaps in our understanding of energy expenditure in a range of contexts, particularly in children. For example, exact measurements of energy expenditure over extended periods of time are not possible. At the other extreme, even small amounts of non-weight-bearing physical activities, such as fidgeting in a sitting position, may account for more energy output than once thought.[31]

More longitudinal studies are necessary as the short-term measurements of energy expenditure in children who are already obese do not always reveal the true relationship between total energy expenditure (TEE) and energy expenditure for activity (AEE) on the one hand, and adiposity during growth on the other hand. Possible differences between obese and lean subjects may also not be revealed. As mentioned previously, the level of physical activity in children and youth today is generally quite low and in many places may still be decreasing, regardless of the individual's level of adiposity.

Obesity does not develop overnight. The condition is the result of long-term metabolic, hormonal, functional, and psychological adjustments related to a different energy balance and turnover in the organism and also based on genetic background. Therefore, ad hoc short-term measurements cannot provide a true picture of any parameter, including a history of the level of physical activity and total energy expenditure during earlier periods of growth. To understand the causes of obesity in a comprehensive manner would require measurements over a long period starting with the very beginning of any increase in weight and deposition of excess fat, and perhaps even the period preceding the development of obesity.

## 5.1 Components of Energy Expenditure

Energy expenditure is comprised of a number of different components. Total energy expenditure (TEE) includes the following:

Basal metabolic rate (BMR): a minimal rate of energy expenditure compatible with life.

Thermic effect of food (TEF), or thermic effect of a meal (TEM): is energy used in digesting, absorbing, storing, and disposing of the ingested nutrients.[391] TEF is usually estimated as 10% of TEE.

Energy spent in physical activity (AEE): activity energy expenditure. Physical activity provides the greatest potential for varying total energy expenditure either by increasing or decreasing TEE (Figure 5.1).

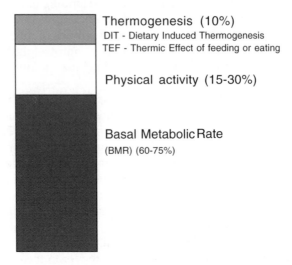

**FIGURE 5.1**
Components of daily energy expenditure in normal subjects.

BMR is usually measured by indirect calorimetry under basal conditions, which in practice means that the measurements are taken during sleep or just after waking. It is also recommended that the individual fast overnight and avoid intense physical activity the preceding day. This methodology is not feasible in subjects living under normal home conditions, and therefore is usually reserved for a laboratory or clinic setting.

A number of regression equations for the estimation of BMR have been developed. The FAO/WHO/UNU Expert Consultation (Rome, 1981) suggested new equations for children and adolescents which were published in the WHO document,[274] and further developed by James and Schofield (Table 5.1).[391] For this estimation of both weight and height, only weight is used for the calculations. The values of BMR are also used for the evaluation

**TABLE 5.1**

Equations for Predicting Basal Metabolic Rate from Body Weight (W) in Children and Adolescents

| Age Range (years) | Kcal.day$^{-1}$ | r | SD$^a$ | MJ.day$^{-1}$ | r | SD$^a$ |
|---|---|---|---|---|---|---|
| *Males* | | | | | | |
| 0–3 | 60.9 W – 54 | 0.97 | 53 | 0.255 W – 0.226 | 0.97 | 0.222 |
| 3–10 | 22.7 W + 495 | 0.86 | 62 | 0.0949 W + 2.07 | 0.86 | 0.259 |
| 10–18 | 17.5 W + 651 | 0.90 | 100 | 0.0732 W + 2.72 | 0.90 | 0.418 |
| *Females* | | | | | | |
| 0–3 | 61.0 W – 51 | 0.97 | 61 | 0.255 W – 0.214 | 0.97 | 0.255 |
| 3–10 | 22.5 W – 499 | 0.85 | 63 | 0.0941 W + 2.09 | 0.85 | 0.264 |
| 10–18 | 12.2 W + 746 | 0.75 | 117 | 0.0510 W + 3.12 | 0.75 | 0.489 |

$^a$ SD, standard deviation of differences between the actual and predicted estimates.
Based on data from Ref. T2.

of TEE using its multiples to characterize the intensity of energy output during various physical activities.

Resting energy expenditure (REE) is usually evaluated on the basis of the uptake of oxygen (indirect calorimetry) under resting conditions in an adequate environment and ambient temperature, after at least 30 min repose. Post-prandial thermogenesis, the thermic effect of food (TEF), or of a meal (TEM) is approximately 10% of TEE (or 0.1 of TEE).

TEE during 1 or more days can also be measured by direct and/or indirect calorimetry in special chambers. Obese adult subjects have been studied under such conditions, but confinement in an isolated chamber for a long period of time is not acceptable for younger children.

TEE can also be measured under normal free-living conditions using doubly labelled water (DLW), a technique that has also been used in studies of obese children.[360,392] AEE can be evaluated as the difference between TEE and (REE + TEF).

Physical activity (PA) is any bodily movement produced by skeletal muscles that results in an increase of energy expenditure.

Physical activity level (PAL) expresses the ratio between BMR and TEE. PAL = TEE during 24 hr/BMR during 24 hr.

Physical activity ratio (PAR) is a similar index relating the values per minute. PAR = TEE min$^{-1}$/BMR min$^{-1}$.

Exercise (E) is a subcategory of physical activity that is structured, repetitive, and purposeful in the sense that improvement or maintenance of physical fitness is often an objective. AEE can be evaluated by direct measurement (calorimetry), or by a procedure suggested by the WHO and James and Schofield.[274,391] The calculation of BMR and the use of multiples of BMR (METs) (Table 5.2) for individual physical activities are in widespread use. An example for a normal child is provided in Table 5.3. Individual evaluation encompasses the ability to consider the time and intensity of workload in activity and/or exercise.

**TABLE 5.2**

Physical Activity Ratios (PAR) of Selected Activities

| PAR | Value Range | Activity |
|---|---|---|
| 1.2 | (1.0–1.4) | Lying at rest, sitting or standing quietly |
| 1.6 | (1.4–1.8) | Washing, dressing |
| 1.4 | | Sitting, playing |
| 2.5 | | Strolling around |
| 2.8 | (2.4–3.3) | Walking on level, speed 3–4 km.hr$^{-1}$ |
| 3.2 | | Walking at a normal pace |
| 4.7 | | Walking uphill slowly |
| 5.7 | | Walking uphill at normal pace |
| 7.5 | | Walking uphill fast |
| 2.8 | (2.4–3.3) | Walking downhill |
| 3.8 | | Cycling, gymnastics |
| 5.1 | | Dancing, swimming |
| 6.7 | (5.9–7.9) | Walking, speed 6–7 km.hr$^{-1}$, football, running, cross-country walking, paddling, etc. |
| 9.0 | (7.9–10.5) | Aerobic dancing, playing tennis competitively |

Based on data from Refs. T2, T3.

**TABLE 5.3**

Examples of the Calculation Used to Derive Energy Expenditure in a 10-Year-Old Girl (Body Weight 33.8 kg)

| Activity | Hours | kcal | kJ |
|---|---|---|---|
| Sleep at 1.0 × BMR | 9 | 435 | 1820 |
| School at 1.5 × BMR | 4 | 290 | 1210 |
| Light activity at 1.5 × BMR | 4 | 290 | 1210 |
| Moderate activity | 6.5 | 690 | 2890 |
| High activity at 6.0 × BMR | 0.5 | 145 | 610 |
| Total expenditure | | 1850 | 7740 |
| Growth | | 65 | 270 |
| Total requirement per 24 hours 1.65 × BMR | | 1915 | 8010 |

Based on data from Ref. T2.

## 5.2 Resting Metabolic Rate (RMR)

RMR can be assessed directly or by using prediction equations. When measured directly, the subject must rest for a minimum of 30 min in an ambient temperature before the measurement is taken. This parameter usually replaces the measurement of BMR that is more difficult to measure in subjects living at home. However, as mentioned above, BMR can be calculated using the regression equations recommended by WHO and James and Schofield.[274,391] As these equations were derived mainly on the basis of measurements in normal-weight children, results must be evaluated with caution when applied to obese children.

The measurements of Kaplan et al.[393] provide some useful working examples. The assessment of REE in pediatric practice using various prediction equations does not apply to obese children. REE was measured by indirect calorimetry and compared with the results of the following prediction equations: FAO/WHO/UNU,[274] the Harris-Benedict (H-B) equation, and two equations of Schofield, one using weight (Scho-WT) and the other using weight and height (Scho-HTWT). The results of a study in children and adolescents (aged 0.2 to 20.5 years) showed that the Schofield HTWT equation predicts REE in children with clinical nutritional problems better than the equations that use weight alone.[393] However, in view of the wide variability in REE measurements in children of various levels of fatness, it is preferable not to predict REE in obese children but to measure it directly whenever possible.

Other measurements in a sample of prepubertal and pubertal children aged 10 to 16 years showed that the indirect calorimetry method (using the ventilatory hood system) did not agree with the results of the calculations using five regression equations. All equations overestimated RMR in obese subjects by 7.5 to 18.1%. Additional regression equations have been derived on the basis of measurements of a further cohort of obese children and adolescents and provided reliable results compared to direct measurements.[394] Figure 5.2 shows the comparison of RMR and BMI in normal-weight and obese children.

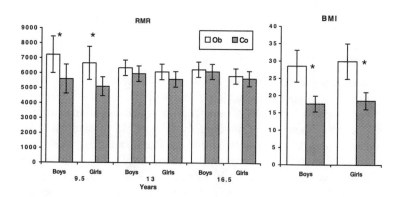

**FIGURE 5.2.**

Comparison of body mass index (BMI) and resting metabolic rate (RMR) in obese (Ob) and normal-weight (Co) boys and girls aged 9.5 to 16.5 years. * indicates ($p < 0.05$). (Based on data from Ref. F10.)

In another study, RMR, BMI, and food intake were higher in obese than normal-weight children (Figure 5.3).[392] When adjusted for fat-free mass, the energy intake was the same in both obese and normal-weight children. The same applied to RMR that did not vary when related to fat-free, lean body mass (FFM, LBM). The main determinant of RMR was fat-free, lean body mass. However, the gender difference remained significant after adjustment for FFM. The adjusted values of RMR decreased slightly but significantly between the age of 10 to 16 years.[395]

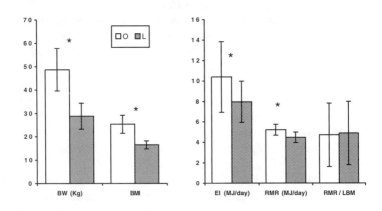

**FIGURE 5.3**
Comparison of morphological characteristics (body weight, body mass index), energy intake (EI), resting metabolic rate (RMR, MJ per 24 hours) in obese (O) and normal-weight (L) boys and girls. * indicates ($p < 0.05$). (Based on data from Ref. F11.)

## 5.3   Thermic Effect of Food

Excess fatness may affect not only RMR but also the thermic effect of a meal (TEM). This phenomenon was studied in a group of obese and normal-weight children aged $8.8 \pm 0.3$ years. RMR was higher in obese than in normal-weight children. As in the above-mentioned study, when RMR was adjusted for FFM, values were no longer significantly different. The thermic response to a liquid mixed meal, expressed as a percentage of the energy content of the meal was significantly lower in obese than in normal-weight children (Figure 5.4).[396] These data indicate that the defect in thermogenesis reported in obese adults originates earlier in life than was previously assumed.

The relationships between REE, diet-induced thermogenesis (DIT, indirect calorimetry), and body fat distribution were analyzed in normal-weight children and obese children distributed in groups of abdominal (WHR > 0.9) and gluteal-femoral obese (WHR < 0.8). No differences in REE and DIT were seen

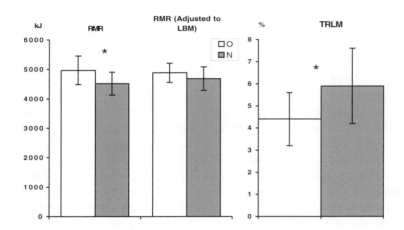

**FIGURE 5.4**

The comparison of resting metabolic rate (RMR) and the thermic effect of mixed liquid meal (TRLM) in prepubertal obese (O) and non-obese control (N) children. * indicates ($p < 0.05$). (Based on data from Ref. F12.)

among children with different types of obesity. Therefore, it was concluded that body fat distribution in obese and normal-weight adolescents has no influence on resting energy expenditure and diet-induced thermogenesis.[397]

## 5.4 Total Energy Expenditure and Physical Activity

Studies of TEE in children, including the energy spent on physical activity (activity energy expenditure, AEE), can be quite difficult. Due to excessive cost, it is unusual to use more sophisticated and costly methods such as the DLW technique for the measurement of TEE on a routine basis, along with measurements of BMR and/or RMR. However, DLW ($^2H_2\,^{18}O$) has been more widely used during the last decade.[360,398]

### 5.4.1 Methods

There is considerable evidence to suggest that physical activity as a youngster has a bearing upon functional status as an adult. Similarly, one might contend that physical activity experiences of children and adolescents play a major role in the development of appropriate lifestyle behaviors in the adult years. The issue of tracking of physical activity behaviors across the growing years and into adulthood is central to the persistence of benefits of physical activity being maintained. One of the limiting factors in our understanding of a range of health issues is the need for valid and reliable measures of physical activity.

A number of methods have been used to measure the physical activity status of children and adolescents. Westerterp groups the available techniques into five general categories: behavioral observation; questionnaires (including diaries, recall questionnaires, and interviews); physiological markers such as heart rate; calorimetry; and motion sensors.[399]

Methods vary in sophistication from the relatively simple and easy to administer self-reporting and monitoring methods to the more costly laboratory-based procedures. The laboratory-based methods are more precise but are not suited to large numbers of individuals while the reverse is true for field methods such as self-reporting and monitoring procedures. Readers are encouraged to access a number of reviews devoted to physical activity assessment in children and adolescents.[400–404] In addition, a recent review of the assessment of physical activity level in relation to obesity provides a useful summary.[399]

There are numerous considerations when choosing a measure of physical activity and these include the reliability, validity, and efficacy of the instrument.[9] Reliability is the extent to which a method produces similar values on 2 or more occasions. Precision and accuracy relate to the ability of a measurement technique to achieve the right answer. Validity in turn refers to the extent to which the method is a true indication of the variable (in this case, physical activity) being assessed.[9]

The energy cost of PA and TEE can be expressed by multiples of BMR METs. This characterizes the intensity of workload related to BMR and therefore, the energy expended. MET values have been derived mostly on the basis of the measurements in adults but have also been used for children.[274] Using this procedure, TEE per day can be calculated. However, during the same physically defined workload, (for example, 2 watts per kg of body weight on a bicycle ergometer), 12-year-old children increased their energy expenditure related to BMR by approximately 29% less than 18-year-old individuals and adults.[405]

Multiples of BMR that characterize the intensity of a workload for adults are higher due to reduction of BMR with aging. Therefore, their use can be misleading when using the WHO procedures for children, especially at younger ages. This phenomenon can partially explain the trend for a higher physical activity level (PAL) in children, especially of preschool age. The transition from resting to active conditions in a young individual is a relatively smaller change than in an older person. However, this principle applies to normal-weight children and less to the overweight and/or obese. Bigger individuals, as a function of their weight, BMI, body composition, and spontaneous physical activity, are more akin to much older individuals.

The BMR to characterize estimation of energy expenditure using the abovementioned procedure should be supplemented by the measurement of young individuals during standardized workloads, deriving more exact multiples of the intensity of each workload. For an approximation of TEE this can still be quite useful.

The DLW method provides a measurement of daily EE and metabolic rate over a timeframe of 1 to 3 weeks. PAL can be evaluated as given previously.

The main advantage of DLW is that it provides a non-invasive method for the assessment of TEE under conditions of normal living. In spite of both the advantages and the disadvantages the technique has been used in both adults and children.[360] The principle involves the oral application of a mixture of $^2H_2O$ and $^2H_2^{18}O$ to enrich the body's water pool with $^2H_2$ and $^{18}O$. The plateau concentration of the isotopes measured 3 to 4 hours after dosage enables the estimation of the water pool, which is used for both DLW calculation and for the estimation of fat mass to lean body mass ratio.

The $^2H$ equilibrates with body water and the rate constant for its disappearance is proportional to water turnover. The $^{18}O$ equilibrates with both water and the bicarbonate pool that is generated from the carbon dioxide appearing as the end product of oxidative metabolism. Their rapid equilibrium is due to carbonic anhydrase reaction, the rate constant for $^{18}O$ disappearance is proportional to the sum of water and bicarbonate turnover. The difference between the two rate constants gives a measure of carbon dioxide production from which energy expenditure can be evaluated using classical indirect calorimetric equations.[360]

The DLW technique is considered the criterion measure or gold standard for the measurement of TEE. Like all measures, the technique has inherent strengths and weaknesses. The major advantage of the technique is its precision, but this needs to be weighed against the substantial cost. As a laboratory-based procedure (at least for assessment of samples) the technique is prohibitive for any large scale, population-based assessment of energy expenditure. Further, the technique provides a gross measure of energy expenditure and is unable to define the nature of the activity or types of activity in which the individual has been involved.

A study by Goran et al.[356] using the DLW technique with 4- to 6-year-old children, quantified associations between energy expenditure, heart rate, resting energy expenditure, and body composition. Findings included a significant association between resting heart rate and energy expenditure. Measures of heart rate and other parameters such as body composition have been considered legitimate options for the measurement of energy expenditure in larger numbers of subjects.

Numerous methodologies have been employed using physiological adjustment as measured by heart rate. Heart rate monitors and derivatives are in widespread use, commonly in conjunction with training programs.[10,406] Other monitors are able to capture heart rate data over an extended timeframe and may register the number of beats in certain bands of heart rate across the measurement period, commonly during the waking hours of the day. The results of these HR measurements form the basis of the estimation of energy expenditure. When HR is correlated with oxygen uptake (by indirect calorimetry) under rest conditions and/or at various levels of workload, an assessment of energy output using individual regression equations of the relationship between HR and $O_2$ uptake is possible.

Other forms of monitoring devices, including mechanical and electronic derivatives, are a range of accelerometers including Tritrac, Caltrac, and CSA. Caltrac is a uni-axial accelerometer as are the Computer Science Application (CSA) and Mini Motionlogger Actigraph. The Tritrac is a tri-axial accelerometer like the movement registration system, the Tracmor.[399] Numerous concerns have been raised regarding the reliability of energy cost measurement of various physical activities using accelerometers; for example, when walking uphill or downhill the incline must be taken into consideration or estimates may be inaccurate.[407]

The use of the Tritrac accelerometer (and deriving METs), along with self-reported physical activity, has enabled physical activity determinants to be derived in obese children. There is a moderate correlation between these two parameters of physical activity (r = 0.46). The difference between the measurements using Tritrac is 1.6 METS and self-reported activity is 2.3 METs. Prediction of activity indicated variance according to factors considered in the hierarchical analysis (socioeconomic level, body composition, fitness, hedonics of child, and adult activity behaviors).[408]

The evaluation of physical activity level using the Tritrac yielded more reliable estimates of the physical activity level in obese children aged 8 to 15 years than a self-reported measure. Correlations between the values of energy output by accelerometer (expressed in METs) and adjusted heart rates (r = 0.71) were significantly higher than correlations between adjusted heart rates and self-reported METs (r = 0.36). Self-reported METs had higher mean standard errors in estimating heart rates, were significantly greater than accelerometer METs, and systematically overestimated accelerometer METs.[25] This means that the information on physical activity levels in obese children using questionnaires may not be objective.

A number of self-report measures are available for use and these vary substantially. The questionnaires usually describe the type, duration, and frequency of daily physical activities that are not always possible to obtain from assessments of TEE by DLW or sums of HR over longer time periods. This is essential for evaluations as only relevant intensity and type of exercise can result in significant changes to morphological and functional variables.

Therefore, an effort has been made to create and validate questionnaires and to evaluate children's activity. Questionnaires may be used simultaneously with the other approaches of energy expenditure measurements. The self-report questionnaires represent the most commonly employed methods of physical activity assessment. Generally, instruments of this type are suitable for individuals over 10 years of age. Assistance is essential from teachers and parents when working with younger children.[409]

The Children's Activity Rating Scale (CARS) with five levels enabled the categorization and discrimination of eight physical activities, and therefore children's levels of energy expenditure. Observers were trained to follow-up young children under field conditions and a satisfactory agreement between the results of observations gained by individual examiners was found. These data demonstrate that CARS can encompass a wide variety of physical activity and levels of energy expenditure. Mean values of energy expenditure for eight activities representing the five levels of CARS were pre-tested by measuring $VO_2$ and heart rates in 5- to 6-year-old children. These values ranged from 1 to 5.2 METs, that is, 14.5 to 80.6% of $VO_2$ max, and heart rate from 89 to 183 beats.min$^{-1}$.[410] This sort of assessment may enable the evaluation of energy expenditure when the use of more sophisticated and expensive methods is not available.[410]

## 5.5 Physical Activity and Energy Expenditure as Related to Fatness

The exact evaluation of physical activity level in individual subjects during growth and living under normal conditions is a problem. Precise and accurate methods such as the DLW technique are too expensive and not available to all researchers. Physical activity epidemiology is essential for the evaluation of the effect of physical activity levels on a child's development and on the prevalence of obesity.[411]

At present, many samples have not been adequately described, or the statistical adjustment was not satisfactory. As a result of recent studies, there are varying positions regarding the relationships between physical activity and fatness, or significant differences in physical activity between lean and obese children. In relation to childhood obesity, the influence of TEE is somewhat unclear as some studies report a reduced TEE[412,413] and others do not.[414,415] An improvement in the existing methods of physical activity epidemiology is necessary.[416]

As mentioned previously, only certain levels of intensity, duration, and type of physical activity and exercise can stimulate changes in body adiposity through an increased energy expenditure (see Chapter 4). Few individuals display a consistent regulation of energy balance and size of body fat stores. There is evidence that low energy output is not counterbalanced by decreased hunger and amended satiety mechanisms in individuals with a genetically determined susceptibility to weight gain and obesity. About 80% of the variance between a subject's RMR can be explained by the amount of lean, fat-free body mass (FFM), and a further 10% is accounted for by fat mass, plasma T3, and noradrenaline levels.[417]

### 5.5.1 Genetic Factors

Some studies suggest that there is a significant genetic component that predisposes both a low level of spontaneous physical activity and an increased deposition of fat. Infants of obese mothers have low energy expenditures that are associated with obesity, whereas no such finding was observed in infants with non-obese mothers.[398,412] In another study, RMR was 6% lower in children with one obese parent than in other children studied.[249] Family membership accounted for 57% of the variance in spontaneous physical activity indicating that a genetic predisposition is involved.[418]

Neonatal adiposity was not significantly associated with parental adiposity and gender and did not predict adiposity later in childhood.[419] However, in a stepwise multiple regression analysis, the daily physical activity level of children and parental adiposity were significantly associated with childhood adiposity. The age or gender of the child did not significantly correlate with childhood adiposity. The increase of parental adiposity or the decrease of daily physical activity level was likely to increase the adiposity in 4- to 8-year-old children.

Genetic factors are assumed to play an important role in RMR and TEM. Measurements in prepubertal children, subdivided according to family history, showed that average RMR was similar in obese children with or without a family history of obesity but higher than in control, normal-weight children. Adjusted for FFM, average RMRs were comparable in all three groups of children. TEM, calculated as a percentage of RMR, was lower in the obese than in control children. These measurements failed to support the view that family history of obesity can significantly influence the RMR and TEM of obese children with obese parents.[420]

Resting metabolic rate (RMR) was studied as a function of body weight in another study of obese children. Measurements showed higher values in obese subjects than in lean children. Child weight accounted for 72 and 78% of the variance in RMR. When parental weight was included, the prediction of RMR did not improve. After 6 months of treatment obese children decreased their percent of overweight but RMR remained unchanged. These data indicate that the RMR does not change when the percent of overweight results from an increase of height and no change in weight.[421]

RMR is a familial trait but the effects can be attributed mainly to familial body size and composition resemblance, that is, FFM and FM. A low level of RMR for a given FFM is a risk factor for increased weight gain and obesity. Based on a meta-analysis, weight-normalized formerly obese subjects have a fivefold greater chance of having a very low RMR when adjusted for body size and composition than matched control subjects who were never obese.[417]

Obese and lean adolescent siblings were compared for RMR (indirect calorimetry), aerobic power ($VO_2$ max in absolute and relative values), and body composition. Obese siblings had an increased amount of stored fat, but similar lean FFM. RMR did not differ among obese and lean siblings. Aerobic power was greater in obese siblings but it was the same when adjusted for FFM.[422]

Energy balance, due to various AEE, plays an important role in the development of obesity during childhood.[423] Results of studies reveal significant relationships between the degree of physical activity and the percentage of fat.[18,61,398] However, some results are controversial and do not confirm these relationships. Measurements of TEE and AEE have shown higher or similar values in the obese than in non-obese children, although obese children were usually more sedentary. Obese children spend less time participating in moderate and more vigorous physical activities than lean children, and their higher energy expenditure was due to a higher energy cost of everyday activities resulting from carrying the extra load of excess fat.[212]

## 5.5.2 Physical Activity in Early Life

The effect of physical activity on adiposity in children has been studied, often since birth and in relation to parental adiposity. Physical activity measures were not associated with neonatal adiposity, nor was neonatal activity significantly correlated with adiposity in later childhood. Two groups of young children at low risk (group N) and high risk of developing obesity (group O) judged by parental obesity, were studied in relation to energy intake. Energy intake was 16% lower in group O. Total energy expenditure (TEE) was determined by the heart rate method.[413]

In many studies, no significant differences in physical activity levels related to overweight have been found. Reduced energy expenditure in early infancy has been associated with the later development of obesity in children born to overweight mothers.

The relationship between energy expenditure and later body composition was studied in healthy children aged $6.67 \pm 0.81$ years with body composition evaluated using a standard deuterium oxide dilution technique. Total energy expenditure had been measured at the age of 12 weeks using the DLW technique. At this age there was a wide variation in total energy expenditure, $71.2 \pm 20.0$ kcal.kg$^{-1}$ body weight, and $91.4 \pm 25.0$ kcal.kg$^{-1}$ FFM.

However, the correlation between energy expenditure at the age of 12 weeks and body fatness was not significant. In addition, the energy expenditure of infants who at any time in later childhood became overweight was not significantly different from the rest of the group. It was not possible to prove any relationship between early total energy expenditure and body fatness at the age of 6.67 years.[424]

Observations in 18-month-old children have shown significant correlations between physical activity levels and caloric intake. Children with a higher caloric intake tended to have lower activity levels. This finding suggests that these two risk factors influencing the development of obesity are likely to occur together in young children.[425] At the preschool age, very active children tended to have a higher food intake than inactive children.[68,426]

Physical activity during growth varies according to age and gender. The level of physical activity is high when BMI decreases during the preschool period and decreases along with the age of adiposity rebound (AR). It may be that all these characteristics are signs of a certain level of maturity for entering primary school. Usually physical activity decreases with increasing age, most commonly after entering primary school. This decrease in activity relates not only to the time spent at school but also leisure time and weekends and during and after puberty.[158] Activity was lower in young females compared to males in a group of African-American high school freshmen as reflected in the Lipid Research Clinic's Physical Activity questionnaires.[427] There appear to be similar trends in physical activity during adolescence.

A significant association between body weight and physical activity ($r = 0.63$) was found in 5- to 6-year-old German children; however, the association between fatness and physical activity was weak ($r = 0.29$).[219] In another study of preschool children using direct observation, motion sensor evaluation, and parental reports, no marked associations between physical activity and weight status, as well as cardiovascular risks such as blood pressure were found.[254] This was not true in a study by Davies et al.[424] who found a significant correlation using DLW between the level of physical activity and adiposity in preschool children.

In a study following TEE (using DLW) in groups of children aged 6 to 8 years with a high and low risk for obesity (with obese or non-obese parents), no significant differences were found.[428] Regression analysis showed that lean FFM, BMR, body weight, and the percentage of stored fat were better predictors of TEE in high-risk children than parental BMI. A trend to greater adiposity characterized the high-risk group, suggesting that these children may be particularly susceptible to the development of obesity later in life. The time spent in active and sedentary activities was assessed by questionnaire (7-day leisure diary) in two groups of normal-weight children aged 6 to 8 years. These children were either at a high (parental BMI > 29.5) or low risk of obesity (parental BMI < 28.2). High-risk children spent significantly more time in active pursuits overall, but were more sedentary on weekends.[428] This may be due to less parental encouragement for sports, resulting in a lack of sufficiently intensive exercise that can influence the somatic and functional development of children.

### 5.5.3   Physical Activity and Adiposity in School Age Children and Adolescents

Numerous studies have been conducted to consider the relationship between energy intake, physical activity, and body fat. White and black girls aged 9 to 11 years enrolled in the National Heart, Lung and Blood Institute Growth and Health Study provide some indicative information. Multivariate regression analyses showed that age, the number of hours of television and video watched, the percent of energy from saturated fatty acids, and the activity-patterns score best explained the variation in body mass index (BMI) and the sum of 3 skinfold measurements in black girls. In white girls, the best model included age, the number of hours of television and video watched, and the percent of energy from total fat.[429] This study indicates that the percentage of stored fat is related to energy intake and expenditure in both black and white girls.

Parameters of body fatness, food intake and composition, and level of physical activity were specified as the most important factors of obesity in Mexican-American girls.[430] These data seem to indicate that the association between activity and fatness only appears at a later age.

The results of the relationships between level of physical activity and body fat vary in some studies with respect to gender. In Swedish adolescents aged 14 to 15 years, a significant relationship was found in boys among the measurements of physical activity level (PAL = TEE/RMR), TEE evaluated by the minute-to-minute monitoring method, RMR by indirect calorimetry, and body composition (evaluated by skinfolds). The same result was not gained in girls.[431]

The etiology of the so-called "low RMR syndrome" is probably hetero-geneous, but low plasma $T_3$ and catecholamine levels and Trp64Arg poly-morphism of the $\beta_3$-adrenergic receptor may be responsible in some cases. Obese subjects with a low value for energy expenditure (EE) over 24 hours achieved a smaller weight loss during dietary treatment than subjects with a high value of 24-hour EE. However, it was assumed that the present lifestyle with physical inactivity might only influence those subjects who are predis-posed psychologically and metabolically to reduced activity, and, therefore, are also susceptible to weight gain and obesity.[417]

TEE (measured by the DLW method) was significantly greater in the obese group than non-obese 12- to 18-year-old adolescents (Figure 5.5).[432] BMR was highly correlated with FFM in both obese and non-obese groups of adoles-cents (r = 0.77, and 0.94, respectively). BMR, using indirect calorimetry and adjusted for FFM, was significantly higher in males than females, and in the obese subjects. The ratios of total TEE/BMR were not significantly different in obese and non-obese groups. These results indicate that BMR and TEE are not reduced in adolescents who are already obese.[432] However, any difference in both TEE and BMR that may have preceded the full development of obe-sity may be a factor. This could only be elucidated by a longitudinal prospec-tive study.

Physical activity levels have been compared in two populations that vary markedly in the prevalence of obesity, Pima Indian children and white chil-dren aged 5 years. TEE and RMR were measured by the DLW method and indirect calorimetry. Different indices of physical activity level were then cal-culated, including AEE = T – (RMR + 0.1 × TEE), and physical activity level PAL = TEE/RMR.

Pima children were significantly heavier and fatter than their white peers of the same age. TEE and RMR were similar in both groups (Figure 5.6) for absolute values after adjustment for body weight, FFM, FM, and gender. Both Pima and white children had PAL levels 20 to 30% lower (1.35 ± 0.13) than currently recommended by the WHO (1.7 to 2.0). However, the calculated indices of physical activity were comparable in these two racial groups.

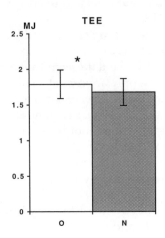

**FIGURE 5.5**
Comparison of total energy expenditure (TEE) in obese (O) and non-obese (N) adolescents. *
indicates ($p < 0.05$). (Based on data from Ref. F13.)

Therefore, the differences in physical activity could not be the cause of obesity in Pima Indian children at the age of 5 years.[433,434]

Some more profound metabolic differences genetically established in Pima Indians may be the cause, along with a suggested higher food intake in this obesity-prone population. Important information for the ever-decreasing physical activity levels in both groups serves as a warning signal for improving the preventive measures for childhood obesity. The time spent in sedentary activities, especially in television viewing by Pima Indian children aged 9.7 ± 2.1 years, predicted weight gain 8 years later at the age of 17.1 ± 1.2 years.[225]

The relationships between the level of physical activity and obesity in older Pima Indian and Caucasian children aged 9.9 and 9.7 years, respectively, were assessed. Pima Indian children were taller, heavier, and fatter. Girls reported significantly lower past-year and past-week sport leisure activities than Caucasian girls and also spent more time watching television. Pima boys also reported lower past-week sport leisure activity than Caucasian boys. In Pima Indian boys, past-year sport leisure activities correlated negatively with BMI ($r = -0.49$) and percentage of depot fat ($r = -0.56$). No similar correlations were found in Pima Indian girls, which was similar to the above-mentioned study.[434]

Children of obese Pima Indian parents were significantly heavier and tended to be fatter with a higher absolute fat mass when compared with the offspring of thin, lean parents. During both normal and overfeeding conditions, the larger portion of variance in 24-hr energy expenditure in a respiratory chamber was accounted for by differences in FFM (54 and 68%,

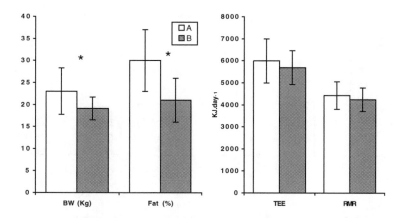

**FIGURE 5.6**
Differences in body weight (BW kg), percentage of stored fat (fat %), total energy expenditure (TEE), and resting metabolic rate (RMR) between Pima Indian (A) and white (B) children aged 5 years. * indicates (p < 0.05). (Based on data from Ref. F14.)

respectively). The differences in the level of spontaneous physical activity accounted for approximately another 19 and 21%.[435]

In a study by Schutz, measurements of energy expenditure by indirect calorimetry showed a linear relationship between body weight and 24-hr AEE.[436] The absolute rate of energy expenditure, especially during weight-bearing activities, is not lower in the obese compared to lean subjects since the hypoactivity does not fully compensate for the greater gross energy cost of a given activity. Similar conclusions were reported by other researchers.[437] However, when discriminating TEE and AEE, the results revealed that in spite of comparable TEE in both obese and normal-weight subjects, the level of activity and energy expended from activity was lower in obese children (Figures 5.7 and 5.8).

The measurement of total daily energy expenditure (TDEE) in free-living conditions (assessed by heart rate using individually determined regression lines at various levels of activity) in obese and non-obese children, aged 9.1 ± 1.6 years and 9.2 ± 0.4 years, respectively, showed higher values of TDEE in obese children. However, the time spent in physical activity was lower in the obese than in the non-obese. This result seemed to be compensated for by a higher energy cost of activity due to higher body weight. In addition, under sedentary conditions, obese children expend more energy than control children.

Energy intake was comparable in both groups, but this lack of difference may be due to under-reporting by obese subjects.[215] Time devoted to sedentary activities was directly proportional to fat mass percentage (r = 0.46, p < 0.050) which suggests the importance of the role of muscular activities in the prevention of deposition of excess fat. TEE was significantly higher in the

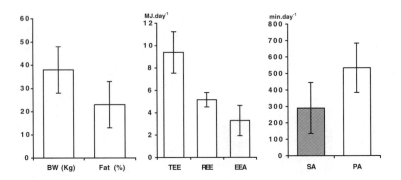

**FIGURE 5.7**
Body weight, percentage of stored fat (fat %), total and resting energy expenditure (TEE, REE), and energy expenditure for activity (EEA), for both sedentary (SA) and nonsedentary physical activities (PA) in 9-year-old boys with broad range of characteristics. Relationship of SA and % fat, r = 0.46 (p < 0.05). (Based on data from Ref. F15.)

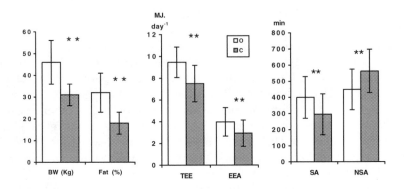

**FIGURE 5.8**
Comparison of body weight (BW), percentage of stored fat (fat %), total energy expenditure (TEE), energy expenditure for activity (EEA, MJ/day), and duration of sedentary (SA) and nonsedentary activities (NSA) in obese (O) and non-obese (C) 8- to 10-year-old children. ** indicates (p < 0.01). (Based on data from Ref. F16.)

obese group than in the non-obese group, and energy expenditure for physical activity together with thermogenesis was significantly higher in obese children.[437]

Higher energy expenditure in obese subjects during laboratory functional testing such as walking and running on a treadmill was found in a group of prepubertal children.[438] At the same speed of exercise during the test, energy expenditure was significantly greater in the obese than in control children. Energy expenditure per kilogram of total and/or FFM was comparable for both groups. Obese children had a significantly larger pulmonary ventilatory response to this workload than did normal-weight control children. Heart rate was comparable in boys and girls combined but significantly higher in obese subjects. These data indicate that walking and running are energetically more demanding for the obese than for normal-weight subjects. Similar results were gained during similar functional testing in other groups of obese children (see Chapter 12).[18] This also helps to explain why obese individuals spontaneously reduce their physical activity levels, especially weight-bearing activities such as running and walking.

In a group of obese and non-obese prepubertal children, TEE was significantly higher than energy intake in the obese children, but comparable to total energy expenditure in the non-obese children. This discrepancy may be explained by the under-reporting of food intake in the obese children, an invalid method in this age group.[439]

An increased intake of sweets found in children of all weight categories indicates that this might be a factor in the increased prevalence of obesity and also dental caries in the growing population, particularly in the industrially developed countries.[440]

A further study of Italian children aged 6 to 14 years showed limited interest in voluntary physical activity and exercise during leisure time, along with incorrect nutritional habits that also concerned subjects enrolled in sport activities.[441] Clearly, an inadequate lifestyle can be detrimental to children from an early age when desirable physical activity and dietary habits and a necessary fitness level should be established. To neglect this critical period would mean the correction later may be more difficult as it is hard to persuade children to take part in activities that are perceived as too arduous and thus unpleasant for them.[442]

Some studies have not shown the expected effect of physical activity. For example, a study in a multi-ethnic sample did not show any differences in physical activity between obese and non-obese girls in grades 5 through to 12. Hispanics and Asians reported lower activity levels than other racial groups. Only 36% of the entire sample and less than one fifth of either Asians or Hispanics met the year 2000 goal for strenuous physical activity, which decreased with age.[443] The time spent participating in games by obese and non-obese Italian children was not different, and the type of game, that is, sedentary or active, was not associated with BMI.[444]

Another study of obese and normal-weight children did not show any between-group differences in daily activities (using a questionnaire). However, sport grades at school were lower and participation in training teams of sport clubs was less frequent among obese than normal-weight children. Obese children were also less fit as judged from the pedaling time in an exercise test on a bicycle ergometer and from the maximum oxygen uptake ($VO_2$ max) related to lean body mass (FFM).[445]

Measurements taken during 2 days did not reveal any differences between obese and non-obese boys and girls physical activity levels, or their attitude toward physical activity. There were no significant relationships between child and maternal activity level, attitude toward physical activity, and adipose level. Obese and non-obese children, with similar levels of physical activity, also showed similar attitudes toward activity, which was unrelated to the maternal factors measured. However, the levels of physical activity were generally low in both obese and non-obese subjects and did not seem to have an important role in their weight control.[446] Unfortunately, measurement was undertaken across a period of time that was too short.

Comparisons between other groups of obese and non-obese adolescents have confirmed the lack of differences in TDEE, measured by doubly labelled water (DLW). This applied to the period of weight maintenance (intake 1.61 × BMR), and also to the period of carbohydrate overloading (2.45 × BMR).[447] BMR measured by indirect calorimetry increased comparably in both obese and non-obese adolescents under such conditions.

In a study of French adolescents aged 12 to 16 years, the relationships between daily energy expenditure (DEE) (evaluated from a long-term measurement of heart rate and whole-body indirect calorimetry), body composition (BIA), and physical activity were examined. Individual relationships between energy expenditure and heart rate were computed and regression equations derived, enabling the evaluation of energy expenditure under free conditions over 5 days, including the weekend. Intragroup variability in DEE, adjusted for differences in FFM, increased during weekends, especially in males. These results were related to the level of physical activity. A decrease in energy expenditure during weekends compared with school days without any physical training was found in 19% of males and 43% of females.[448] This indicates the passive character of leisure time in adolescent subjects.

Groups of fifth graders, subdivided according to level of obesity, were examined with respect to TDEE using DLW, RMR, and body composition (tertiles of subscapular plus triceps skinfolds). No differences in FFM between the groups were revealed, while the highest tertile group weighed 14 kg more than the lowest. Mean energy expenditure using either day was nearly identical (Figure 5.9). No differences in RMR, energy expended in activity, or TDEE among the three groups were observed. A reduction in RMR or TDEE could not explain differences in obesity in these prepubertal children.

However, the fact that the heaviest children expended the same amount of energy in activity and had the same TDEE as the leanest while weighing 14 kg more, indicates that the obese children had reduced activity.[414] This could be explained by the greater energy demands for the same movement due to excess fat load interfering especially during dynamic, weight-bearing activities.

Studies using DLW have shown that as a group, obese children consume more energy and have higher TEE than lean children. In many follow-ups, energy intake was reported as the same, and sometimes lower in obese children. Therefore, it was assumed that energy imbalance is due particularly to a decreased TEE and cannot explain the deposition of excess fat. However, under-reporting of food intake in the obese and higher energy efficiency in subjects predisposed to developing obesity were also considered. This ques-

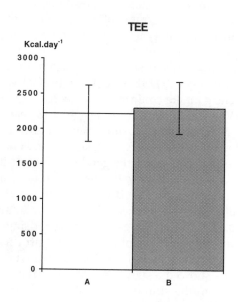

**FIGURE 5.9**
Daily total energy expenditure (TEE) in groups of obese pre-pubertal children from highest (A) and lowest (B) tertiles of body weight and fatness. (Based on data from Ref. F17.)

tion requires further research focused on complex longitudinal studies evaluating simultaneous and repeated energy intake and output along with BMI and body composition changes.

Additional recent results show comparable energy expenditure in obese and normal-weight children after adjustment for body size. Therefore, at least on a group basis, there do not appear to be any defects in energy metabolism that would predispose obesity.[228,414,449] However, a low level of physical activity is associated with increased body fatness in some cross-sectional studies, and, more importantly, in some longitudinal studies in both normal-weight and obese children.[18] These findings indicate that a low level of physical activity is important in the development of pediatric obesity and that intervention programs with increased exercise are essential for its rectification, especially in subjects with low physical activity levels.

### 5.5.4 Longitudinal Studies of Physical Activity, Fatness, and Cardiovascular Risk

The Amsterdam Growth and Health Longitudinal Study (AGAHLS) showed that the development of fat is fairly predictable, especially based on repeated assessments of the level of physical activity. This study is the longest study executed repeatedly on the same subjects, from 13 to 27 years of age. The protocol includes measurement of 4 skinfolds, dietary intake (cross-check dietary history interview in a timeframe of the last 3 months), and physical activity level (standardized activity interview based on a questionnaire, retrospective over the previous 3 months).

The results showed a sharp decrease in energy expenditure from the age of 13 years from approximately 4500 METs per week to 3000 METs at the age of 27 years. Data on dietary intake confirmed the decrease of energy per kg of body weight from about 225 kJ per day at the age of 13 years to about 155 kJ at the age of 27 years. The energy turnover was higher in males than in females during adolescence, with energy intake 15% and energy output 20% higher in boys. At the age of 23 years, the gender difference in energy intake was reduced to 10%, and the difference in energy output disappeared.

Low stability coefficients were found for physical activity (0.34: 0.19 to 0.49), but higher coefficients were revealed for dietary intake (0.55: 0.45 to 0.64) and fat mass (0.63: 0.56 to 0.71). Somewhat surprisingly, fat mass was negatively related to daily energy intake. The longitudinal relationship between fat mass and physical activity corrected for dietary intake for the ages of 13 and 27 years showed a significant negative relationship when fat mass was estimated from the sum of 4 skinfolds, but not when estimated from the values of BMI.[450] Therefore, this unique longitudinal study involving the same subjects provides much more reliable results and also reinforces the effect of physical activity and exercise on body adiposity.

## 5.6 Social Class, Fatness, and Physical Activity

Social class affects the prevalence of obesity and participation in regular exercise. In lower socioeconomic areas the rate of overweight and obese children was up to 23% higher while enrollment in sports activity was low. In contrast, in higher social class regions, the rate of overweight and obese children was lower and the rate of children involved in sports was higher.[105]

Observations in preschool children from low-income families showed that during free-play periods, 58% of time was devoted to sedentary activities and only 11% to vigorous physical activities. Children's BMI, teacher-rated type A behavior, parent-reported mother and father BMI, parents' vigorous activities, and family history of cardiovascular diseases (CVD) were the independent variables studied. The multiple regression of moderate-intensity activity was significant; family cardiovascular risk, parent vigorous activity, and father's BMI accounted for a significant amount of variance. The results indicate that the parental role in modeling physical activity for their young children may extend beyond the confines of their home.[451]

## 5.7 Concluding Remarks

Further studies on energy metabolism related to pediatric obesity are needed. Such studies should include repeated and longer-lasting measurements of RMR, physical activity levels, and other parameters related to TEE. The DLW method is very expensive and the measurements, in spite of the new information provided, are limited given their non-specificity and the relatively short timeframes of studies. Therefore, there is insufficient time to explain long-term changes in body composition and fatness as related to energy expenditure and physical activity during growth using such a technique. In addition, obese children are less active even during participation in the "same" sport or exercise activity program as reported in their questionnaires compared to normal-weight children.[24]

It is possible to speculate that longer-lasting and more exact measurements of physical activity and its character, and energy output preceding increased fatness at the beginning of obesity in children, might reveal some differences that could explain the enhanced deposition of fat in inactive subjects.

Physical activity levels have been decreasing during recent decades in all groups of individuals. Therefore, one might conclude that at present, both obese and non-obese children display low levels of physical activity. As the average BMI of the adult population has been increasing it could be suggested that even growing subjects who are lean at present may become overweight or obese in adulthood, provided poor lifestyle behaviors are maintained.

The results of studies to date indicate that children, particularly those of obese parents and those with low levels of physical activity, are predisposed to obesity, especially when an inadequate diet is also present. The classic adage of the multi-factorial origin of childhood obesity, including physical inactivity, seems to be valid in spite of contradictions regarding the relationship between activity and fatness presented in some studies.

Carrying an excess load of stored fat increases the energy cost of the same dynamic activity; for example, running on a treadmill with load results in a higher energy cost than without a load when completing the same exercise.[391] The higher energy cost of dynamic activities and lower mechanical efficiency in the obese increase the strain and discomfort of any physical activity. This is the most common reason for the spontaneous reduction of such activities when measured repeatedly during prolonged periods of time.[450,452]

# 6

## Evaluation of Functional Status

Levels of physical fitness and physical performance are among the most important characteristics of the human organism. There are different indicators of functional capacity, the most important being cardiorespiratory fitness and endurance, motor and sensorimotor development, muscular strength, and motor skill and coordination. Psychological factors also play a significant role in functional performance.

Appropriate levels of physical fitness and performance may be considered essential ingredients for a meaningful standard of participation in sport and athletic activities, rather than essential ingredients of the functional status of all individuals. For example, a particular standing in cardiorespiratory fitness and skill would thus concern all individuals. Functional characteristics and capacity to perform daily living tasks with ease may be far more important criteria than performance capabilities and body size.

The evaluation of functional status in marginally malnourished children from some developing countries has demonstrated that in certain functional characteristics, especially those concerning the cardiovascular and respiratory systems, such individuals were on a higher level than normally fed children from industrially developed countries.[18] Obese children may also have a range of sub-optimal functional characteristics.[18,53,57,68,316]

Physical fitness has been defined as an ability to carry out daily tasks with vigor and alertness without undue fatigue, and with ample energy to enjoy leisure time pursuits and to meet unforeseen emergencies. Numerous other definitions of fitness exist but all largely express the same sentiments. Physical fitness is partly conditioned genetically and is also related to health status. Fitness can be increased significantly by the process of adaptation to various types of physical activity and exercise that stimulate the individual systems related to physical performance.[389]

Physical fitness is comprised of numerous components. An adequate level on one of the components of fitness does not necessarily mean a corresponding adequacy in another. This is particularly the case in obese children. Excess fat does not always interfere with individual functional characteristics in the same manner, so the level of physical performance and fitness in the young obese individual is modified in a characteristic way, not always negatively. This chapter outlines some of the more important issues in relation to the functional status of an individual and considers both their development and evaluation.

Locomotor ability and movement characteristics of children include indices of cardiorespiratory function, flexibility, muscular strength, endurance, and agility. Cardiorespiratory capacity is most frequently linked with general health maintenance; it is an important limiting factor in the performance of aerobic tasks in both weight-supported tasks such as riding a stationary bicycle and activities such as walking and running.

## 6.1 Cardiorespiratory Function

### 6.1.1 Criteria and Methods

Cardiorespiratory function can be evaluated by different tests. It is commonly assessed through measurements of aerobic power expressed as the oxygen uptake during a maximal workload ($VO_2$ max) on a treadmill or stationary bicycle, in both absolute ($ml.O_2^{-1}.min^{-1}$) and relative values, that is, values related to total and/or lean, fat-free body mass ($ml\ O_2^{-1}.min^{-1}.kg\ BW^{-1}$ and/or $LBW^{-1}$). The capacity to transfer oxygen to the working tissues, mainly skeletal muscles, depends on the efficacy of the heart muscle, and vascular and respiratory systems. Therefore, the peak value of oxygen uptake during a certain period of time (one minute) of workload gives the best information on the level of aerobic power and the cardiorespiratory efficiency of the individual.

Evaluation of aerobic fitness using absolute values of maximal oxygen uptake ($VO_2$ max) can be misleading since it can be quite high even in obese subjects, and does not always reveal the 'true' level of physical fitness. As this test measures $O_2$ during a dynamic, weight-bearing workload, it is necessary to consider body weight, especially its total value, including stored fat. $VO_2$ max is therefore related to total and/or lean body mass. However, relating $O_2$ to lean, fat-free body mass is also not logical as it is not possible to execute the workload without one's own fat weight; work performance must be realized with the simultaneous loading of an excess inert mass. A similar parallel may be to exercise with a suitcase or a knapsack equivalent to the excess weight.[391]

The level of performance achieved must also be taken into account. When evaluating aerobic power, it is desirable to consider the conditions during which it was achieved; for example, the distance covered and the speed or slope of the treadmill. During the bicycle ergometer test, level of performance can be expressed in physical terms ($Watts.min^{-1}$). Real performance is more important in everyday life than a theoretical value of the consumed $O_2$.

Simultaneously, other variables such as $CO_2$ output, respiratory quotient (RQ), ventilation (in absolute values and related to total and lean FFM), breathing frequency, and blood pressure can be assessed. Individual parameters are commonly expressed over 1 min. More recent studies with newer technology enable breath-to-breath analysis of all the parameters mentioned.

Functional capacity of the cardiorespiratory system is often evaluated during other types of workload; for example, during a standard workload (equal to various proportions of $VO_2$ max such as one third, one sixth, etc.), or at the level of $PWC_{170}$ (physical working capacity at the level of 170 beats per minute).

DuRant et al.,[453] in assessing the value of working capacity indices in children, found that $PWC_{170}$ discriminated among underweight, normal, and overweight children. The finding was indicative of overweight and obese children scoring lower on $PWC_{170}$ than normal-weight children. In contrast, the results from other indices tended to overestimate the capacity of overweight children, equating them with normal-weight children. The submaximal $PWC_{170}$ is an appropriate regimen for the assessment of aerobic capacity.

Some contention surrounds the choice of the most suitable ergometer procedure to employ in $PWC_{170}$ estimation. These concerns have related to the initial loading, load increments, number of workloads, and duration and frequency of pedaling. Cognizant of these concerns, the following protocol was used by the author: physical working capacity ($PWC_{170}$) was ascertained following heart rate response to exercise at three successive workloads on a mechanically braked Monark cycle ergometer following an appropriate warm-up and familiarization with equipment. Three workloads were utilized with an initial load of 1 watt per kg of body weight ($1 W.kg^{-1}$) and two further increments of 0.5 or 1 watt depending on the heart rate reached with each load lasting 2 min. Subjects pedaled at a rate of 60 rpm (range 58 to 62). The seat of the cycle ergometer was adjusted to the position of maximum comfort for each subject. Data on the above-mentioned workloads were used to ascertain both $PWC_{170}$ ($kpm.min^{-1}$ and $Watts^{-1}$) and $PWC_{170}$ ($kpm.kg.^{-1}min^{-1}$ and $Watts.kg^{-1}$).

Aerobic power is differentiated from anaerobic power (the capacity to work involves a period under anaerobic conditions, i.e., with absence of oxygen), and therefore is an important part of cardiorespiratory fitness. Ventilatory threshold (VT, or anaerobic threshold AT), is defined as the greatest oxygen uptake at which pulmonary ventilation stops to increase linearly with increasing exercise intensity and starts to take a steeper slope. This measure is also used to evaluate the efficiency of the cardiorespiratory system and overall level of physical fitness and performance. Detailed descriptions of these functional measurements are provided in a number of textbooks on exercise physiology.[389,454] In many studies, approaches are used simultaneously to provide a more accurate characterization of different aspects of cardiorespiratory fitness.

## 6.1.2   The Effect of Age, Gender, and Body Composition

Reviews of the epidemiological studies on physical fitness and physical activity in normal-weight children show significant developmental trends and gender differences. Some comparisons show that aerobic power ($VO_2$ max) related to body mass remains stable from 6 to 16 years in boys. However, when comparing different groups in individual age categories, some developmental trends might be obscured because of the lack of homogeneity of subjects in these groups. Longitudinal studies during which repeated measurements of individual characteristics with increasing age are taken show developmental trends. Such studies are rare due to the difficulty of preserving the same groups over a number of years. A longitudinal study on adolescent boys showed an increase in aerobic power ($VO_2$ max.min$^{-1}$.kg body weight$^{-1}$ and/or kg lean body mass$^{-1}$) until 14 to 15 years and then a decline. The decline is less or not apparent in subjects enrolled in regular sport training.[18]

Meaningful comparisons between different studies can be limited, even when considering a single parameter such as cardiorespiratory function. Groups of children tested using different protocols and procedures and at various chronological and maturational age and degrees of obesity, make comparisons awkward. For example, treadmill protocols may use different speeds and workloads and may or may not use a slope. Moreover, these procedures are not always described in detail in the literature. Therefore, it is only possible to consider the conclusions. To directly compare the individual values is difficult due to the methodological differences mentioned and may give spurious conclusions. Therefore, wherever possible, a more detailed description of individual studies is given in this volume.

Normal weight girls have lower aerobic power than boys by approximately 25%, which usually decreases during prepubertal and pubertal periods. Reports on physical activity have shown that boys are about 15 to 25% more active than females.[455] This review indicated that older youth and especially girls are at an increased risk of obesity, mainly due to a sedentary lifestyle.

## 6.1.3   The Effect of Obesity

Figure 6.1 shows a comparison of body composition and aerobic power for normal-weight and obese boys. Obese boys of the same age were slightly taller and heavier in total lean and fat body mass. The absolute values of $VO_2$ max.min$^{-1}$ were the same in both groups.[18] This result was also found in other studies.[422,456] However, when maximal oxygen was related to total and/or lean body mass, the values were significantly lower in the obese. The peak level of maximal oxygen uptake was achieved in obese boys after a shorter period of running on a treadmill at a lower speed, with the performance achieved being worse in the more obese children.

Similar measurements of maximal aerobic power ($VO_2$ max) (Figure 6.2) using an open circuit during a workload on a treadmill and stationary bicycle

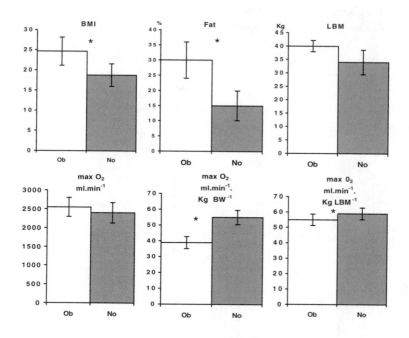

**FIGURE 6.1**
Comparison of body mass index (BMI), percentage of stored fat (%), lean fat-free body mass (LBM, kg), aerobic power expressed as oxygen uptake during maximal workload on a treadmill in absolute values as related to total and/or lean, fat-free body mass in obese (Ob) and normal-weight (No) boys. * indicates ($p < 0.05$). (Based on data from Refs. F6, F18.)

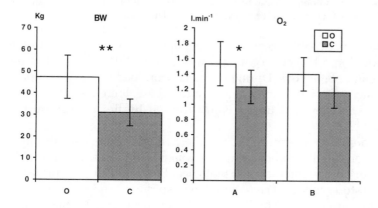

**FIGURE 6.2**
Comparison of body weight and oxygen uptake during maximal workload on a (A) treadmill (2% slope) and a (B) stationary bicycle in obese (O) and control, normal-weight (C) pre-pubertal children aged $9.5 \pm 0.8$ years. * indicates ($p < 0.05$); ** indicates ($p < 0.01$). (Based on data from Ref. 19.)

showed higher absolute values in obese children aged 9.5 ± 0.8 years as compared to normal-weight control children of the same age in test A. When expressed per kilogram of fat-free mass, the differences disappeared.[456] Results related to total body mass were not given in this study.

Measurements in obese Tunisian girls showed lower values of maximal oxygen uptake per kilogram of body weight along with a lower BMR, energy expenditure, and physical activity level (Figure 6.3), with a markedly increased energy intake.[457]

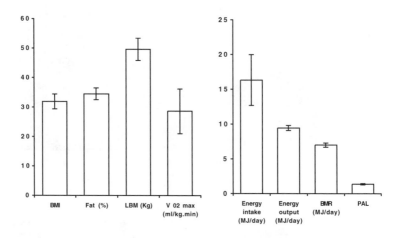

**FIGURE 6.3**
Body mass index (BMI), percentage of stored fat (% fat), lean body mass (LBM, kg), aerobic power (oxygen uptake during maximal workload related to body weight, $VO_2$ max.$kg^{-1}$), energy intake and output, basal metabolic rate (BMR), and physical activity level (PAL = 1.35) in obese Tunisian adolescent girls. (Based on data from Ref. F20.)

Performance characterized by oxygen uptake evaluated during a standard workload on a bicycle ergometer was significantly different in normal-weight and obese boys. During the same workload, the oxygen uptake and heart rate were significantly higher in the obese, therefore, the same performance was executed under conditions of higher energy output (see Chapter 12).[18]

It is rare in the literature to find international comparisons from studies with a consistent protocol, but this was possible in the 1960s within the framework of the International Biological Program (IBP).[405] This large international study followed somatic, cardiorespiratory, and motor development of a population aged 12 to 55 years. It is not surprising that such large international studies have not been repeated.

Aerobic power was evaluated in another study during an incremental treadmill test in obese and non-obese prepubescent girls aged 7 to 12 years. Open circuit calorimetry was used and maximal oxygen uptake ($VO_2$ max.kg body weight$^{-1}$) was significantly lower in obese subjects (23.0 ± 3.9 ml.kg$^{-1}$.min$^{-1}$) compared to normal-weight controls (36.0 ± 0.9 ml.kg$^{-1}$.min$^{-1}$). Exercise tolerance was longer in non-obese girls, although this result was not statistically significant. These data also indicate that excess body weight, due to increased fatness, diminishes cardiopulmonary performance and attenuates exercise tolerance in prepubescent obese females compared to other subjects.[458]

Similar observations were found in other groups of obese children aged 9 to 14 years in which gas exchange was assessed during exercise. Maximal oxygen uptake (VO$_2$ max) as related to total body weight was significantly lower in obese subjects than in normal-weight children. Ventilatory anaerobic threshold (VAT) as a percentage of VO$_2$ max was similar in both groups. A significant correlation was found between VAT and VO$_2$ max in both obese and normal-weight children. The habitual level of physical activity was lower in obese subjects compared to controls. These results show that the level of physical fitness is reduced in obese children. Fitness can be assessed by the measurements of VAT, which does not require a maximal workload and is therefore suitable for the evaluation of subjects with exercise intolerance.[459]

Other measurements revealed lower aerobic power (VO$_2$ max ml$^{-1}$.min$^{-1}$, VO$_2$ max.ml$^{-1}$.kg$^{-1}$ body weight) and reduced physical working capacity (PWC$_{170}$). Both of these parameters were significantly lower than in normal-weight children.[460] Measurements in Russian children showed that those with moderate, average, or slightly higher body mass had the highest level of physical working capacity PWC$_{170}$.kg body weight$^{-1}$. With increasing weight, a decrease in working capacity was apparent and was most pronounced in obese subjects.[461]

The relationship between functional capacity and the content of stored fat, ranging from normal to gross obesity was assessed in adolescent females. Skinfold thicknesses correlated significantly with the absolute values of maximal oxygen uptake. That is, the higher body weight and fatness, the higher maximal oxygen uptake in absolute values, but significant negatively with oxygen uptake per kg of body weight and treadmill endurance time ($r = 0.49$ and 0.42, respectively).

Obesity did not affect submaximal walking economy.[462] These results indicated that increased fat levels increase oxygen uptake during a workload but functional fitness, i.e., the performance achieved, declines because of the inert load created by excess stored fat.

In another study of obese girls aged 7 to 11 years, no relationship was proved for VO$_2$ max (assessed on a bicycle ergometer test) and the percentage of deposited fat (DXA). Significant correlations were found for VO$_2$ max and leg lean mass and/or total lean body mass. These data suggest that aerobic power is mainly dependent on lean, fat-free body mass when not using weight-bearing exercise on a treadmill.[463,464] However, in other studies, a significant negative relationship between VO$_2$ max and body fatness was found.[18] The relationships, however, appear to be most significant when the range of assessed values is sufficiently large. In homogeneous groups they may not be apparent at all.

Obese children often display abnormal reactions to exercise but their real lack of fitness is also sometimes questioned. In obese subjects aged 9 to 17 years, size-independent measures of exercise, i.e., the ratio of $O_2$ uptake ($VO_2$) to work rate during progressive workload, the temporal response of $VO_2$, carbon dioxide output ($VCO_2$), and minute ventilation (VE) at the onset of exercise were used. The ability to perform external mechanical work was corrected for $VO_2$ max at unloaded pedaling (change in $VO_2$ max, i.e., delta $VO_2$ max) and in anaerobic threshold (delta AT).

On average, children's responses were in the normal range. However, in one third of the obese children tested, values of delta $VO_2$ max or delta AT of more than 2SD below normal were found. With increasing age, no increase of delta $VO_2$ max or delta AT was found in obese children and adolescents, which is usual in normal-weight children. Although the response time of $VO_2$ max was normal (with regard to predicted values), those for both $VCO_2$ and VE were prolonged.[465] These results indicate that not every obese child is unfit and that testing cardiorespiratory responses is indispensable for selecting subjects with more serious functional impairment. The effect of excess fat on functional capacity seems to be dependent on the nature of the individual at the onset of obesity.

Thai children aged 9.2 years with differing degrees of adiposity were evaluated using the following tests: evaluation of maximal oxygen uptake ($VO_2$ max during submaximal stationary bicycle testing), vital capacity, 50-m run, flexibility (sit-and-reach), abdominal strength, and endurance (30-s sit-ups). The usual gender differences were seen, i.e., better results in boys except for flexibility. However, gender differences in fitness levels were not apparent in obese groups unlike in normal-weight children. The performance level varied significantly according to the degree of obesity, especially in the $VO_2$ max test.[466]

Oxygen uptake and energy output measured by open circuit spirometry during walking at four different speeds was assessed in obese boys and girls. Energy output was related to total and lean FFM (measured by hydrodensitometry). ANOVA analysis revealed significant differences in the energy output between the speed conditions. There was no significant difference between genders such as the amount and distribution of fat (see Chapter 4).[18]

A nonlinear increase in energy output with increasing speed indicated a decreasing efficiency with increasing speed of walking. Biomechanical factors may be important in this respect. These factors include the extra energy output needed to accelerate the extremities and trunk, increased energy output due to increased inertia, and increased upper-body forward lean to maintain balance at faster speeds of movement. An increased load in the form of excess fat may be responsible for this lower efficiency.[467]

The level of cardiovascular fitness was evaluated in groups of children aged 8 to 13 years with high and low adiposity (evaluated by 3 skinfolds: triceps, subscapular, and suprailiac). Physical working capacity ($PWC_{170}$) was used for the evaluations. The most important predictor of cardiovascular fitness in high adiposity children was the physical activity score computed for each child from a 2-day observation period. Age, BMI, and physical activity scores accounted for 38% of the variance in $PWC_{170}$.[468]

Measurements of VAT in children aged 4 to 16 years on a treadmill showed significantly lower values in obese children compared to normal-weight peers. The habitual level of physical activity assessed by questionnaires was 27% (p < 0.01) lower in the obese compared to healthy controls. Strikingly lower ventilatory thresholds in the obese children may cause obese children to avoid moderate or strenuous exercise because of the higher degree of effort needed. This mechanism is also assumed to be essential for the maintenance of obesity during childhood.[469,470]

Oxygen uptake ($VO_2$ max) and carbon dioxide output ($VCO_2$) were measured in obese children aged 11 ± 3.8 years during a workload on a treadmill. Analysis of respiratory gas exchange was performed by measuring breath-by-breath. The BMI of the obese children was 25.0 ± 0.20. To eliminate the effect of body weight, the slope of $VO_2$ vs. $VCO_2$ was evaluated. This slope was calculated below the ventilatory threshold (S1) and above the ventilatory threshold (S3). Comparison of the results showed that S3 was significantly steeper in the obese than in normal-weight children in a comparable age range (10.8 ± 2.2 years). The steepest values for S3 were found in the subjects with the highest degree of obesity. This approach has limitations since, in a large proportion of subjects (48%), the VT could not be achieved.

However, these measurements again demonstrated that cardiorespiratory exercise function in obese children is reduced, especially during dynamic, weight-bearing exercise.[471] From these results, it follows that obesity interferes with athletic activities, mainly those with a dynamic performance component and of an aerobic nature, such as running and cycling.[339-341]

In studies undertaken by the authors, obese subjects were grossly disadvantaged in some movement tasks, recording lower scores on $PWC_{170}$ than normal-weight subjects even following correction for body weight. Obese subjects also scored appreciably higher 600-m run times than lighter counterparts and the ability to balance in the stork stand test was inferior. The relatively short duration tasks of a standing broad jump and a shuttle run were less of a problem for obese subjects. Significant positive correlations were found between both height and sitting height and standing broad jump, indicative of the advantage gained via body dimensions favoring linearity. Significant negative correlations were found between body weight and $PWC_{170}$ ($kpm.kg^{-1}.min^{-1}$), sum of three circumferences and $PWC_{170}$, and sum of 4 skinfolds and $PWC_{170}$.

As shown by Hills, in the obese group only a limited number of high correlations between physical and motor fitness variables were found compared to the lighter group. Both groups showed a strong association between grip strength and most measures but correlations were stronger in the normal-weight group. The most significant relationship was between the strength measure and body mass (0.662 vs. 0.864). Similar findings were seen for all other measures in the normal-weight group except $PWC_{170}$ ($kpm.kg^{-1}.min^{-1}$). The relationship between cardiorespiratory working capacity and many anthropometric and body composition measures was pronounced in this group.

The results of this study indicate the greater working capacity of normal-weight prepubertal children compared with obese children and support the evidence derived from similar studies of older children. Obese children, due to their greater fat content, showed an operational disadvantage in $PWC_{170}$ kpm.kg$^{-1}$.min$^{-1}$ and negative correlations between $PWC_{170}$ and body weight. The results have implications for the involvement of obese children in aerobic physical activity by adding objective evidence in contrast to the many generalized claims made by other studies regarding movement capacity and quality in this population.

Thoren et al.[472] postulated that the additional weight carried by children at lower levels of obesity may be sufficient to provide a training effect that could enhance their physical fitness status, but such a benefit would only be possible through regular physical activity. The possible training effect would relate to the slight overload stress provided by the additional adipose tissue being transported. As will become evident in the following sections, training with an appropriate exercise prescription can provide significant positive effects on movement capability.

Ward and Bar-Or have described the lack of habitual physical activity that too often characterizes the obese individual as secondary inactivity.[473] Unfortunately, this level of inactivity contributes to a withdrawal from the physical activity setting which, if left unchecked, can lead to further inactivity. It is this cycle of inactivity and increased adiposity that is recognized as the major factor in registrating subnormal physical working capacity. As the level of obesity increases, mobility of the obese child becomes more difficult and compounds the already vulnerable physical condition of the individual. With further worsening, any advantages gained via fat-free weight increase would be outweighed by the increased inactivity.

Physical activity is important during childhood for developing the functional capacity of the cardiopulmonary system; progressive but slight reductions in level of activity in the obese mean that they are predisposed to inadequate development of this system.[2]

## 6.2　Lung Function Measurements

The development of obesity leads to deterioration in a number of indices of lung function including vital capacity and maximum ventilatory volume (MVV). Obese individuals frequently complain of breathlessness on mild exertion and are more susceptible to chest infections, the heavier chest wall serving to impede normal respiratory movements. Improvement in exercise tolerance and a feeling of well-being can be gained through weight reduction.

Lung function can be evaluated in greater detail by measuring forced expiratory flow and MVV. These values are often reduced by obesity to between 60 and 70% of predicted normal values. In Singapore, the more obese children had significantly lower values for each test of lung function. The results seem to indicate a narrowing of small airways and increased respiratory inertia possibly due to excessive accumulation of fat in the chest wall and abdomen leading to respiratory limitation.[474]

Comparisons with predicted normal values for height, gender, and body surface area (BSA) revealed significantly reduced values (mean% predicted) in the obese with respect to a range of values. Residual volume (RV), total lung capacity (TLC), minute ventilation (VE), and resting energy expenditure (REE) were increased. These results show altered pulmonary function due to obesity during growth, characterized by a reduction in diffusing capacity, ventilatory muscle endurance, and airway narrowing. The changes may reflect extrinsic mechanical compression on the lung and thorax, and/or intrinsic alterations within the lung.[475]

Spirometry was performed in a group of obese children before and every 3 minutes after a workload on a treadmill. The majority of obese children had at least a 15% fall in at least one of the three monitored pulmonary function parameters. The same result was observed in less than half of the normal-weight children. The mean percentage falls in forced expiratory volume (FEV) and forced expiratory flow ($FEF_{25-75\%}$) and was significantly greater in obese children than in the controls. The pattern of bronchospasm, which appeared soon after workload, was consistent with that found in the asthmatic population. The degree of fall in $FEF_{15-75\%}$ significantly correlated (0.55, $p < 0.005$) with triceps skinfold thickness. These results reveal that bronchospasm of the smaller airways occurs more frequently in obese children and is related to subcutaneous fat. This might contribute to the avoidance of exercise and increased workloads in obese subjects due to bronchial hyper-reactivity; however, this result requires further consideration.[476]

In children with mild obesity, pulmonary volumes are within the normal range. In severe obesity, the main factor is decreased distensibility of the chest wall, which becomes worse over time, and is the cause of alteration in ventilatory volume, flow, and transfer factors.[477]

Expiratory reserve volume (ERV) of the lungs and its relation to vital capacity (ERV/VC) was examined in a group of prepubertal boys and girls. The relationship of these respiratory parameters to percentage of body fat was assessed using regression analysis. The regression for preadolescent boys and for adult men was similar but this was not so for girls. In this group (girls), the expiratory reserve volume increased with increasing fatness (ERV/VC) × 100 = 29.3 + 0.19 fat%, ($r = 0.48$, $p < 0.03$). In all groups there was no correlation with age or height. In contrast to adults in whom body weight correlates significantly with the above-mentioned parameter, no such relationship was seen in younger subjects.[478] Spirometric data showed positive dependence of lung function on BMI in girls with increasing values of BMI. This was not the case in boys.[479]

Pulmonary function tests, polysomnography, and multiple sleep latency tests showed abnormal results in obese children. Forty-six percent of obese subjects had abnormal polysomnograms; there was a positive correlation between the degree of obesity and the apnea index, and an inverse correlation between the degree of obesity and the degree of sleepiness on multiple sleep latency tests. These results reveal that obese adolescents have a high prevalence of mild sleep-disordered breathing. Obstructive sleep apnea syndrome improved after tonsillectomy and adenoidectomy.[480]

Another study of adolescents aged 10.3 ± 4.4 years, with a history of morbid obesity and breathing difficulty during sleep, showed that 37% of the group had marked abnormalities (apnea, hypopnea, excessive arousal levels, or abnormalities in gas exchange). A sleep history questionnaire showed that all patients snored. Pulmonary tests indicated that 28.5% of subjects had a restrictive defect and 47% of subjects possessed obstructive changes. Multiple regression analysis revealed a significant association between weight, age, and gender, and any physiological measure on the polysomnogram. Most of the abnormal polysomnograms were only mildly abnormal during adolescence, but, in two cases, the abnormalities were so severe they required clinical intervention.[481]

## 6.3   Blood Pressure, Cardiac Function, and Obesity

The Amsterdam Growth and Health Study revealed that longitudinal measurements of body fat percentage in the early teenage years seems to be the most important cardiovascular disease indicator in predicting risk levels in young adults. The amount of physical activity measured in young adulthood is the only behavioral parameter to show a significant interrelationship with other cardiovascular disease risk.[452]

Systolic and diastolic blood pressure were significantly elevated in the obese as compared to normal-weight control children (Figure 6.4).[482] Another study in Italian children aged 6.6 to 14.4 years with a wider range of BMI followed weight, height, waist and hip circumferences, and blood pressure. Insulin sensitivity was evaluated by an Insulin Tolerance Test (ITT). The results of this study suggested that blood pressure in children is more closely related to body fat distribution and insulin resistance than to weight excess.[483]

Blood pressure in healthy boys and girls aged 4 to 18 years increased regularly with advancing years and was always more closely correlated with height and total body weight than with age. This association became much stronger during puberty in males. Correlation with body height was not found after puberty but the correlation with body weight remained and increased. In children whose weight in relation to height was greater by 20% or more, the risk of increased blood pressure was a multiple of 2.5 in boys and 2.0 in girls.[484] However, the extent to which the increase in blood pressure is

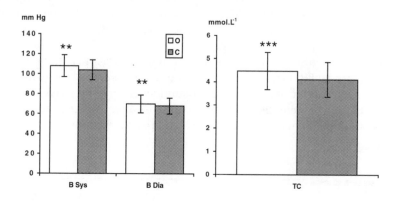

**FIGURE 6.4**

Comparison of systolic and diastolic blood pressure (B Sys, B Dia), and total cholesterol (TC) in obese (O) and control, normal-weight (C) children. ** indicates (p < 0.01); *** (p < 0.001). (Based on data from Ref. F21.)

due solely to excess weight and fatness, instead of to other possible factors such as the level of maturity and early development of other tissues (muscle, bone), needs to be studied in greater detail.

In adults, significant correlations between blood pressure and the level of obesity have been reported. In childhood, some studies reveal the same findings; however, exploratory analysis indicates an occasionally strong but quite variable relationship between blood pressure and BMI, which differs by age, gender, and the particular blood pressure measure under consideration.[485]

A 3-year longitudinal study followed self-reported behavior and height, weight, skinfold, blood pressure, and BMI in a sample of matched cases. Data were analyzed according to ethnicity, age, and gender; a greater proportion of females were obese as school seniors. Overweight trends for each of the four groups by ethnicity and gender were stable over the period of the study. Later, a marked increase in obesity among black females was found. Blood pressure correlated significantly with percent of ideal body weight, skinfold thickness, and BMI, indicating that increasing obesity is associated with an increase in blood pressure in both black and white subjects.[486] The positive relationship between fatness and blood pressure becomes more apparent when obesity has been established over a longer period of time. The hypothesis that the early onset of obesity is associated with obesity later in adolescence is supported by these results and is indicative of a persistent health risk.

The effect of obesity on echocardiographic parameters (the thickness of the interventricular septum and of the posterior wall, end diastolic left ventricular internal dimension, and left ventricular mass) was studied in groups of Japanese children aged 6, 12, and 15 years. Left ventricular parameters were normalized for height. Significant correlations between the indices of obesity and left ventricular internal dimension or left ventricular mass were revealed. The obesity index was more strongly correlated than BMI with posterior wall thickness and left ventricular internal dimension. The most important finding concerned the significant effect of obesity on left ventricular parameters as early as 6 years of age.[487]

These results confirm that cardiac function is significantly influenced by excess weight and fatness, especially when initiated at an early age. In growing overweight individuals, increased insulin levels may be a risk factor for the accumulation of increased left ventricular mass after correction for growth, which is not dependent on obesity level, blood pressure, or insulin.[488]

## 6.4   Hematological Parameters

Plasma hemostatic measures, D-dimer, fibrinogen, and plasminogen activator inhibitor-1 (PAI-1) were evaluated in obese boys aged 7 to 11 years. Boys had significantly greater fibrinogen and D-dimer concentrations than girls; black children had significantly greater fibrinogen and D-dimer concentrations than whites. Fibrinogen was positively associated with the percentage of stored fat ($r = 0.40$, $p < 0.01$), subcutaneous abdominal tissue ($r = 0.40$, $p < 0.01$), total fat mass ($r = 0.42$, $p < 0.01$), and BMI ($r = 0.41$, $p < 0.01$). PAI-1 was positively associated with visceral adipose tissue ($r = 0.49$, $p < 0.01$), subcutaneous abdominal adipose tissue ($r = 0.32$, $p < 0.01$), FFM ($r = 0.50$, $p < 0.01$), and insulin ($r = 0.61$, $p < 0.01$). D-dimer was positively associated with the percentage of stored fat ($r = 0.40$, $p < 0.01$), subcutaneous abdominal adipose tissue ($r = 0.37$, $p < 0.05$), total amount of stored fat ($r = 0.40$, $p < 0.01$), and BMI ($r = 0.43$, $p < 0.010$). Multiple regression analysis revealed that fibrinogen, gender and the higher percentage of stored fat explained significant independent portions of the variance.

Significant predictors for PAI-1 were higher amounts of visceral adipose tissue and FFM. The significant predictor for D-dimer was ethnicity. General adiposity and visceral adipose tissue may play a role in regulating plasma hemostatic factors in obese children. Increased fatness of the individual is associated with unfavorable concentrations of hemostatic factors that, in turn, are implicated in cardiovascular morbidity and mortality later in life.[489]

In healthy adults, a positive correlation of white blood cells (WBC), the percentage of stored fat, and leptin was reported. This relationship was also analyzed in children aged $10.3 \pm 3.2$ years. BMI, sum of skinfolds, ideal body weight percent, arm fat area, and body fat measured with BIA, were correlated with WBC, lymphocytes (L), and neutrofils (N). Spearman rank correlation coefficient and stepwise variable selection analysis were performed. Simple linear regression analysis showed an inverse correlation of WBC with age and direct correlation for body weight percent and BMI. N correlated significantly with body weight, percent of ideal body weight, sum of skinfolds, arm fat area, body fat mass, and BMI. Using stepwise variable selection analysis, WBC correlated with percent of ideal body weight and N with BMI alone. These results agree with those found for the adults. It is possible that the relationship between WBC and percent body fat may be mediated, in part, through the effect of leptin which is directly involved in proliferation of hemopoietic stem cells.[490]

## 6.5 Physical Performance and Motor Abilities

A number of studies have found that increased body fatness has a negative influence on children's physical performance, particularly in activities requiring the body to be projected through space as in jumping. Earlier studies of the performance of adults have also highlighted the inverse relationship between body fat and the ability to move total body weight. Åstrand and Rodahl maintained that such a relationship is due to the fact that body fat adds to the mass of the body without making a contribution to force-generating capacity, subsequently becoming additional weight to be moved during tasks that involve weight bearing.[389] Although the disadvantages of the condition have often been mentioned, much of the evidence has not been quantified and has resulted in considerable subjective reporting of movement capacity.

### 6.5.1 Motor Skill

For the most part, motor skills are age and gender dependent with the efficiency of movement progressively improving throughout childhood and into early adolescence. Motor skill development is also highly influenced by environmental influences. Risk factors that negatively impact on performance levels include previous injury, decreased endurance fitness, and level of adiposity.[491] In preschool children, the performance level of jumping on the spot and in the 20-m dash was significantly worse in those who are overweight compared to those of normal weight (Figure 6.5).[61]

Motor skills consist of a number of specific but interrelated components that include agility, flexibility, and speed, each of which has a bearing upon performing physical activity tasks.[61,389] Generally, the efficacy of movement improves progressively during the childhood years with development highly dependent on environmental influences. Some of the factors affecting motor skill development include motivation, interest, practice, training, and body characteristics. One might expect that the obese individual, who is ridiculed because of body size and form and who is more likely to voluntarily reduce habitual physical activity, would exhibit inadequacies in the performance of motor tasks (standing broad jump, sit-and-reach, flexed arm hang, shuttle run, plate tapping).

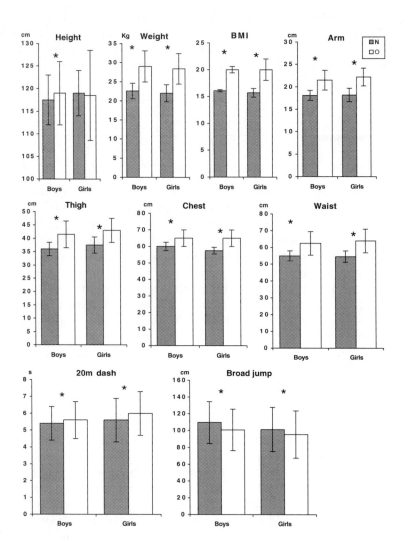

**FIGURE 6.5**
Comparison of morphological characteristics (height, weight, BMI, arm, thigh, chest, waist circumferences, (cm)) and motor performance (20-m dash, broad jump) in normal-weight (N) and overweight (O) 6.4-year-old children. * indicates ($p < 0.05$). (Based on data from Refs. F18, F22.)

Motor performance involving individual limbs and/or smaller muscle groups, and all types of performance which do not require the manipulation of one's own weight in space, are influenced much less in the obese than other modes of dynamic, weight-bearing workloads.

## 6.5.2 Flexibility

Gender comparisons have traditionally recognized that females are more flexible from 5 years of age to adulthood. Reasons cited include differences in activity patterns, limb length, and muscle mass. The reduced physical activity of obese individuals, as well as the presence of greater amounts of adipose tissue, has contributed to suggestions that the obese have reduced joint flexibility.

Impaired general physical condition, inactivity, and related decreased flexibility are commonly reported in sedentary individuals. Individuals who are more active and who are better performers of physical tasks also tend to be more flexible. Borms has suggested that a limited range of motion can result in lower work efficiency and limited movement and that quality and aesthetics of movement are aspects often overlooked.[492]

Docherty and Bell reported a high and consistent relationship between measures of flexibility and anthropometric measures of linearity and found mostly similar results between sexes.[493] Krahenbuhl and Martin assessed the relationship between body mass and flexibility characteristics and found that flexibility decreased as body surface area increased.[494]

Most studies of children's fitness have assessed flexibility using simple measures such as the sit-and-reach test rather than more comprehensive and objective analyses of the range of motion of major joints. Further, only a limited number of studies have considered the effect of body fat on flexibility and the results of these studies are inconsistent. Therefore, utilization of a comprehensive flexibility protocol with obese prepubertal children, along with a test of agility, a component of fitness that relies partly on flexibility, is warranted.

## 6.5.3 Strength

Strength is related to parameters of body size such as height and weight. Watson and O'Donovan reported that many human performance variables are more highly related to the cube of height than to body weight. In growing children, the relationship between size and muscular strength is so great that it probably obscures other more subtle influences such as those differences due to variation in body shape.[495] Obese children are superior to non-obese children in measures of back and grip strength. Grip strength serves as a good indicator of absolute strength and it increases monotonically with body weight and percent body fat. However, excess fat does not appear to negatively influence this strength indicator.[496]

Laubach and McConville[497] showed that strength was negatively related to skinfold thickness, while Lamphiear and Montoye[498] found strength more highly related to biacromial diameter, upper arm circumference, and triceps skinfold thickness than other measures.

Back strength is one of the few items that is superior in obese children.[499,500] This is logical as muscle strength is related to the muscle and lean body mass of the individual. A static workload not requiring weight bearing over a distance is not influenced by an excess load of stored fat and may be even higher due to greater lean body mass in the obese.[18]

The obese group was also inferior to the normal group in stepping up and down on a stool where body weight produces a considerable overload on the cardiorespiratory system. Wear and Miller suggested that the relationships found may be due partly to indirect factors other than excess weight itself, such as lack of physical activity which may affect performance.[501] In studying children, Palgi et al.[502] and Gutin et al.[503] found a significant relationship between percent body fat and slower run times over 1 to 2 km, results that support the disadvantage of transporting additional body fat in running tasks.

## 6.6 The Effect of Obesity on Motor Performance at Different Ages

Motor abilities can be influenced by excess weight from a very early age. Groups of normal-weight and obese babies were compared and a delayed gross motor development was found in the obese. A significant correlation was found between excessive weight and gross motor delay. Over the following year, both weight and motor development reverted to normal in the majority of infants.[504] It was suggested that a comprehensive evaluation of the motor-delayed overweight infant be performed before concluding that the delay in motor development might be caused by other factors, not just an increased body weight and fatness.

The potential deteriorating effect of excess fat on dynamic performance increases with age and the longer the duration of obesity. In preschool children, the effect of increased weight and BMI is only apparent in some areas such as broad jump and the 20-m dash (Figure 6.5), and much less so in other measured variables.[61] The significant effect of increased weight and fat is most marked during puberty.

Sawada found inferior performances in the 50-m dash, running and jumping, repeated side-step jumping, and vertical jumping.[505] Sawada noted that half of the obese group experienced difficulty in chin-ups, results that were similar to those reported in an earlier study by Wear and Miller.[501]

Obese boys aged 12 to 14 years were tested in 19 physical fitness and motor ability items and body fatness was evaluated using 6 skinfolds and BIA. Obese boys had significantly poorer results in the 1500-m run, 5-min run, 50-m run, running long jump, and many other variables. Obese boys were superior in back strength only. These data confirm previous studies on the differentiated effect of excess fatness on physical performance, which has the most negative influence during dynamic workloads of aerobic, weight-bearing activity.[18,158,189,396,405,457]

The association between fitness and fatness was examined in girls aged 7 to 17 years. The measurements included 5 skinfolds, the sit-and-reach test, sit-ups, flexed arm hang, and motor performance items such as standing broad jump and vertical jump, arm pull strength, flamingo stance, shuttle run, the plate-tapping step test, and $PWC_{170}$. Age-specific partial correlations between fatness and each fitness item, controlling for stature and weight, showed that subcutaneous fat accounted for health-related fitness of the variance in each of the items. The most important items for health-related fitness were the step test and $PWC_{170}$. The fattest girls had generally poorer levels of physical fitness compared to lean girls.[340,506,507]

Gender differences in fitness levels as well as the amount of fat and its distribution were not apparent among obese boys and girls.[18] This might be one of the reasons for the undifferentiated physical performance levels between genders. The performance level varied significantly according to the degree of obesity, especially in $VO_2$ max tests, the 50-m run, and sit-up test.[466]

Levels of motor abilities and coordination influence those of physical activity. Similarly, visual coordination difficulty is also considered a possible cause of problems obese children have during exercise, which may result in the preference for sedentary behaviors.[508]

# 7

## Food Intake

Increased energy intake has long been considered the single most important factor in the pathogenesis of obesity. Energy excess which is ingested or "economized" during the organism's metabolic processes due to hormonal, biochemical, etc. characteristics of the individual, or which is simply not used contributes to enhanced deposition of fat. The composition of food and the relationship between individual components of food items also have an important role in an increased adiposity level.

However, many studies in both adults and growing obese subjects have not shown any significant differences between the food intake of obese and normal-weight subjects. As is the case in similar studies on physical activity status or energy expenditure (EE), research has been undertaken in subjects who are already obese and often in a maintenance or steady period of obesity rather than during a dynamic phase. Similarly, observation periods in such studies are generally very short, rarely lasting longer than 1 week.

### 7.1 Methods

Food intake can be evaluated using a number of procedures. Food can be evaluated directly by weighing, but this is only possible under special conditions (in a metabolic unit, hospital, or when funding permits an appropriate number of dietitians). The use of questionnaires, food diaries (inventory method), interviews, and/or a combination of these methods are more common. The nature and comprehensiveness of the questionnaires and the duration of the analysis period can vary. Most common time periods are 1 week or a representative 3- to 4-day block of time including at least 1 day of the weekend. Telephone interviews seeking information on one previous day of a study have been used on occasion. A comprehensive description of methods is not the function of this volume but may be found in numerous textbooks on nutrition.[509,510]

## 7.2   Development of Food Behavior in Early Life

As early as the 1930s, it was demonstrated that when given choices of nutrients children select an adequate diet, without adult supervision. These children grew well and were healthy despite patterns of intake at individual meals that were not predictable and were also highly variable. A later study of young children from 2 to 5 years of age in which 24-hr food intake was measured for 6 days showed a great variability in energy intake at each of the individual 6 daily meals. However, the total daily energy intake was relatively constant for each child. The mean coefficient of variation for each child's energy intake for individual meals was 33.6%, but for total daily energy intake it was 10.4%. In most cases, a meal high in energy was followed by low energy intake at the next meal, or vice versa.[206]

These findings seem to indicate the existence of satisfactory mechanisms to preserve an adequate energy balance. However, this might only apply when food intake is well balanced in macro- and micronutrients and only when satiety mechanisms with regard to energy balance in the organism are involved. When highly attractive foodstuffs with a high energy density are available, this ability can be compromised and inadequate food intake can occur, which, over time, could result in obesity. The effect of the family and the whole environment of the child, including mass media and television, can play a significant role.

The early periods of growth are particularly important in the development of appropriate eating habits. Eating behavior has to be viewed as a complex phenomenon involving the coordination of cognitive, social, motor, and emotional development, which are under the regulation of both central and peripheral factors.[511] Besides providing necessary biological substrates for growth, development, and maturation processes, food intake and eating habits are also important for social interactions, such as the formation of the mother–infant relationship which plays an essential role at the beginning of an individual's life.

In the U.S., dietary patterns have changed in children aged 2 to 10 years during the period from 1978 to 1988. The results indicate that the intake of macronutrients remained fairly stable during this period and exceeded RDAs. Daily vitamin and mineral intake was lower in 1988 which was the case for the majority of subjects studied.[512] Food intake and the composition of the diet have also changed over time in various countries. A further study in U.S. children showed that food consumption patterns have changed along with health and demographic profiles during recent decades. These changes often do not follow RDAs and health promotion trends; they are considered a link with the increasing prevalence of obesity.[513]

A number of factors can modify an individual's food behavior from early childhood. The suckling of infants was measured twice in a laboratory during the first month and its effect on the development of early adiposity was followed in a group of healthy infants. Multiple regression analysis revealed that parental education and a measure of feeding behavior, that is, the interval between the bursts of suckling, accounted for 18% of the variance in triceps skinfold measures at 1 year of age. A lower level of education of the parents and shorter intervals between the bursts were associated with greater adiposity.

Other variables, such as the pressure of suckling and the number of reported feedings per day, accounted for 21.5% of the variance in skinfold thickness at 2 years of age. Fewer but larger feedings and higher suckling pressure were associated with greater adiposity. These data indicate that greater adiposity in early age is related to a vigorous infant-feeding style. That is, suckling more rapidly at higher pressure, with a longer suck and burst duration and a shorter interval between bursts of suckling, causes higher energy intake. The differences in feeding style could also be genetically endowed. In this study, breast-feeding protected children against early adiposity only to the age of 6 months.[514]

Body size and food ingestion behavior are related to different risks of obesity during the first 2 years of life, that is, obese and lean mothers. Of all the risk factors for the development of obesity, including maternal and paternal BMI, gender, feeding mode (breast, bottle, or mixed), 3-day food intake, nutritive sucking behavior during laboratory test feeding, and parental education, nutritive sucking behavior was revealed to be higher in the high-risk group with obese mothers at the age of 3 months. In this sample, infant food intake and nutritive sucking behavior at 3 months of age contributed to measures of body size at 12 and 24 months.

As mentioned in conjunction with the development of BMI (Chapter 4), the effect of early diet is undisputed. A follow-up study of nutrition and growth in French children from 10 months to 8 years of age showed a positive correlation of BMI at the age of 8 years with energy intake at the age of 2 years. However, this correlation became insignificant when adjusting BMI at 2 years. As mentioned in Chapter 4, the percentage of energy as protein ingested at the age of 2 years correlated positively with BMI and subscapular skinfold at the age of 8 years, after adjustment for energy intake and parental BMI. The percentage of energy contributed by protein at the age of 2 years was also negatively associated with the age of adiposity rebound.

Therefore, the higher the protein intake at 2 years of age, the earlier the adiposity rebound and the higher subsequent BMI level. Protein intake at the age of 2 years was the only nutrient associated with a fatness development pattern in following years. A high protein intake increased body fatness at the age of 8 years via an earlier adiposity rebound (AR). The association between protein intake and obesity is also consistent with increased values of body height and generally accelerated growth of obese children. This might also be related to the role of IGF-1 and other hormones.[114,201]

A high-fat, low-protein diet such as human milk is adapted to a high-energy demand for growth in early childhood that may not always be the case with bottle-feeding. Bottle-fed children become obese more often in later years than breast-fed children. A high-protein diet in early childhood could therefore increase the risk of obesity along with other co-morbidities later in life.[201] A comparison of the age of rebound and BMI development as related to diet in various countries with different nutritional habits and RDAs also contributes to these conclusions.[292]

---

## 7.3    Food Intake and Obesity

As indicated above, there is surprisingly little evidence that the obese over-eat. This parallels the limited evidence that the obese are more sedentary. Some studies even show a decreased energy intake in the obese when compared to normal-weight children. Understanding of the biological basis of obesity has grown rapidly during the last decade and this work has particularly concerned the identification of a novel endocrine pathway involving the adipose tissue-secreted hormone leptin and the leptin receptor in the hypothalamus. Plasma leptin levels are regulated *inter alia* by feeding and fasting and may play an important role, not only in food intake, but also in the utilization of energy and deposition of fat in the organism (see Chapter 9).[59]

In a group of white and Mohawk children aged 4.2 to 6.9 years, TEE was measured using the doubly labelled water (DLW) method. In addition, mothers completed the Willet food-frequency questionnaire to report the usual dietary intake of children. Total energy intake assessed by the food-frequency questionnaire was significantly higher than TEE. Over- and underestimation of energy intake was not related to the gender or body composition of children. It was concluded that use of such questionnaires significantly overestimate energy intake of children.[516] This study also confirms the methodological problems concerning food intake analysis in young children (see Chapters 1 and 3).

Energy intake in two groups of young children with a low (Group N) and high risk of obesity (Group O) as judged from parental obesity was assessed. Energy intake was 16% lower in Group O as assessed by dietary record along with TEE, ascertained by monitoring heart rate. The energy intakes of all children together, and also in Group N, showed the usual wide variability and absence of correlation with body size; however, in Group O, a significant relationship between body weight and height with energy intake was found ($r = 0.5$).[413] Along with elevated fat mass and serum lipid levels, an increased energy intake (two to three times) compared to normal-weight children was found by Lahlou et al.[515]

In a group of Italian obese and non-obese children aged $10.1 \pm 2.1$ years, energy intake was the same. When expressed in relation to total and/or FFM, energy intake was lower in the obese than in the non-obese children ($189.5 \pm 74.5$ vs. $292.0 \pm 109.2$ kJ.kg body weight$^{-1}$.day$^{-1}$, $p < 0.001$, or $251.9 \pm 91.2$ vs. $333.0 \pm 122.6$ kJ.kg fat-free body mass$^{-1}$.day$^{-1}$). Composition of the diet was comparable for both groups. Obese children ate more protein than controls, in particular, from animal origin ($14.6 \pm 3.7$ vs. $13.6 \pm 3.0\%$ of energy). The animal/plant ratio was $2.4 \pm 1.7$ vs. $2.1 \pm 1.1$, $p < 0.05$). Intake of saturated fats and cholesterol was comparable in both groups. No correlation was found for the intake of nutrients and percentage of body fatness at the age of 10 years.

Obese children were also significantly less active than controls but no difference was found in obese vs. non-obese children in relation to the time spent in sport activities only, both at school and during leisure time. These differences in physical activity may explain, at least partly, those in body fatness.[214]

Eating style and its relationship to children's adiposity were examined in children aged 3 to 5 years who attended a university preschool setting. Children completed controlled, two-part meals, reflecting children's ability to precisely adjust food intake in response to changes in the diet's energy density. An eating index, reflecting this ability to regulate energy intake, correlated with morphological characteristics of children. These correlations showed association between fat stores and responsiveness to energy density cues. Pearson's correlation coefficients revealed that children with greater body fat stores were less able to regulate energy intake accurately.

The most important predictor of children's ability to regulate energy intake was parental control in the feeding situation. Mothers who were more active in controlling their children's food intake had children who showed less ability to self-regulate energy intake ($r = -0.67$, $p < 0.0001$). These observations suggest that the optimal environment for children's development of self-control of energy intake is not when healthy food choices are provided, but when children are allowed to assume control of how much they consume.[517] This might also contribute to preventing development of increased body adiposity in early life.

In another study, food intake was assessed in obese and normal-weight children, aged 7 to 11 years. An interview and a food dictionary were used during the 2 days prior to the study and on 1 holiday, along with a week-long questionnaire. Food intake in obese children did not exceed that of children with normal body weight, rather, it was lower (Figure 7.1).[518] The studied group consumed approximately 15% of energy as proteins, 35% as fats, and 50% as carbohydrates, and no difference was noted between obese and normal-weight children. The percentage of carbohydrates was lower, and that of proteins and fats higher than RDAs. A significant increase with age was noted for protein and fat intakes, along with a significant reduction in carbohydrates. These deviations concerned the majority of both obese (70%) and normal-weight children (80%).

Measurements in a study by Forbes and Brown showed that the energy required for weight maintenance in a group of adolescent and adult subjects of widely varying body size was directly proportional to body weight ($r = 0.92$).[519] Greater lean body mass and larger energy demands for carrying an increased load of excess fat explained the increased energy requirement in the obese.

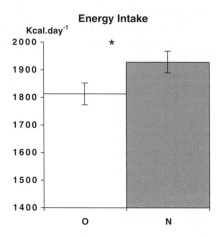

**FIGURE 7.1**

Comparison of energy intake in obese (O) and normal-weight (N) children. * indicates (p < 0.05). (Based on data from Ref. F23.)

## 7.4    The Effect of Diet Composition and Eating Behavior

Composition of the diet, especially fat content, is particularly important in early childhood. Essential fatty acids provide the substrates for arachidonic acid, docosahexaenoid acid, and their metabolites which are essential for an adequate maturation of the central nervous system, visual development, and intelligence.[520]

There is still only limited evidence on the relationship between the composition of a child's early diet and the development of chronic diseases in later life. However, the essential role of individual nutrients in particular periods of growth and development have been more frequently documented in recent studies and analyses.[201,212,521,522] The effect of protein in early life on adiposity development was mentioned in Chapters 3 and 4, and will be also considered in Chapter 8.

Composition of the diet was compared in obese and lean subjects in a group of 8- to 12-year-old children.[522,523] There were no differences in energy, fat, calcium, iron, Vitamins A and C, thiamin, and riboflavin intakes between groups. A study of Spanish obese and non-obese adolescents showed no difference in energy intake of adolescents; however, obese subjects derived a greater proportion of their energy from protein (19.8% vs. 16.4%) than non-obese controls. The proportion of energy from fats was also higher in the obese (45.4%) than in the non-obese (38.7%) and the obese also consumed greater amounts of cholesterol.[524] This study also confirmed that it is necessary to check and manage the diet not only for total amount of energy but also for various macro-components.

Dietary intake of children 7 to 14 years of age in a small Italian community showed a higher intake of protein (up to 15.8% of energy) with an increased animal/vegetable protein ratio (1.5 to 2.1). Intake of fats was higher than 35.9% of the daily energy and the polyunsaturated/saturated fatty acid ratio was low, ranging from 0.3 to 0.5. Intake of cholesterol exceeded the recommended level (231 to 347 mg per day) and the daily intake of total carbohydrates was also low (45.3 to 48.5% per day). Crude fiber intake increased with age from 2.8 g to 4.5 g per day. A comparison of dietary intake of obese and non-obese growing subjects did not, however, reveal any significant differences.[123]

The effect of fat intake on fat mass was studied in white and Mohawk children 4 to 7 years of age, along with body composition (BIA, skinfolds) and energy expenditure based on physical activity level. Before statistical analysis, FM was adjusted for FFM and intake of fat was adjusted for non-fat food intake. No influence of gender or ethnicity on fat intake was found, and no influence of ethnicity on the relationship between fat intake and fat mass. Adjusted mean intakes for the groups of children based on parental obesity status are presented in Figure 7.2.

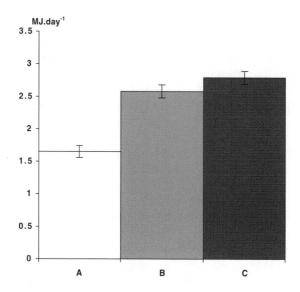

**FIGURE 7.2**
Adjusted mean values ($\times \pm$ SE) of fat intake or nonfat intake in children with a non-obese father and mother (A), obese father and non-obese mother (B), and obese father and mother (C). A significant relationship between fat mass and fat intake, $r = 0.48$, $p < 0.01$, was revealed. (Based on data from Ref. F24.)

An influence of maternal obesity on dietary fat intake of children and a significant correlation between fat mass and fat intake in boys, but not in girls when adjusted for physical activity and energy expenditure, was revealed. According to the results of this study mothers may contribute to the development of obesity in their children by influencing the dietary fat content of boys. Dietary fat intake contributes to obesity independent of physical activity and energy expenditure.[525]

Imbalances in the contribution of macronutrients to total energy intake appear more marked in overweight and obese Spanish individuals, with a greater proportion of their energy intake coming from fats and a lower percentage of their energy from carbohydrates. No differences in total energy intake were found among these overweight and normal adolescents. Moreover, obese subjects had significantly larger intakes of cholesterol. The situation was worse in females who consumed 50% of their energy from fat, 21.9% from proteins, and only 27.5% from carbohydrates.[524] The most significant result of this study is confirmation that diet composition, rather than energy consumption, was the main factor responsible for obesity in both young women and men. A high-fat and low-carbohydrate diet was associated with leptin levels.[526]

A study by Tucker et al.[527] showed that the percentage of body fat in children aged 9.8 ± 0.5 years varied according to their diet composition. Children's energy intake was positively related to their adiposity. The percentage of energy from fat was also positively related to adiposity before and after controlling for potential confounding variables (fatness, fitness, physical activity, and parental body mass). The percentage of energy derived from carbohydrates was inversely related to adiposity under the same conditions. This study confirmed again that composition of the diet and the relationships between individual macronutrients play an essential role in the development of obesity.

The percentage of body fat correlated positively with intakes of total, saturated, monounsaturated, and polyunsaturated fat, and negatively with carbohydrate intake and total energy intake adjusted for body weight in boys and girls aged 9 to 11 years.[528] The associations remained for the intake of all mentioned nutrients after adjustment for energy intake, resting energy expenditure (REE), and physical activity. These results also confirm that composition of the diet, particularly the ratio of fats, may play an important role in the development of children's obesity, independent of total energy intake, REE, and physical activity.

In further studies it was shown that both total energy intake and the composition of the diet are positively associated with the development of obesity, especially saturated fats. Many studies have shown an intake of fats exceeding 30% of energy intake and therefore recommend a lower ratio of fats in the diet. However, this mainly concerns children over 2 to 3 years of age.[529]

In infants and younger children, fats are indispensable because of their high-energy needs and limited dietary capacity. The proportion of fat in children's diet is thus dependent on the age of the child, and should not be severely decreased at an early age.

Reduced fat diets in young children are problematic. Children who were placed on a very low fat diet due to hypercholesterolemia showed marked growth and development problems.[202,530] Therefore, the definition of appropriate fat intake for any child must be made with great caution. However, it is very common for the intake of fats to be too high, exceeding 30% of energy intake during later childhood. This should be rectified to prevent obesity by using the appropriate RDAs.

Measurements of dietary intake and composition in obese children have showed that the percentage of dietary lipids correlated directly with serum level of triglycerides (TG), and inversely correlated with HDL-C. The percentage of dietary carbohydrates was inversely correlated to TG and ApoB/A1 and directly correlated to basal insulin. The prevalence of dyslipoproteinemia and hypertension was significantly higher in the families who showed hyperinsulinemia. Patients who reported a dietary animal/plant lipid ratio of greater than 1 also showed a significantly higher prevalence of cardiovascular disease in their families.

From these observations, composition of the diet seems to have greater importance than excessive energy intake in regard to dyslipoproteinemia, which along with the excess weight, plays the main role in obesity-related diseases.[382]

Another study of Italian children and youth confirmed inadequacies of energy intake, macronutrient distribution, and preference for inadequate foodstuffs in youth. More than two thirds of children consumed more than 70 g of soluble sugars per day, while 10% of them exceeded 150 g per day. Results showed that snacks account for 34% of the total daily energy intake, and an imbalance in energy distribution of macronutrients. Evaluation of weight self-perception revealed that only 62% of adolescents were able to correctly match perception of their body weight with actual measurement. The majority of youth consumed a regular breakfast but only rarely was it nutritionally adequate. Obesity prevalence reached almost 30%.[531]

## 7.5 Eating Behavior and Food Preferences

Food preferences in 3- to 5-year-old children were related to parent's weight status and skinfold thicknesses; children who preferred fat had heavier parents. Fat preferences were significantly related to triceps skinfold measurement ($r = 0.61$, $p < 0.01$). On the other hand, epidemiological studies provide evidence that sugar consumption as well as total carbohydrate consumption is associated with leanness.[532]

The most marked relative changes in the composition of diet and nutritional patterns have occurred in the countries of the Third World. For example, in southern Africa, urban black 5-year-old children consumed a low fat

(30% of energy), high carbohydrate (61% of energy) diet in 1984, but a typical Westernized diet in 1995 (fat 41%, and carbohydrate 52% of total energy).[533]

As mentioned previously in Chapter 3 and this one, high fat consumption accompanying acculturation is assumed to be one of the causes of the increasing prevalence of obesity in many populations. Similar changes in fat ingestion (but also of sugar) were assessed in Canadian Inuits, in New Guinea, and Samoa (Chapter 2), and were connected to an increasing prevalence of obesity, diabetes, and cardiovascular diseases.[172]

Recently, more evidence has emerged about increased susceptibility to these diseases by immigrant groups coming to northern Europe due to a changed food intake, composition of the diet, and patterns of eating. As mentioned in Chapter 2, conditions related to overnutrition such as obesity, cardiovascular diseases, and diabetes, are most often considered in this respect.[534]

Evaluation of eating behavior in obese Italian prepubertal and adolescent girls aged 9.9 ± 0.88 and 15.56 ± 1.61 years showed an increased food intake in both groups. When compared to RDAs, the energy intake was higher in 36% of obese girls in the younger group and in 46% in the older group of obese girls. Protein intake was increased in 78% of the younger and in 66% of adolescent obese girls. Decreased calcium intake was also found in the majority of obese girls in both age groups. Total cholesterol was increased in 33% of the younger and 23% of the older obese girls.[535]

During recent years, the role of fruit juices and their intake, which does not correspond to the optimal needs of children, was considered as a possible factor contributing to obesity. Excess fruit juice consumption was reported and excess energy intake may be due to children's preference for foods with a sweet taste.[536]

Morbid obesity, defined as body weight exceeding 100% of reference weight, has been reported in the U.S. and also from some European countries, such as Austria. Twenty-two adolescents with a BMI of 32.5 ± 3.9 were divided with respect to the onset of obesity; that is, subjects became obese between the 9th and 11th year (1) and those who were already considered obese as infants (2). In group (1), insulin, total cholesterol (TC), LDL-C, and triglyceride levels were higher than in group (2). The majority of these adolescents had an energy intake 20% higher than the normal-weight children, ate more restaurant meals such as pizzas, noodles, and pasta, and less vegetables and fruit. Family doctors and pediatricians, and/or parents and caregivers never tried to rectify the preferences of these children.[537]

## 7.6 Thermic Effect of Food and Obesity

Some studies showed that the thermic effect of food (TEF) was similar and did not significantly change in groups of obese and normal-weight children during overfeeding.[447] However, insulin and 3.5.3-triiodothyronin levels did increase significantly, but did not differ between the groups. Plasma norepinephrine (NE) and urinary excretion of 4-hydroxy-3 methoxymandelic acid (VMA) did not increase during overfeeding. TEF did not appear to be reduced in obese adolescents; therefore, facultative TEF does not appear to be a significant factor in weight maintenance during adolescence.[447]

However, Maffeis et al.[538] showed that the thermic effect of a meal (TEM) compared to the mixed liquid meal (at an energy level corresponding to 30% of the 24-hr pre-meal resting metabolic rate) was significantly lower in obese children compared to control children (Figure 7.3).[538] This was found in spite of higher test meal energy in the obese.

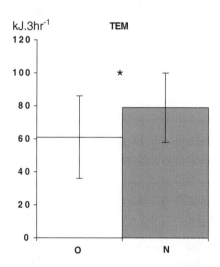

**FIGURE 7.3**
Comparison of the thermic effect of mixed liquid meal (TEM kJ.3hr$^{-1}$) in pre-pubertal obese (O) and control, non-obese (N) children. * indicates ($p < 0.05$). (Based on data from Ref. F25.)

The following study, executed under resting conditions and after exercise, showed that thermogenesis was significantly greater in a lean relative to an obese group. The percentage of fat mass was the best predictor of TEF at rest and during post-exercise recovery. Absolute basal energy expenditure was higher in the obese than in lean adolescents and no significant differences were observed between groups in relation to basal energy expenditure per kg of fat-free body mass. Therefore, even when lean and obese adolescents are comparable with respect to fat-free mass, thermogenesis is blunted in obese subjects (Figure 7.4).[539]

Post-meal (chocolate milkshake) energy expenditure (TEM) was compared in normal (BMI = 17.8) and obese (BMI = 35.9) adolescent girls. Cumulative TEM was calculated as the integrated area under the TEM curve with resting

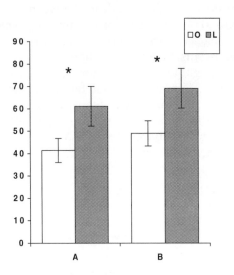

**FIGURE 7.4**

Comparison of thermogenesis after a test meal in obese (O) and lean, normal-weight (L) 15-year-old subjects under rest (A, kcal.3 hours$^{-1}$) and post-exercise (B) conditions. * indicates ($p < 0.05$). (Based on data from Ref. F26.)

metabolic rate (RMR) as baseline. The meals resulted in a greater rise in insulin and glucose for the obese compared to the non-obese subjects, and a significant increase of TEM for both groups. The cumulative TEM was 61.9% greater for the non-obese when expressed relative to body mass, and 33.2% for the non-obese when expressed relative to the fat-free body mass. Expressed relative to the meal, the TEM was 25.5% less for the obese. These observations support an energy conservation hypothesis for obese female adolescents.[540]

## 7.7   The Role of Food Consumption Patterns in the Development of Obesity

The role of metabolic and/or behavioral daily rhythms with regard to food intake was also studied in obese children.[541] Daily energy consumption and the distribution of intake over the waking hours was studied in a group of children aged 7 to 12 years, divided into 5 corpulence categories. No difference in the estimated daily energy intake was observed between corpulence groups; however, the distribution of intake during the waking hours was different. Obese and fatter children ate less at breakfast and more at dinner than their lean peers. Lunch and dinner, which are usually the largest meals of the day, represented a higher ratio of daily intake in fatter and obese children. The energy value of breakfast and afternoon snacks was inversely related to the degree of corpulence of children.

These observations do not exclude hyperphagia during other periods of the observation; however, a possible contribution of disturbed metabolic and/or behavioral cycles in the development of overweight was suggested.[541] Therefore, these results confirm the old notion that to prevent obesity, it is recommended that breakfast be eaten, a greater proportion of daily intake be ingested during the first half of the waking hours, and, correspondingly, one should eat more modestly at the end of the day, with an early dinner.

A multiple regression analysis in Italian schoolchildren used relative weight as the dependent variable, and age and the percentage of the energy intake ingested at breakfast, morning snack, lunch, afternoon snack, dinner, and post-dinner snack as independent variables. The study showed that overweight was positively correlated with food intake at dinner and negatively correlated with an afternoon meal.[542]

Obese and overweight children were also compared in another study, particularly with regard to eating breakfast. The energy profiles of the obese subjects were more imbalanced than in normal-weight subjects. A significant difference was found between the amounts of energy supplied by carbohydrates. Obese children had less satisfactory breakfast habits which could contribute to poorer food choices over the rest of the day, and, in the long term, to an increased risk of obesity.[543]

A study in preschool children showed that the overweight subjects had a lower consumption at lunch than normal children when the high carbohydrate pre-loads (fruit juice, banana, 30 min before lunch) were tested. High protein pre-load (chicken meat) had no effect on lunch consumption. When energy intake derived from food consumption was analyzed, the same tendency for food consumption was revealed.[544] These data show a different response of overweight children to the high carbohydrate pre-loads consumed before lunch, especially in children aged 24 to 36 months.

Italian adolescents often show disorders of dietary behavior predisposing them not only to obesity but also to anorexia nervosa. Recommendations for improving their diet concern promoting regular breakfast, a balanced intake of animal and vegetable foods, and increased calcium intake to maximize bone density.[545] Later development of osteoporosis, especially in women, is related to early intake of calcium and balanced food (U.S. RDAs, 1989). Dairy products, vegetables, and especially enriched cereals constitute a basis for an adequate diet during this period of development.

The inevitable undesirable effects of a Westernized lifestyle in Japan negatively influenced eating habits, causing irregular timing of food intake and a reduction of physical activity. The increasing number of working mothers also promotes the eating of processed food and thus increased intake of energy in the form of fat.[546] Education systems attempting to promote optimal nutrition and lifestyle practices are often overwhelmed by the effect of the mass media. Most commercials for fast food products do not consider health promotion; however, such foods are attractively packaged, readily available, and easy to prepare for the whole family.

Eating behaviors including duration and rate of consumption were measured during 2 lunch meals in obese and normal-weight children aged 11 years. The obese children ate faster and did not slow their eating rate toward the end of the meal as much as normal-weight children. The obese also indicated they had less motivation to eat before lunch than normal-weight children. A deficient satiety signal or an impaired response to such signals in obese growing subjects may possibly explain the above-mentioned differences.[547]

Eating behavior has also been compared in obese and normal adolescents using several tests with vanilla drinks. No significant differences were found with respect to the absolute amount of the drink and/or energy intake consumed. However, differences were assessed in the amounts prior to and after the tests indicating greater sensitivity and higher responsiveness to external stimuli in the obese.[548]

Food intake can influence gastric electrical activity as measured by electrogastrography (EGG) as well as being related to nutritional status and adiposity. Electrogastrographic power normally increases post-prandially. However, when normal and obese children aged 6 to 12 years were assessed using EGG, the response to a mixed meal was not affected by BMI values. Gastric electrical rhythm and rate and gastric power were also not influenced by age and gender.[549]

Another factor often cited for its contribution to the development of childhood obesity is between-meal snacking. A study in Antigua indicated that children consume significant amounts of food between main meals.[550] While some of the components of snacks had an adequate nutritional value, most were undesirable and could play a major role in the deterioration of health.[550]

Behaviors and concerns related to weight were measured by questionnaire in fourth-grade children attending a rural school in central Iowa. Weight-related behaviors and concerns increased with increasing weight-for-age and BMI and were more prevalent among girls than boys. The frequency of drinking diet soft drinks was positively correlated with weight-for-age and BMI and tended to increase with an increase in weight-related behaviors and concerns. Girls were more likely than boys to report a desire to be thinner, whereas boys were more likely than girls to want to be taller. The desire for less body fat was more significantly associated with an increase in the frequency of weight-related behaviors and concerns than with the frequency of drinking diet soft drink, weight-for-age, and BMI.[551]

REE, RQ, plasma glucose, and insulin concentrations were studied in obese children with respect to the effect of different kinds of meals. These parameters increased sooner, and were steeper and higher with the liquid meal (LM) than with the three consecutive small meals (SM) in obese boys and girls aged 12.7 ± 0.6 years. The magnitude of TEF was greater after the LM than the SM. These results indicate that frequency of food consumption influences the immediate thermogenic response as well as changes in the respiratory quotient; glycemia and insulinemia followed simultaneously.[394,554] This may also be related to the development of adiposity.

## 7.8 Utilization and Oxidation of Macrocomponents

Fat may not be handled in the same way in prepubertal normal-weight and obese children. Post-absorptive fat oxidation expressed in absolute values was significantly higher in obese than in non-obese children, but not when adjusted by analysis of co-variance with FFM as the co-variate (Figure 7.5). In obese children and in the whole group, fat mass and fat oxidation were significantly correlated (r = 0.65; p < 0.001). The slope of the relationship indicated that for each 10 kg of additional fat mass, resting fat oxidation increased by 18 g per day. The higher post-absorbtive rate of fat oxidation in obese children as compared to non-obese subjects may favor achievement of a new equilibrium in fat balance, opposing further increases of the adipose tissue.[552]

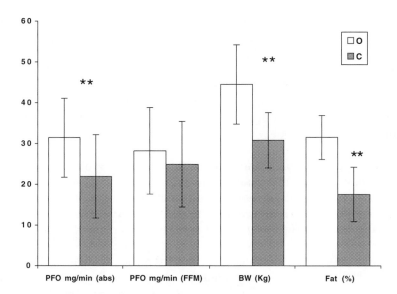

**FIGURE 7.5**
Comparison of morphological characteristics and post-absorptive fat oxidation (PFM mg.min⁻¹) in absolute values and as related to fat-free, lean body mass (FFM) of obese (O) and normal-weight (C) pre-pubertal children. * indicates (p < 0.05); ** (p < 0.01). (Based on data from Ref. F27.)

Oxidation of the individual items of fat, that is, of exogenous (meal intake) and endogenous fat (lipolysis) and their ratios was considered in children with a wide range of BMIs.[553] The relationship between adiposity and fat oxidation during the post-prandial period after a mixed meal was also examined. The use of stable isotope ($^{13}$C)-enriched fatty acids added to a mixed meal and indirect calorimetry rendered possible the differentiation between exo- and endogenous sources of fat oxidation. During the 9-hr post-prandial period, children oxidized an amount of fat comparable to that ingested in the meal. Exogenous fat represented the average 10.8% (0.9%) total fat oxidation.

Endogenous fat calculated as the difference between total fat oxidation and exogenous oxidation represented 88.2% (0.9%). Significant correlations between endogenous and total fat oxidation ($r = 0.98$, $p < 0.001$), and total and endogenous fat oxidation ($r = 0.73$, $p < 0.001$) were found.

Exogenous fat oxidation expressed as a proportion of total fat oxidation correlated significantly with the degree of adiposity ($r = 0.6$, $p < 0.01$). The relationship can be considered a protective mechanism to prevent further increase in fat mass in the organism, and hence to maintain fat oxidation at a sufficient rate under conditions of exposure to exogenous fat in a meal.[553]

Similar results were gained in another study of Hungarian children with higher oxidation rates of fat in obese as compared to normal-weight peers. Both fat-free, lean body mass and fat mass were important determinants of the rate of oxidation of fat.[554]

The effect of obesity on carbohydrate oxidation (exogenous compared with endogenous carbohydrate) after the consumption of a mixed meal was studied in obese and normal prepubertal children aged 8 years.[555] Total carbohydrate oxidation was calculated by indirect calorimetry (hood system), whereas endogenous carbohydrate oxidation was estimated from carbon dioxide production ($VCO_2$), the isotopic enrichment of breath $^{13}CO_2$, and the abundance of $^{13}$C carbohydrate in the meal ingested. The time course of $^{13}$C in breath was measured over 570 min and followed a similar pattern in both groups.

Although total carbohydrate oxidation was not significantly different between both groups, exogenous carbohydrate utilization was significantly greater and endogenous carbohydrate oxidation was significantly lower in obese compared with control children of normal weight. The rate of carbohydrate oxidation was positively related to the body fat of the children ($r = 0.68$, $p < 0.01$).

This study suggests that in the post-prandial phase, a smaller proportion of carbohydrate oxidation is accounted for by glycogen breakdown in obese children. Sparing of endogenous glycogen may result from decreased glycogen turnover already present at prepubertal age.[555]

Energy expenditure (EE, measured by indirect calorimetry) was also followed at rest and after an oral sucrose load of 3 g per kg of body weight in overweight girls aged $14.54 \pm 0.38$ years. Food-induced thermogenesis (FIT) was evaluated by computing the area under the curve of the EE response and above resting EE during the first 3 hr after the sucrose load. Resting energy expenditure (REE) (kcal.day$^{-1}$) was higher in the overweight subjects. When REE was related to fat-free mass (FFM), the values were lower in the obese children than in the normal-weight children.

A linear correlation between REE and FFM was evidenced in both control and overweight subjects (r = 0.78 and 0.68, respectively; $p < 0.05$ and 0.001). Actual REE in the obese children was significantly lower than the values predicted from regression equations of REE on FFM in controls to the actual FFM in obese children. FIT (food induced thermogenesis) was identical in overweight and normal-weight subjects, regardless of whether it was expressed in absolute value, as a percentage of energy intake, or standardized by FFM.[556]

# 8

## Biochemical Characteristics

### 8.1 Serum Lipids, Lipolysis, and Body Adiposity

Nutritional status and adiposity are significantly associated with a number of biochemical parameters including serum lipids and lipoproteinemia. Commonly, total cholesterol (TC), high-density lipoprotein (HDL-C) and low-density lipoprotein cholesterol (LDL-C) and triglycerides are assessed. Apolipoprotein A1, B, and E have been analyzed in studies of obese children and youth less frequently.

In the Bogalusa Heart Study, 3,311 children and young adults, grouped according to gender, age, and race from a biracial community, were examined. A significant positive relationship between ponderosity and LDL-C was found in older age groups (that is, 22 years) but was absent in the younger age groups. It could be speculated that such relationships might appear later in life, after a longer period of increased weight and fatness. A significant negative association was found between ponderosity and HDL-C, which was particularly apparent in males at the age of 22 years.[557]

As a measure of central obesity, subscapular skinfold thickness correlated similarly with serum lipoproteins. This enabled the elaboration of a regression model using the subscapular skinfold to predict serum lipids.[558] Similar relationships between serum lipid level and obesity were found in Japanese children.[559]

In other studies, a positive relationship between serum lipids and fatness was found in preschool children. The percentage of fat correlated significantly with the serum levels of total cholesterol (TC) and triglycerides (TG) in children aged 4.7 years, indicating the importance of adiposity and dyslipoproteinemia in early age.[61,68,303] DuRant et al.[411] showed that more favorable serum lipid and lipoprotein levels were associated with lower levels of fatness and higher levels of cardiovascular fitness in children aged 4 to 5 years. Physical activity appeared to have an indirect association with serum lipid and lipoprotein values through its relationship with higher fitness levels and lower body adiposity. Similar relationships were reported by Gutin.[264]

Correlates of the serum level of HDL-C were examined in black and white girls aged 9 to 10 years in the framework of NHLBI Growth and Health Study. Each 10 millimeter increase in the sum of 10 skinfolds was associated with a decrease of 1.4 mg.dL$^{-1}$ of HDL-C, and each unit increase in the triceps/subscapular skinfold ratio was associated with an increase of 2 mg.dL$^{-1}$ LDL-C. In addition, each 10% increase in polyunsaturated fat intake was associated with an increase of 3.4 mg.dL$^{-1}$ HDL-C. The associations of sedentary activity and sexual maturation with HDL-C were mediated by the differences in adiposity. HDL-C serum levels were, on average, 3.6 mg.dL$^{-1}$ higher in black compared to white girls.[560] Aerobic conditioning is used to modify dyslipoproteinemia and the health risks of atherosclerosis. Without a reduction in excess fat, health cannot be effectively promoted.[561]

Obesity among Greek adolescents was associated with unfavorable lipid profiles, similar to other countries. Adolescents living in urban areas had a significantly higher level of total and LDL-C but this was more consistent with lower socioeconomic status. There was evidence that TC, LDL-C and HDL-C levels were significantly affected by qualitative aspects of diet as evaluated through a food-frequency questionnaire.

The results of this study also reveal that a traditional Mediterranean pattern of living and eating in the rural areas of Greece is associated with a favorable lipid profile in adolescents. This may explain the very low incidence of coronary heart disease (CHD) in this part of Europe.[562]

The serum lipid level of children in Milano, Italy was also comparable to other west European data, but higher than in southern Italy where dietary intake and body fatness are generally lower. This is related to a lower socioeconomic level. In obese children, higher levels of ApoB, triglycerides (TG), total cholesterol (TC), and LDL-C, and lower levels of HDL-C were seen. The values were higher in obese boys than in obese girls. An assessment of dietary intake showed the significant effect of nutritional factors. A higher TC/HDL-C ratio was found in children on the lower quartile of polyunsaturated fatty acid intake.[563]

The increased prevalence of risk factors, as characterized by an unfavorable profile of serum lipids for later atherosclerosis, was also found in other child populations with increased obesity, for example, in Poland[564–566] and the Czech Republic.[567,568] Significantly lower serum HDL-C levels were found in the obese when compared with normal-weight boys (Figure 8.1).[569]

A study of Polish children revealed that in boys there was a significant association between BMI and atherogenic lipid profile, that is, positive correlations of BMI with TC, LDL-C, TG, and a significant negative correlation with HDL-C. In girls, a significant negative correlation was found for BMI and HDL-C.[565]

Another study of obese children aged 10 to 11 years showed higher values of Apo B and a lower Apo A-1/B ratio. Significant correlations were found between Apo A-1 and physical fitness, triceps skinfold thickness, birth weight, physical fitness and triceps skinfold, and between Apo A-1/B ratio and triceps skinfold thickness. When both obese and normal-weight children

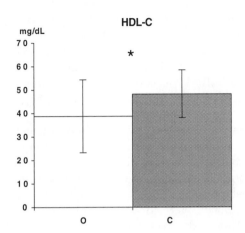

**FIGURE 8.1**
Comparison of serum level of HDL-C (mg/dL) in obese (O) and control, normal-weight (N) boys 5.3 to 9.9 years old. * indicates ($p < 0.05$). (Based on data from Ref. F28.)

were grouped together, a correlation was found between BMI and TC, Apo B, and the Apo A-1/B ratio. Multiple regression equation analyses indicated a significant positive contribution to the Apo A-1 level by HDL-C and physical fitness, and negatively with birth weight.[570]

The prevalence of obesity in Austrian children is 19% at the age of 7 to 9 years and 29% at the age of 15 to 19 years in boys. There is a decrease in prevalence in girls from 16 to 13% in the same age intervals. TG levels were within the normal values in both obese and normal-weight children; however, in the non-obese, TG serum level was significantly lower. No significant differences were found in TC, HDL-C, and LDL-C between obese and non-obese children and adolescents; however, a higher TC/HDL-C ratio was found in the obese subjects.[121]

In another study of obese children aged up to 17 years, the relationship between serum lipids, the level of obesity, and waist-to-hip ratio was evaluated.[571] In boys, TG increased and LpA1 (which is a lipoprotein particle containing only Apo A-1) decreased with the overall obesity. In obese girls, TG and insulin increased, and LpA1 decreased with upper body fat distribution. However, in a multivariate analysis, these correlations were found only in boys.

An Italian study showed a 28% obesity percentage; 23% of the young were hypercholesterolemic and 21% had hypertriglyceridemia. Hypertension was not revealed. The high percentage of obese and hyperlipidemic primary school children indicates a serious health risk and the need for intervention.[572] In Belgian children aged 6 to 12 years, increased levels of TC and TG were seen, along with a marked prevalence of obesity in the sample studied. In girls, TC correlated positively with the energy density of saturated fat, cholesterol and protein intake, and negatively with the polyunsaturated/satu-rated ratio of fat intake and energy density of carbohydrate intake. No such relationships were observed in boys. In addition, no relationships between TG and nutritional factors were observed in either gender. In boys, TC and TG correlated positively with BMI while in girls, this relationship was observed for TG and BMI. It was concluded that environmental and family factors have a different effect with regard to gender, being more pronounced in girls.[573]

The effect of obesity and fat patterning on lipoproteinemia has also been studied in Japanese children and youth.[574] In boys, anthropometric indices of obesity correlated with risk factors of atherosclerosis; strong correlations were observed among the indices of overweight, adiposity, and body fat dis-tribution. In contrast, only the indices of body fat distribution, but not those of overweight or adiposity, were correlated with serum biochemical indices in the obese girls. This study indicated that body fat distribution is signif-icantly related to certain biochemical complications of childhood obesity, and androgenic fat patterns induce metabolic derangements during growth and development.

Another study of obese adolescents aged 11.0 to 13.8 years concerned serum lipids and fat distribution characterized by the waist-to-hip ratio and triceps/subscapular ratio. A fat tolerance test was also executed. The results were evaluated in two subgroups of obese subjects, divided according to the type of obesity, that is, peripheral and/or central. Post-prandial lipemia did not differ between obese and non-obese adolescents. Higher post-prandial lipemia concentration was observed in subjects with a central pattern of fat distribution compared to those with a peripheral distribution. These data also confirm that the occurrence of lipid metabolism disturbances during growth may depend more on the type of fat distribution than on its total amount in the organism.[575]

Lipolytic activity of the adipose tissue of obese children is decreased. *In vivo* lipolysis that reflects the mobilization of lipid stores from the sub-cutaneous adipose tissue shows decreased sensitivity to epinephrine in childhood onset obesity. As an *in vivo* index of lipolysis, glycerol flux was measured using a non-radioactive tracer dilution approach, and plasma free-fatty acids (FFA) concentration. At the basal state, obese children had a 30% lower rate of glycerol release per unit of fat mass than did control children. To study lipolysis regulation, epinephrine was infused stepwise at fixed doses. In lean children, glycerol and FFA increased 246 to 249% of basal val-ues, in obese children, only 55 to 77%. The resistance of lipolysis to epineph-rine did not show any relationship with the Arg64 polymorphism of the beta-(3)-adrenoreceptor gene.[576]

Since the study was executed in obese children during the dynamic phase of fat accumulation, the observed resistance to catecholamines might possi-bly be causative rather than the result of obesity. Decreased mobilization of TG may contribute to the increased accumulation of lipids in adipocytes. Reduced lipolysis and decreased sensitivity to epinephrine might be also related to reduced physical activity in the obese. This problem was also studied in an experimental model.

## 8.2 Uricemia and Obesity

The relationship between uricemia and adiposity was examined in adolescent girls. It was shown that both dietary factors and clearance of uric acid (CIU, which was not influenced by an increased intake of water) appear to be responsible for hyperuricemia in young obese individuals.[577]

## 8.3 Protein Metabolism

In prepubertal children, obesity is associated with an absolute increase in whole-body protein turnover that is related to an increased lean FFM. Both of these factors contribute to the explanation of the higher resting energy expenditure in the obese compared to non-obese children (Chapter 5). A significant relationship was found between protein synthesis and FFM ($R = 0.83$, $p < 0.001$) and protein synthesis and resting energy expenditure ($r = 0.79$, $p < 0.005$).[578]

## 8.4 Mineral Metabolism

Mineral metabolism may also be altered. During an oral glucose tolerance test (OGTT), serum calcium and phosphorus decreased, and serum parathyroid hormone (PTH) and calcitonin (CT) increased less in obese than in non-obese children. When obese children received a diet with a high carbohydrate content, changes in mineral metabolism occurred, which were characterized by a secondary increase of PTH and 1,25(OH)2D3. Calcium decreased and PTH and CT increased less markedly during OGTT. Bone mineral content (BMC) measured by a photon absorptiometer and BMC/bone width ratio were lower in obese than in non-obese children.[579]

Along with other biochemical variables, the parameters concerning mineral metabolism and some hormones were changed in a group of obese children (who were on a diet rich in energy and carbohydrates) aged 8 to 11 years. In basal conditions, alkaline-phosphatase (AP), osteocalcin (OC), parathyroid hormone (PTH), calcitonin (CT), and 1,25 dihydroxyvitamin D3 (1,25 (OH) 2D3) levels were significantly higher, along with increased levels of glucose, immuno-reactive insulin (IRI); 25-hydroxyvitamin D3 (25OHD3) levels were lower in obese children when compared to controls. Urinary excretion of calcium (Ca/Cr) and phosphorus (TmP/GFR) were lower in obese than in non-obese children. Hydroxyproline (OH-P/Cr) and cyclic AMP (cAMP/GFR) were higher in obese children.[579]

## 8.5    Total Antioxidant Capacity and Lipid Soluble Antioxidant Vitamins

Total antioxidant capacity (TAC) is decreased in obese children. Reduced plasma levels of lipid soluble antioxidant vitamins (α-tocopherol and β-carotene) were also demonstrated in obese children as compared to controls.[580] The differences remained significant after correction for lipemia.[580,581] Reduced plasma concentrations of main lipid-soluble antioxidants may increase the risk of cardiovascular diseases in obese children and youth. Reduced values of serum levels of fat-soluble antioxidants in obese children were also confirmed in the NHANES III study.[582]

# 9

## Hormonal Characteristics

Hormonal activities are essential for the maintenance of normal body composition. Disturbances in hormonal secretion and clearance have often been considered the main causes of increased body fatness, particularly in those who are very obese. However, hormonal abnormalities are rare. Many of the features that characterize obesity and relate to hormonal function are considered to be secondary and may have resulted from a changed overall metabolic status of an obese individual.

Many studies have considered the hormonal profile of growing children, including those who are obese. Most studies in growing children simultaneously describe levels of hormones and their mutual associations, as related to the characteristics of obesity. Comparative studies involving children are difficult as mentioned previously. This difficulty is compounded by the different stages of sexual maturation of the individuals who are being studied.

Obese children as a group are characteristically taller than children who have a normal body weight. In most cases, these differences are only temporary and the normal-weight children usually catch up to their obese peers with increasing age and maturity. A number of hormones and their interactions are affected by increased adiposity and are also related to the temporarily accelerated growth of the obese.

### 9.1 Insulin-Like Growth Factor (IGF)

IGF displays a wide range of metabolic effects. The prevailing component of IGF in plasma is bound to a specific binding protein (BP). It is presumed that BP modulates the biological activities of IGF. BP3 is regulated by growth hormone (GH) and has a high affinity for IGF. The GH-independent BP1 and BP2 show lower affinities.

The results of another study suggest that in prepubertal and early pubertal girls, IGF-1 concentration in blood is related to overall body size. Along with sexual maturation, this relationship between IGF-1 and somatic size diminishes, and relationships between IGF-1 and both fatness and physical fitness start to appear.[583]

The study by Bideci et al.[584] showed significantly increased values of IGF-1 in obese children, but IGFBP-3 levels did not differ from the control group. IGF-1 and IGFBP-3 levels were significantly higher in obese pubertal children than in the prepubertal ones. A positive linear correlation was found between BMI and IGF-1 levels (r = 0.51, p < 0.05). Therefore, Bideci et al.[584] suggested that obesity had a considerable effect on IGF-1 levels during growth.

Increased linear growth with a normal or high insulin-like growth factor (IGF-1) level is apparent in spite of low growth hormone (GH) secretion during the prepubertal period. In a study of children with simple obesity and normal children with shorter stature, it was revealed that peak levels of GH in the growth hormone releasing factor (GHRF) test were significantly lower in children with simple obesity. There was also a significant positive correlation with sigma IGFBP-1. With pubertal stage matching, serum GHBP and IGF-1 levels were significantly higher in children with obesity than in the other group of normal-weight children. The results of this study lead to the hypothesis that increased dietary intake and hypernutrition during growth cause hyperinsulinemia that increases GH receptor and IGF-1 secretion despite low GH secretion. Hyperinsulinemia may also increase free IGF-1 by lowering IGFBP-1.

These two mechanisms are supposed to be nutrition-related hormonal changes and can explain the temporary accelerated growth of obese children. The increased IGF-1 may contribute to the decreased GH secretion due to negative feedback in simple obesity during childhood.[585]

Free forms of IGF-1 in circulation are normal in children with simple obesity.[586] Increased values of IGFBP-3 along with increased insulin were found in obese children in which IGF-1, free IGF-1, free IGF-1/IGF-1, and IGFBP-1 levels were not significantly different from non-obese children. A negative correlation of IGFBP-1 and insulin level in obese children was also found. This study indicated that normal growth in obese children might be maintained due to normal IGF-1, increased IGFBP-3 levels which are stimulated by increased insulin levels or nutritional factors, or by an increased responsiveness to GH.[587]

Obese girls aged 15.0 ± 1.0 years, with a mean BMI of 31.1 ± 3.8 kg.m$^{-2}$ were examined with regard to the above-mentioned parameters. The following associations, using Spearman's correlation coefficients adjusted for age were revealed. IGF-1 correlated with body height, fasting insulin, and BP3 levels. In contrast with recent data on adults, no relationship was found with BMI, WHR, and blood lipids. IGF-2 correlated with insulin and BP3 levels. BP1 and BP2 negatively correlated with BMI and insulin, and positively with SHBG levels. The ratio BP1:BP2 was related to TC and LDL-C. Furthermore, BP2 showed a negative correlation with WHR, TG, and uric acid levels. Studies provided new insight into the physiological role of IGF; their BP, BP1, and BP2 seem to be insulin-regulated. They are associated with several metabolic parameters, possibly due to their modulation of IGF-1 metabolic actions. High BP1 and low BP2 levels appear to reflect a higher atherogenic risk, which is increased in obese subjects.[836]

Fasting serum levels of insulin-like growth factor 1 (IGF-1), IGF binding protein-3, and type 1 pro-collagen C-terminal peptide (PICP) were assessed in groups of obese children and adolescents at different stages of puberty. The effect of insulin, GH, and weight loss was also studied.[589] The growth velocity (GV) was greater in obese boys and girls than in controls during the prepubertal phase. Puberty development had a significant effect; that is, it was lower in obese girls at pubertal stage II and in obese boys at stage III. PICP increased during puberty with a more rapid decrease occurring later in obese girls and in control subjects with normal weight. Prepubertal values were higher in the obese but were later reduced at pubertal stages IV to V when compared to control subjects. GV was the only anthropometric variable that correlated with PICP. IGF-1 serum values increased significantly in puberty and were higher in the obese than in controls at stage I for both genders. IGFBP-3 values were higher in the obese than in controls at stages I to III in boys, and I and II in girls; however, no gender differences were observed. No differences were evident in the IGF-1:IGFBP-3 molar ratio between the two groups. A positive correlation between IGF-1 and IGFBP-3 was observed in prepubertal but not in pubertal subjects with normal weight.[589]

Fasting insulin values correlated with IGFBP-3 in the obese, accounting for 24.8% of the variation in prepubertal subjects and 17.1% in pubertal subjects. No relationship was revealed in normal-weight subjects. In prepubertal control subjects with normal weight, PICP and standard deviation score (SDS) of BMI correlated with IGF-1, and the SDS of BMI correlated with IGFBP-3.[589]

In obese pubertal subjects, no significant correlations were revealed, but PICP and SDS of BMI accounted for 14.3% of the variation in the IGF-1:IGFBP-3 molar ratio. These results demonstrate that IGF-1 and IGFBP-3 are influenced by age, gender, sexual development, and nutritional status. An influence of insulin on IGFBP-3 serum levels was observed in the obese. The relationship of IGF-1 to PICP in normal-weight subjects and the IGF-1:IGFBP-3 molar ratio to PICP in the obese support the concept that IGF-1 influences skeletal growth. The increased IGFBP-3 serum values in the obese suggest a possible role in controlling the growth stimulus induced by nutritional status.[589]

Insulin-like growth factor binding protein-1 level (IGFBP-1) was found to be strongly associated with insulin sensitivity and fatness in early prepubertal children aged 9.8 to 14.6 years. Insulin sensitivity, IGF-1, and obesity are important predictors of IGFBP-1 levels in pubertal children. IGFBP-1, which is suppressed by insulin, may increase free IGF-1 levels and thus contribute to somatic growth in obese children. Similar mechanisms may appear in pubertal children where growth acceleration and insulin resistance occur simultaneously.[590]

In contrast, a study by Saitoh et al.[591] showed that the fasting IGFBP-1 level was suppressed in prepubertal obese children ($22.1 \pm 18.4$ µg.l$^{-1}$, $p < 0.001$) compared to control children ($76.0 \pm 62.9$ µg.l$^{-1}$). However, obese children had normal insulin levels. IGFBP-1 level may be a useful predictor for the early identification of the development of insulin resistance in prepubertal obese children.[591] The results of Attia et al.[592] suggest that the compensatory hyperinsulinemia that characterizes adolescent obesity chronically suppresses levels of IGFBP-1. Low IGFBP-1 concentrations may serve to increase the bio-availability of free IGF-1 which may then contribute to low circulating GH, total IGF-1, and IGFBP-3.

Significant positive relationships were found between BMI and somatomedine-C/insulin-like growth factor-1 (SM-C/IGF-1), between immunoreactive insulin (IRI) and SM-C/IGF-1, and between BMI and IRI. These data seem to indicate that SM-C/IGF-1 in obese children is regulated by IRI dependent on BMI; this regulating effect of insulin may be important in obesity since human growth hormone (HGH) production of stimulating factors is reduced.

## 9.2   Growth Hormone

Obesity is associated with a decrease in growth hormone (GH) synthesis and excretion and an increased GH clearance, along with high insulin and insulin-like growth factor 1 (IGF-1) levels which may interfere in the complex interactions of various hormones.[593]

Previous studies have shown an exponential decline in the calculated daily secretion rate of GH as a function of age in healthy men. There is also a significant negative correlation between the daily GH secretion rate and indices of obesity, for example, BMI. For each increase in BMI of 1.5 $kg.m^{-2}$, there is a 50% decrease in the amount of GH secreted per day. At puberty and across the span of adulthood, gonadal steroid hormone concentrations in blood positively determine GH release.

Urinary growth hormone (U GH) excretion in obese children was significantly lower than in normal-weight children before and after puberty in spite of comparable normal height. GH levels significantly increased at puberty in obese children although the pubertal increase was significantly lower (1.7 in both sexes) than in normal children (2.5-fold increase in boys and 2.3 in girls). A multiple regression analysis showed that age, gender, and pubertal stage contributed to the variation in U GH levels.[594] A study by Bona et al.[595] provided the reference values for U GH excretion in children. A blunted GH response to provocative stimuli and reduced nocturnal GH concentrations were found in obese as compared to age-matched normal-weight children, both before and after puberty.

As shown in a study on prepubertal children with exogenous obesity, the GH-IGF axis was significantly altered even when most changes in the peripheral IGF system appeared to be independent of the modifications in GH secretion.[596] Serum concentration of the high-affinity growth hormone binding protein (GHBP) was increased in obese children and adolescents. GHBP correlated significantly with percent body fat, waist and hip circumferences, body weight, WHR, and with serum leptin concentration, uric acid, insulin, cholesterol (TC), LDL-C, LDL-C:TC ratio, triglycerides, and height standard deviation scores. Age, gender, and stage of puberty had no effect on GHBP. Multiple regression analysis using age, gender, anthropometric variables, fat percentage, and waist circumference as independent variables revealed significant associations between GHBP and leptin, triglycerides, TC, and LDL-C, LDL-C:HDL-C ratio.[597]

Waist circumference, an indicator of abdominal body fat mass, is a major determinant of GHBP levels during childhood, while leptin may be one candidate for a signal linking adipocytes to the growth hormone receptor-related GHBP release. Increased serum GHBP levels may further reflect metabolic abnormalities in obese children and adolescents. Circulating leptin levels decreased during a treatment program that resulted in a reduced weight.[597]

A comparison between groups of short-to-normal weight and obese children showed a similar response of GH to GH-releasing factor. The neuroregulation of GH release appears to be similar in normal-weight and obese peri-pubertal children.[598]

GH-secretory bursts and mean serum GH concentrations are proportional to serum estradiol and testosterone. Body composition and especially visceral adiposity appear to be dominant negative determinants of GH production, since the relationships between GH secretion and age, testosterone, or sleep are all attenuated or abolished by adiposity.[599]

## 9.3 Insulin

Insulin resistance and hyperinsulinemia coexist in preadolescent boys and girls with moderate and severe obesity.[600] A study of obese adolescents by Rocchini et al.[601] consistently showed a significantly elevated fasting insulin concentration and abnormal insulin response to an oral glucose tolerance test, along with significantly higher systolic and diastolic blood pressure and elevated 24-hr urinary sodium excretion. Significant correlations were also found among fasting insulin, body weight, and blood pressure.

Insulin-stimulated glucose uptake measured at two physiological levels of hyperinsulinemia was reduced in obese subjects compared to non-obese subjects. Defects in oxidative and non-oxidative glucose metabolism were revealed in all obese preadolescents at the higher infusion rate using an euglycemic hyperinsulinemic clamp. The ability of insulin to inhibit lipid oxidation was impaired in obese subjects at two levels of hyperinsulinemia (180 and 480 mmol). Increases in basal and glucose-stimulated insulin levels during the hyperglycemic clamp reflected the reductions in glucose uptake during the insulin clamp in obese preadolescents.

Fasting, circulating insulin was assessed in white and black adolescents aged 11 to 18 years, along with C-peptide as a noninvasive measure of insulin secretion by beta cells.[602] C-peptide:insulin ratio served as an indicator of hepatic insulin extraction, and insulin-to-glucose ratio as a measure of insulin sensitivity. BMI was positively related to insulin and C-peptide, and inversely with a C-peptide-to-insulin ratio in both ethnic groups of adolescents in this study. Both increased insulin secretion and decreased insulin clearance contributed to hyperinsulinemia in obese adolescents.

In prepubertal obese children, both immuno-reactive and bio-active GH concentrations were low. Therefore, nutritional factors and insulin may contribute to sustaining normal growth by modulating several components of the IGF-IGFBP system.[603] Another study hypothesized that over-nutrition causes hyperinsulinemia, which increases growth hormone (GH) receptors and IGF-1 secretion despite low GH secretion. Hyperinsulinemia may also increase free IGF-1 by lowering IGFBP-1. These two mechanisms are supposed to be the hormonal changes related to nutrition in children with simple obesity and can also explain the growth of children with simple obesity. The increased IGF-1 may contribute, due to negative feedback, to reduced GH secretion in obese children.[604]

The development of hyperinsulinemia and insulin resistance was examined in children with obesity lasting various periods of time and with continuous weight gain, compared to normal-weight children. Early in the evolution of obesity, insulin and C-peptide responses to a normal meal were increased by 76 and 80%. The first insulin peak was higher and occurred later in the obese subjects than in normal-weight children. The obese children had more insulin peaks within the 6-hr period after the lunch than normal-weight children. In contrast, fasting plasma insulin and C-peptide levels remained normal during the initial years of obesity then increased progressively and significantly with the duration and degree of obesity.[605]

Insulin sensitivity, evaluated as the rate of glucose uptake during a three-step hyperinsulinemic euglycemic clamp, was comparable in obese and normal children. Initially higher than normal in obese children, the maximal rate of glucose uptake decreased with both obesity duration and age of children, indicating the progressive development of insulin resistance.[605]

Insulin sensitivity was markedly lower in obese prepubertal children compared to a lean group of peers, whereas glucose effectiveness was higher in a study by Hoffman and Armstrong.[606] Hepatic insulin resistance was also higher in the obese with an increased insulin secretion over the first 19 min following glucose, although plasma glucose levels were higher (Figure 9.1). Results show that obese prepubertal children have peripheral and hepatic insulin resistance. The increases in glucose effectiveness and insulin secretion may be compensatory responses to these defects in insulin secretion.

Gonzales et al.[607] studied circadian rhythms of insulin and cortisol in obese and non-obese children. Hyperinsulinemia was confirmed in the group of obese children; the plasma cortisol levels were higher in male obese and control children. No correlation was found between body fat and cortisol and/or

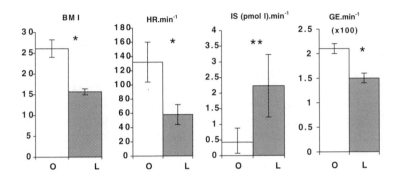

**FIGURE 9.1**
Comparison of BMI, hepatic insulin resistance (HIR), insulin sensitivity (IS), and glucose effectiveness (GE) in obese (O) and lean (L) pre-pubertal children. * indicates ($p < 0.05$) **($p < 0.01$). (Based on data from Ref. F29.)

insulin levels. Both normal-weight and obese children showed circadian rhythms. The rhythm for cortisol was similar in both normal and obese children; however, the insulin rhythm was disturbed. The acrophase was delayed 2 hr when values for both genders were evaluated together, but only by 1 hr when obese girls were evaluated separately. The acrophase of cortisol and insulin rhythms in both obese and control groups is delayed in relation to the degree of obesity. The circadian rhythm of cortisol and insulin in both obese and control groups are not dependent. The alterations cited were not related to the duration of obesity in children. Radetti et al.[608] found that insulin secretion in obese children is pulsatile as in adults, and its secretion pattern is related to body weight.

Increased values of insulin appear in the saliva of obese compared to normal-weight children. Insulin was investigated along with glucose, total protein, and amylase activity in the saliva of normal and obese children following a meal. Considerable variability in the values of these parameters was found in different subjects and all values were higher in obese children than in normal-weight children. The concentration of insulin and the other parameters were, on average, higher than the maximum insulin level in normal children, and in some of the obese children, they were more than four times higher. The progressive hypersecretion of insulin may thus promote an increased predisposition to type II diabetes mellitus at a later age.[609]

Impaired glucose tolerance, hyperinsulinemia, and insulin resistance are the most important metabolic complications of obesity. These characteristics can eventually result in non-insulin-dependent diabetes (NIDDM).[610] Even if values are within the normal range, relatively increased glycemia and high insulinemia may be considered in untreated obese children as a metabolic adjustment to insulin resistance and to intracellular glycopenia.

## 9.4    Steroid Hormones and Sexual Maturation

Altered steroid metabolism has been found in obese children when compared to normal-weight peers.[611,612] There was a trend for higher secretion of steroids in obese children than in non-obese children but the differences were greatly reduced when the excretion rate was related to total body weight. Correlations were sought between body weight and the excretion of certain steroid groups, such as C2105 corticoid metabolites and compounds representing the androgen line, androsterone, ethiocholanolon, and dehydroepiandrosteron. In normal-weight children, the correlations between these parameters were significant.

No significant correlation was found in obese children regardless of whether steroid excretion was related to body weight, body surface, or BMI. A relationship between body weight and ideal weight, and the excretion of cortisol metabolites was revealed in both genders. In contrast, with regard to androgen excretion it was shown only for boys already in puberty. For all nine groups of steroid compounds evaluated in this study, there was a stronger correlation between the excretion rate and the anthropometric parameters in the prepubertal groups than in children with the markers of pubertal development. The differences in steroid secretion point to certain alterations of adrenal function in obese children[611] but do not support the expectation of any significant disturbances in their steroid metabolism. The study of Chalew et al.[613] showed that the integrated concentration of cortisol was reduced in obese children.

The study by Juricskay and Molnár indicated that the excretion of cortisol metabolites increased along with the increased excretion of androgen metabolites and pregnenediol, a metabolite of pregnanolon. There was a trend for increased excretion of all steroid groups, which in certain cases was significant. Wide variability was also observed in the steroid excretion in obese children. In about one third of the obese children studied there was hypersecretion of some components of the steroid spectrum. This phenomenon was more frequent in boys.[611,612]

Hyperphagia and obesity are the characteristics of hypercortisolism. A single-dose dexamethasone suppression test was performed on obese children to rule out hypercortisolism. It was shown that a single dose of dexamethasone significantly increased the high leptin levels in obese children. Therefore, it was hypothesized that glucocorticosteroids up-regulate leptin levels in humans.[614]

Klein et al.[615] showed that in the prepubertal or early pubertal stages of growth and development obese children had similar estradiol levels and equivalent bone ages at a younger chronological age than non-obese children. Leptin levels did not correlate with estradiol level or bone age.[615]

Menarche is related *inter alia* and to a certain level of fat deposition during puberty in girls. The changes in circulating concentrations of leptin could be a hormonal signal that influences gonadotrophin secretion. A study of adolescents and young adults aged 13 to 19 years with significant variability in the level of fatness showed that in perimenarcheal and young adult girls, LH and FSH responses to GnRH were negatively correlated with BMI and circulating leptin. Decreased LH and FSH responses to GnRH were associated with increased adiposity and hyperleptinemia. These data are consistent with a direct neuro-endocrine negative effect of excess leptin on the central reproductive system in obese girls. In boys of comparable adiposity, no influence of BMI or leptin on gonadotrophin concentrations was revealed. This is another aspect of the sexual dimorphism characterizing human leptin physiology.[616]

Precocious puberty in obese children may be related to excess weight. Bone age may often be advanced along with accelerated growth. A group of obese children was studied when undergoing an ACTH stimulation test during which they received an intravenous bolus of 250 micrograms of Cortrosyn. Blood samples were taken at 0 and 6 min for 17-OHprogesterone, 217-OHpregnenolone, dehydroepiandrosterone, androstenedione, and cortisol levels. In two of the overweight children there was a suspicion of congenital adrenal hyperplasia, but these subjects did not differ from the other obese subjects with regard to linear growth rate and degree of skeletal maturation. Normal weight children displayed all measured values within reference ranges.[617]

Menarche is a key biological marker of maturity in girls. In a study by Stanimirova et al.[118] menarche occurred in Bulgarian obese girls at the age of 12.1 ± 1.30 years of age, with height of 154.5 ± 5.35 cm, body weight 57.20 ± 5.00 kg, and total body fat 32.27 ± 2.12%. Menarche occurred approximately 7 months earlier than in non-obese girls. These results provide further confirmation of the link between obesity development and physiologically mediated parameters of growth.

## 9.5 Beta-Endorphin and Somatostatin

The relationships between plasma beta-endorphin, insulin concentration, body fat, nutritional parameters, diet history for energy and macronutrient intake of overweight or obese prepubertal children aged 5.8 to 9.6 years have been investigated. Obese children were characterized by significantly higher average concentrations of beta-endorphins along with increased insulin as compared to normal-weight children. An analysis of concentrations in relation to the percentage of body fat revealed that beta-endorphin concentrations increased more with increasing fatness than insulin concentrations. A significant positive correlation between beta-endorphin and insulin levels was only noted in the obese subjects. In addition, there was a significant positive correlation between beta-endorphin levels and energy and macronutrient intake in this group. In both groups the percentage of energy from fat correlated positively with beta-endorphin concentrations.

Energy and fat intake showed a significant positive correlation with insulin levels in both groups. These results indicate that the level of beta-endorphins may be useful as an indicator of appetite in overweight and obese prepubertal children whose food intake has not yet been restricted.[618]

There is relatively little information on somatostatin concentrations in obese children and their responses to a meal. Following mixed meal ingestion, the reaction of somatostatin was the same as in the normal-weight control children. Although integrated insulin response over 180 min was higher in this group, the integrated somatostatin response did not differ from controls. After an oral glucose load, no change in circulating somatostatin concentrations was found.[619]

## 9.6   Leptin

The role of leptin in childhood obesity and specifically during puberty and adolescence has received considerable attention in the recent past.[620,621] Leptin, a recently defined hormone, is the product of the adipose tissue-specific ob gene and is involved in the regulation of metabolic processes and the deposition of fat.[622,623] Leptin provides information to the central nervous system on the energy stored in the body deposits of fat and appears to function as a link among adiposity, satiety, and physical activity.

The identification of the ob gene and its adipocyte-specific protein leptin has provided the first physiological links to the regulatory system controlling body weight. In experimental animals, specifically the (ob/ob) mouse, extreme obesity is attributed to mutation in the gene encoding leptin that has profound effects on appetite and energy expenditure. Until recently there was limited equivalent evidence on the role of leptin in the control of stored fat in humans.

Present knowledge reveals that the leptin system is highly complex. It is well known that leptin is involved in a range of physiological processes in a manner far transcending the initial lipostatic content. Leptin is produced in white adipose tissue and also brown fat, the placenta, and fetal tissues (heart, bone, and cartilage). Leptin is still widely described as a satiety factor but also has a stimulatory effect on energy expenditure, and therefore interacts with both components of energy balance.[624,625]

Physiological factors which influence leptin include fasting, exercise, and exposure to the cold, each of which causes a fall in ob-gene expression and a corresponding reduction in the circulating level of leptin. However, the nature of the leptin complex may reduce its potential as a target in the treatment of obesity. The administration of human recombinant leptin seems to provide only limited effects.[625]

Leptin is known to decrease food intake and increase energy expenditure in ob/ob mice. Variants of the ob gene were not found in humans and relatively little is known about the action of leptin on food intake and energy expenditure in humans, although circulating leptin concentrations are positively correlated to body fat stores.[625] Leptin exerts its central effects through several neuro-endocrine systems, including neuro-peptide Y, glucagon-like peptide-1, melanocortin, corticotrophin releasing hormone (CRH), and cocaine- and amphetamine-regulated transcript (CART).

Obese subjects have significantly higher serum leptin concentrations than normal or lean individuals (Figure 9.2).[515] Body fat mass correlates significantly with serum leptin concentrations in newborns, children, and adults. Females who are characterized by an increased percentage of stored fat also have higher serum levels of leptin. Circulating leptin concentrations change under conditions of extreme variations in energy intake such as fasting or overfeeding.

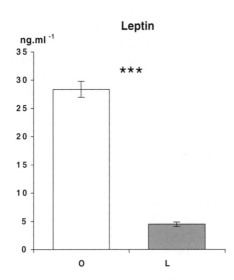

**FIGURE 9.2**
Leptin levels in obese (O) and normal-weight (L) children (ng.ml$^{-1}$). *** indicates (p < 0.001). (Based on data from Ref. F30.)

Measurements in white and black children and adolescents (aged 9 to 20.5 years) showed significant sex-by-race interaction on serum leptin levels, adjusted for subscapular skinfold thickness and age. Girls had serum leptin levels that were on average 2.15 times those of boys. There was an age-by-sex interaction, with serum leptin concentrations decreasing with age in boys but not in girls. A strong inverse relationship between serum testosterone levels and serum leptin levels in boys appeared to explain the effect of age.[626]

Newborns with intrauterine growth retardation have significantly lower serum leptin levels than those with normal growth, and leptin levels were only positively correlated with BMI in a study by Jaquet et al.[627] These data indicate that the development of adipose tissue and the accumulation of stored fat are the major determinants of fetal and neonatal serum leptin levels. Sexual dimorphism was evident *in utero*. In female fetuses, higher levels of leptin were found during the last weeks of gestation, and this was consistent regardless of growth status at birth. At this time, subcutaneous fat is already deposited in significant amounts and can vary according to the term, gender, or metabolic status of the mother.[18,53,55]

In the study by Hassink et al.,[628] leptin was also present in all newborns (mean concentration 8.8 ng.mL$^{-1}$, SD = 9.6). In this study, serum concentration also correlated significantly with newborn weight and arm fat. Comparisons with older children indicated that leptin levels in newborns cannot be explained by adiposity alone; for example, there was no correlation between leptin and insulin. Leptin was also present in all mothers (mean value 28.8 ng.mL$^{-1}$, SD = 22.2 ng.mL$^{-1}$). Leptin concentration correlated with pre-pregnancy BMI, BMI at the time of delivery, and arm fat. In addition, maternal leptin correlated with serum insulin but there was no correlation between maternal and newborn leptin concentrations.

A number of newborns (13%) had higher levels of leptin than their mothers. These results seem to indicate that leptin plays an important role in intrauterine and neonatal development and that the placenta provides a source of leptin for a growing fetus.[628]

In other studies, birth weight correlated with cord leptin levels. Gender differences in plasma leptin concentration was present at birth in umbilical cord blood, then at the age of 4 weeks. Plasma leptin levels at 4 and 14 weeks were lower than leptin concentrations observed in umbilical cord plasma, and an increase of its values was observed during this period of growth.[629] Maffeis et al.[630] confirmed that female newborns have significantly higher serum leptin levels in cord blood than males. IgF-1 was significantly lower in newborn males compared to females while insulin and cortisol did not differ. Also in this study, birth weight correlated with leptin concentration in newborns (r = 0.56, p < 0.001). When gender was taken into account in the statistical analysis, the concentration of circulating hormones (insulin, cortisol, IGF-1, S-HBG) did not independently affect leptin inter-individual variability.[630]

As mentioned before, leptin correlates with the indicators of body mass and neonatal cord leptin concentrations correlate significantly with birth weight and BMI, but gender differences were absent with regard to cord blood leptin. Maternal obesity had no effect on cord leptin, whereas exogenous maternal steroids increased neonatal leptin concentrations.[631] These findings indicate the importance of fetal and neonatal periods for the development of leptin levels along with BMI.

Significantly higher serum leptin concentrations were found in obese Finnish children when compared to normal-weight children during the first 5 years of life, but serum concentrations of leptin did not show any significant relationship to dietary parameters or serum lipids in normal-weight children of the same age. The results also suggested that serum leptin concentration expresses a greater amount of body fat and it may also play a role as a predictive factor for childhood adiposity.[632]

The results of an ongoing prospective study on characteristics of leptin after long-term storage describe its relationship to body weight from birth to old age in a population-based sample of Swedish women. The group was first examined at the ages of 38 to 60 years and re-examined 24 years later. Low values of self-reported birth weight were related to higher leptin levels in adulthood ($p < 0.01$), after controlling for age and adult weight. This might be related to the findings of Barker[186] and others who have indicated low birth weight as a risk for the later development of diseases including obesity.

Prospective analyses showed that high leptin levels in 38- to 46-year-olds predicted subsequent long-term weight gain ($p = 0.003$), although the opposite (but non-significant trend) was seen in women initially aged 50 and older. This study indicated that leptin values from frozen serum could serve to predict the risk of increased weight gain later in life in women 38 to 46 years old. Retrospective analysis on birth weight values also suggested that leptin resistance in adulthood might have a fetal origin.[633]

A longitudinal study of plasma leptin levels in Australian children who were assessed at the age of 12 and 18 months, and for a proportion of the group at the age of $10.1 \pm 1.6$ years has been done. The results showed that the baseline leptin continued to predict greater values of BMI percentile change over time and remained a potentially useful indicator of an increasing weight gain.[634]

Leptin levels were significantly higher in children in prepuberty and at early stages of puberty and did not correlate with estradiol levels or bone age.[615] The relationship between serum leptin levels and energy expenditure was also studied in Pima Indian children aged 5 years. Body composition was assessed by isotopic water dilution, total energy expenditure (TEE), and resting metabolic rate (RMR) using doubly labelled water (DLW) and indirect calorimetry. Total physical activity was evaluated as the ratio of TEE/RMR. Serum leptin levels correlated significantly with TEE, both in absolute values and when adjusted for body size, and with physical activity level. Significant and positive correlations were found for serum leptin level and the percentage of stored fat, and these correlations were similar after adjusting for the percentage of body fat in both boys and girls.[635]

As shown in experimental models with laboratory rodents, defects in leptin or its receptor in the hypothalamus result in obesity development. Leptin administration can cause weight loss in both ob/ob mice and in normal-weight control animals. However, this has not yet been replicated in humans. These observations suggest that humans may be resistant to endogenous leptin levels.[636]

The measurements of serum leptin concentrations in obese children aged $14.5 \pm 1.2$ years showed mean values of $21.1 \pm 12.1$ ng.ml$^{-1}$. At a given BMI level, a one- to fourfold range of leptin plasma levels was noticed. Seventy-five percent of these values were out of the range of mean $\pm 2$ SEM. Age, gender, and/or gender maturity stage do not appear to explain these marked differences. BMI correlated significantly with leptin levels ($r = 0.79$; $p < 0.001$). These data suggest that the biological background as reflected by low or increased leptin concentrations in severely obese children is heterogeneous and cannot be explained by single factor analysis.[637]

Serum leptin levels increase during growth and development; this increase continues in girls during sexual maturation but decreases in boys. Suppression of testosterone increased leptin levels in boys and the resumption of puberty was associated with decreased leptin levels. In girls, serum leptin levels did not change with the alteration of the pituitary-ovarian axis and were permanently higher than in boys. Serum leptin levels were also significantly higher during the night.[638] There is a hypothesis that leptin could contribute to the regulation of GH secretion.[639] Forward stepwise regression analysis selected the change in total body fat in young females over a 6-month period as the most powerful determinant of the percent increase in the nocturnal leptin concentration.[640]

Measurements in girls showed higher serum levels of leptin (Figure 9.3).[515] This applies even after correction for the differences in body fat mass. In a multiple regression analysis with age and body mass index (percent body fat) as fixed variables, testosterone had a potent negative effect on serum leptin levels in boys, but not in girls. Argente et al.[596,641] also found a marked variation of serum leptin levels in boys and girls which significantly depended on the maturational stage. Along with progressing puberty, leptin increased permanently in girls and decreased in boys. In obese children, leptin levels were markedly increased and a significant correlation of leptin and BMI was again found.

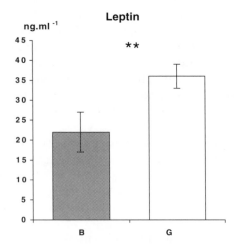

**FIGURE 9.3**
Leptin levels in obese boys (B) and girls (G). ** indicates ($p < 0.01$). (Based on data from Ref. F30.)

*In vitro* experiments using newly developed human adipocytes in primary culture showed that both testosterone and its biologically active metabolite dihydrotestosterone are able to reduce leptin secretion into the culture medium up to 62%. Using the semi-quantitative reverse transcriptase-PCR method, testosterone was found to suppress leptin mRNA to a similar extent. These results indicate that apart from the differences in body fat mass, the higher androgen concentrations in obese boys are responsible for the low leptin serum concentration when compared with obese girls.[642] A critical leptin level is obviously needed to maintain menstruation.[643]

Another study by Ellis and Nicolson confirmed a significant positive relationship for serum leptin and BMI.[644] The percentage of fat and fat mass was gender dependent and not influenced by ethnicity. At each degree of sexual maturation females had higher levels of leptin than males and this difference remained significant when leptin was normalized for fat mass. In boys and girls, the mean leptin:fat mass ratios were relatively invariant during sexual maturation and no differences were observed between the oldest children with the highest degree of sexual maturation and in young adults. The finding of a higher average serum leptin and leptin:fat mass ratio in girls at pre-pubertal ages may suggest that there are gender differences in leptin synthesis, clearance rates, bio-activity, and/or leptin transport.

Along with the elevated serum leptin levels and increased fat mass, the follow-up of obese and lean children revealed an increased intake of energy (two to three times) compared to normal, lean children.[515] Obese children had higher leptin levels even when they were normalized with fat mass. Gender differences, that is, higher serum levels of leptin in girls and a significant correlation between leptin and fat, were also seen in this study. It appears that serum leptin reflects but does not halt fat deposition in obese children. When serum levels of leptin were normalized to body adiposity, leptin in females was found to be increased independently by obese status, sexual maturation, and being female.

Leptin was also positively associated with percent fat intake and negatively associated with percent carbohydrate intake. These results show that a high-fat, low-carbohydrate diet was related with leptin levels, and circulating leptin was positively associated with several cardiovascular risk factors.[526] Correlations between serum leptin levels, BMI, and percentage of fat were also found in diabetic children, but insulin dependent diabetes was not associated with higher leptin concentrations.[645]

Other studies have confirmed significant relationships between leptin and age, gender, level of pubertal development, BMI, and insulin.[628] Serum leptin levels were four to five times higher in obese children and adolescents compared to normal-weight children of the same age.[588,589] Using partial correlation analysis in subjects subdivided according to gender and pubertal stages, log values of serum leptin and fasting insulin values, adjusted by age and standard deviation scores for BMI, correlated significantly with a weaker correlation in boys than in girls. In obese children, leptin concentrations correlated better with total insulin area (TIA) under the curve during a glucose tolerance test (evaluated before the therapeutic program started) than with fasting insulin level.

Caprio et al.[600,646] found a significant correlation between serum leptin levels and subcutaneous fat deposits in children and adults. Surprisingly, a weaker correlation was found with visceral fat mass. In this study, leptin levels remained unchanged under both euglycemic and hyperglycemic hyperinsulinemic conditions in both obese and non-obese subjects. As apparent early in the development of juvenile obesity, leptin levels are increased and more closely related to subcutaneous fat mass. Acute elevations of insulin concentrations do not affect circulating leptin levels.

Two very severely obese children who are members of the same pedigree had very low leptin levels in spite of markedly increased stored fat. In both, a homozygous frame-shift mutation involving the deletion of a single guanidine nucleotide in codon 133 of the gene for leptin was found. The severe obesity in these congenitally deficient children provides the first genetic evidence that leptin is an important regulator of energy balance in humans.[647] Another study of extremely obese German children, however, did not show leptin deficiency mutation.[648]

The hypothesis that juvenile obesity in humans may be caused by leptin resistance mediated through genetic variations in isoforms of the hypothalamic leptin receptor was tested. Obese Danish men with a history of juvenile onset obesity were followed. The results of this study showed that it is unlikely that mutations in the coding region of the long isoform of the leptin receptor are a common cause of juvenile-onset obesity.[649]

Research in the area of hormonal activities in obesity during the growing years has been extensive, with important information gained in recent years. However, definite conclusions on the pathogenesis, treatment, and prevention of childhood obesity have not been defined yet.

# 10

## Psychosocial Aspects of Obesity

### 10.1 Psychosocial Determinants of Obesity

There is a range of psychosocial ramifications of being overweight or obese but little consensus regarding the etiology of these problems. We do not know, for example, whether these problems are innate characteristics of the obese, or caused by others through social pressures to be thin, or the use of restricted dietary practices.[650]

Dietz has claimed that the most prevalent consequence of childhood obesity is psychosocial.[651] While there are widespread examples of discrimination against people of all ages who are fat, the most potentially damaging consequence may be the psychological well-being of obese children. Obese children are consistently rated by their peers as lazy, dirty, ugly, cheats, and liars.

Studies that have considered preferences for various forms of disability, including obesity, have consistently shown that children and adults rated obesity lowest. Generally, children with other disabilities were considered unfortunate victims of the environment whereas the obese were considered "responsible" for their plight. Many obese adults disliked drawings of obese children because the images reminded them of their own situation.

The social stigma associated with the obese individual's ungainly appearance is one of the least recognized and understood problems with which such individuals must cope.[49] In countries where the favored body size and shape for a male is a tall, lean, and an athletic build, the obese individual is often ridiculed and made to feel like a social outcast. This is particularly true for children and adolescents.

In addition to the social stigma, obese individuals commonly report a fear of participating in social activities, sports, and recreational activities. Many obese individuals dread being on view in public places and wearing a swimsuit or sport clothes. The obese child is potentially more sensitive and therefore vulnerable to the comments of his or her peers. Such individuals may avoid physical activity and many social contacts wherever possible. The need for a degree of self-esteem and self-worth is critical to being a well-balanced individual. If these traits are damaged or missing, obese individuals may consider themselves ugly and unattractive to the people around them, which leads to unhappiness and depression. This scenario perpetuates a vicious circle whereby misery and discontent with physical appearance can precipitate the use of food as solace and a corresponding increase in weight and further discontent.[54,409,652,653,656]

Other examples of social discrimination include the findings of a large study by Gortmaker et al.[654] This group obtained follow-up data on a nationally representative sample of men and women who were 16 to 24 years old at baseline. Seven years later, women whose BMI was greater than the 95th percentile showed the following characteristics: They had completed fewer years at school, had higher rates of poverty, and were less likely to be married than those who had been normal weight 7 years earlier. The work of Lissau and Sorensen found that the strongest predictors of the development of later obesity were indices of parental neglect, and not level of education or parents' occupations.[655]

In the 1970s Bruch contended that social attitudes toward the body, a preoccupation with physical appearance, and an overwhelming emphasis on beauty in our society were contributing factors to mild forms of body image distortion in non-obese individuals during growth.[657] These factors are intimately related to widespread condemnation of overweight and obesity as undesirable and ugly. This illustrates the psychological and social context in which young people with a weight problem find themselves.

Stunkard has also indicated that obesity can be triggered by psychological problems. This is of particular concern for children and adolescents.[656] The tendency to overeat and satisfaction in eating highly processed foods containing a high proportion of fat and/or sugar can originate from stress at school or in the family. For example, separation or divorce of parents, stress of exams, or a disruptive time with peers may all be prompts to overeat. In addition, Bruch identified the difficulties faced by obese children who have over-protective parents.[657] Such parents were more likely to use food as a comfort rather than in response to hunger. Wadden et al.[658] found no association between measures of anxiety or depression and weight category in high school girls (mean age of 15.8 years). But, consistent with other studies,[49,350] overweight girls in this sample were significantly more dissatisfied with their sizes and shapes and more of them were attempting to lose weight.

The psychological ramifications of such circumstances are too often not considered in the prevention, treatment, and management of obesity. A psychological evaluation of the situation and an appropriate psychosocial approach as an adjunct to the treatment of an obese child are important starts and perhaps keys to a successful and lasting result.

Recent research also indicates that the adult preoccupation with weight, restrictive dietary practices, and other harmful methods of weight regulation is also common in the childhood and adolescent years.[653,659–662] In order to prevent distorted attitudes about food, weight, and exercise there is a need to determine what motivates these attitudes, when they first begin to emerge, how they evolve over time, and which individuals are most vulnerable.[663]

Extensive research has assessed body image and weight-control practices of different populations but like many other areas of study there has been considerable variability in the assessment protocols employed. Therefore, the interpretation of results in many instances reflects the assessment methodology utilized as much as the data collected, or the varying statistical procedures utilized to interpret the data. As a result, to adequately assess psychological characteristics such as body image and weight-control practices, the efficacy of the assessment protocols used must be considered.

Research devoted to analyses of weight- and eating-related issues has largely concentrated on female populations[664–667] and to a lesser degree on gender differences in early adulthood.[668] Considerably less work has involved adolescents and younger children and few studies have focused on differences between individuals categorized on the basis of body composition or satisfaction with physical appearance.[653]

## 10.2 Definition of Body Image

Body image is the picture one has of his/her own body.[669] It is a self-concept construct that has been conceptualized in various ways. As a result, a range of related terms with differing connotations has evolved. These include body percept, body concept, body-ego, body ideal,[670] body schema,[671] body boundary,[672] body awareness, body identity, body structure, body self, and social body concept.[657] While the term body image is recognized as a generic label, its interpretation has been dependent upon the individual researcher's definition.[673]

Body image is acknowledged as a complex, dynamic, and multidimensional aspect of the personality.[674] Consequently, there has been considerable criticism of Schilder's simple definition, contending that it is too imprecise.[669] However, no suitable alternative has been advanced. Lack of agreement in defining the concept and resultant rival approaches in methodology have contributed to difficulties in measuring body image.[675] This remains the most criticized feature of body-image research.[676–679]

Fisher categorized research dealing with body image issues into nine primary focal areas.[680] These include the perception and evaluation of body appearance; accuracy of perception of body size, body sensations, spatial position, and body boundaries; distortions associated with psychopathology and brain damage; responses to body damage; cosmetic alterations; and sexual identity of one's body. The most pertinent of these to overweight and obesity and a consideration of weight-control practices, are perception and evaluation of physical appearance and accuracy of perceptions of body size.

Do all obese individuals have a body-image disturbance? Some people might contend or suggest that this is true but it is not the case. Dissatisfaction with the body is not always a central factor. Some obese individuals (more particularly adults) are able to look at their bodies in a realistic manner and recognize the need to diet and exercise without significant emotional involvement. Others do not regard their extra body fat as undesirable, either for cultural or personal reasons.

## 10.3 Appearance-Related Body Image

Body image has both self-perceptual and subjective (attitudinal and affective) components.[681–682] Garner and Garfinkel proposed that body image could be separated into two elements: body image distortion and body dissatisfaction.[682] Body-image distortion was considered indicative of a perceptual deficit while body dissatisfaction results from a disturbance in thoughts and feelings about the body. Therefore, it is often associated with a desire to alter physical appearance.[681,683–685] Williamson added an alternative conceptualization of body-size dissatisfaction,[686] which was composed of two constituent parts: body-size distortion and preference for thinness. Thus, body-image disturbance could result from a cognitive inability to assess body appearance (body-image distortion) or body size (body-size distortion) accurately. Alternatively, disturbance could result from a subjective evaluation that the body does not meet the ideal (body dissatisfaction) and in particular the lean ideal (preference for thinness).

### 10.3.1 Body-Size Distortion

Body-size distortion involves a perceptual disturbance in which an individual seems unable to assess his/her body size accurately. Body-size distortion was first studied by Slade and Russell.[687] They noted a greater body-size overestimation in anorexic subjects compared to controls. Others suggest that size overestimation is not specific to eating-disordered populations.[688,689] However, it has been suggested that a cognitive inability to accurately assess body size may be an important diagnostic criterion in discriminating between excessive dieting and disordered eating practices.[681]

### 10.3.2 Body Dissatisfaction

Body dissatisfaction represents an attitudinal or affective dimension in which one expresses a certain level of satisfaction with the body or specific body parts.[682] Body dissatisfaction is associated with various problematic eating attitudes and behavior patterns including dietary restraint, weight preoccupation, binge eating, and the risk of developing eating disorders.[690]

In the assessment of disordered eating behaviors, body dissatisfaction is the best predictor of dietary restraint.[691] Streigel-Moore et al.[692] noted that body dissatisfaction more accurately predicted students whose eating symptoms worsened during their first year of studies than perceived stress, ineffectiveness, perfectionism, and competitiveness. Cognizant of research concerning attitudes toward exercise, body dissatisfaction may also influence motivations for exercise, with individuals dissatisfied with physical appearance more likely to exercise for weight-control and to improve muscle tone.[48,529,652,653,693,694]

### 10.3.3 Preference for Thinness

The third type of body-image disturbance proposed by Williamson et al.[695] is indicative of an individual's "ideal body size," or a body size that is used as a standard for judging satisfaction with current body size. Research suggests that individuals who intensely fear weight gain prefer a body size which is significantly thinner than those who do not have such fears.[695,696]

### 10.3.4 Body-Size Dissatisfaction

Dissatisfaction with body size may be the strongest predictor of overall body dissatisfaction and associated weight-modifying behaviors.[551,666] Delineation of the concept into separate components has enabled research in appearance-related body image to assess perception of, and attitudes toward, physical appearance in different populations. However, there has been a bias in the research toward the assessment of certain populations. Females of all ages have been more commonly studied than males, and adults and college students have been more regularly assessed than children and adolescents. Consequently, there is still a paucity of data considering gender differences across childhood and adolescent years. Because adolescence is a period commonly associated with the emergence of disordered behavioral patterns such as anorexia and bulimia nervosa (and obesity),[697] an understanding of age and gender differences in the appearance-related body image of children and adolescents is important.[653]

## 10.4 Relevance of Psychological Accompaniments of Physical Growth during Childhood and Adolescence

During childhood, physical growth changes are characteristically slow and gradual. The small changes in appearance and increases in height do not generally require wholesale revisions to the image a child has of his or her own body. Similarly, through most other stages of life the body changes imperceptibly and so does one's body image.

In contrast, the more rapid changes during the adolescent period, such as increase in size, changes in body proportions, primary and secondary sex characteristics, and facial appearance mean that minor adjustments in body image are not sufficient for some individuals. It is important to mention that while adjustment and coping with changes in body image are important for many young people, body image is not of uniform importance and significance to adolescents across the entire period of growth. Adolescence is a period when self-awareness of appearance and body shape becomes more important. However, this self-awareness can appear much earlier, for example, at the beginning of the school years, and may result in a deterioration of food habits and or physical activity participation. The effect of mass media, e.g., television, may be important.

The hormonal activity that occurs during puberty contributes to observable bodily changes, the most obvious being those of secondary sexual characteristics. Despite the commonality of physical changes, there are individual differences in the onset and rate of change during this period. Social comparison during puberty is particularly relevant in young people so the timing of puberty may be a more important aspect of pubertal development than actual pubertal status.[698,699]

Pubertal timing is usually defined as a measure of an individual's relative development in comparison with the maturation status of the reference group.[700] Richards et al. reported that behavior patterns are influenced more by 'social age' than chronological age.[701] Thus, for school children, the reference group would most likely be other students within the same grade.

Early researchers postulated that personality adaptation is affected by body shape, which influences the impression a person makes on others and how one views oneself.[702] Bernstein suggested that the 'bio-psychosocial phenomenon' of body image is an individual's view of him/herself not only physically, but also physiologically, sociologically, and psychologically.[703] Thus, it has been argued that during late childhood and early adolescence, self-awareness is particularly intensified due to the complexity of changes. These include physical changes, the increase of introspection, the importance assigned to physical traits by the peer group, and the increased tendency to compare oneself with culturally determined standards.[667,698]

Statistical analysis of school performance of obese children in Spain showed that obese children of both genders had significantly better results than normal-weight children. This observation may be explained by the additional time spent in academic pursuits compared with being physically active. It is also possible that obese children attend school more diligently in order to be better accepted by their peers and to counterbalance their negative body image.[704]

In a group of black, inner city school children, 35% were obese according to triceps skinfold thickness criteria. Behavioral characteristics were assessed using the Child Behavior Checklist (CBCL) and the hyperactivity sub-scale of the Connor's Parent's Questionnaire. Obese children were more likely to have abnormal scores. CBCL sub-scale scores showed a higher "sex problem" score in obese girls. There was a significant trend for obese boys and girls to have higher CBCL sub-scale scores. These data supplement the limited information on obese children and are consistent with previous findings suggesting subtle behavior differences in obese children. Also the proportion of obese children placed in special education or remedial class settings was twice that for children with normal body weight.[705]

Psychological functioning and its association with the changes in BMI during 1 year were evaluated in boys and girls aged 9 years. Increases of BMI were significantly associated with unfavorable changes in physical activity attitudes, activity preferences, perceived physical activity competence, self-concept, and body image. There was limited support for the hypothesis that overweight children are more sensitive to changes in body shape than children with normal weight. The data illustrate that growing obese individuals are overly concerned with body weight and shape.[706]

Personality and intelligence were followed up in obese Chinese children aged 9.8 years.[707] While the prevalence of childhood obesity in China is only approximately 1 to 3%, this does represent a large absolute number of the population. The system of one child per family may be contributing to this problem as single children might be spoiled more frequently which contributes to the development of obesity early in life. In this study children with severe obesity had significantly lower performance on a score of IQ (Wechsler Intelligence Score) than control children with normal weight. Simultaneously, a significantly higher EPQ psychoticism score (Eysenck Personality Questionnaire) was found in severely obese children. These results seem to indicate that obesity has more serious consequences in a population less adapted to hyperalimentation and obesity than in other populations. Children with a milder degree of obesity did not show the same results.[707]

A study of Chinese children also confirmed other abnormalities in the obese. Assessments showed a greater increase in baseline secretion of insulin and C-polypeptide in obese subjects than in controls. Total IQ, speech IQ, and operational IQ along with thyroid function were relatively lower in the obese than in controls, and gonad development and maturity took place earlier in the former than in the latter.[622] It can be speculated that the Chinese subjects were not entirely obese due to overeating and energy imbalance, but their obesity pathogenesis was caused, at least in part, by an endocrinological deviation. Similar findings in other child populations have not been replicated.

In a special study it was revealed that patients with the early onset of obesity demonstrated a greater frequency and higher levels of emotional distress and psychiatric symptomatology than those with late onset of obesity. The findings of this study support the belief that obesity is associated with greater internal psychological conflicts. Therefore, childhood obesity can also serve as a predictor variable for possible psychological problems and disturbances in obese populations in later life.[708]

In addition to the biological changes that characterize adjustment at puberty, psychological adjustments occur in relation to physical changes. At the perceptual level, individuals and their peers react to bodily changes that are observable and make comparisons based on these observations. Due to individual variability in biological maturation, there are common changes noticed in all young people but at the same time there are extensive differences related to the rate of change and to genetic diversity. Each individual alters his or her mental image of their body form as it changes and similarly, responds to social reactions that these bodily changes elicit. Social responses will also have a great bearing on one's psychological state. This will depend on where in the range one is perceived, from approval to disapproval, admiration to ridicule, acceptance, or rejection.[679]

Adolescence is a period of physical and psychosocial change that for many involves a stressful re-evaluation of self-concept and interpersonal relationships.[709] Well before the onset of puberty, in fact during the younger elementary school years, individuals understand that thinness in women, and athletic leanness in men, are considered physically attractive and socially acceptable.[710] There is also evidence that body dissatisfaction and dieting increase at the time of puberty.[660] Early maturing females display these attitudes and behaviors before others.[691]

## 10.5 Sociocultural Influences

Body image is influenced by culturally defined standards of physical attractiveness. Fallon and Rozin suggested that body image includes the perception of cultural standards, perception of the extent to which one matches the standard, and the perception of the relative importance that members of the cultural group and the individual place on the match.[711]

Physical appearance is important because it determines to a large extent the initial attraction to others, and is a key factor in how individuals are judged. Although the physically attractive 'ideal' may vary across cultures and historical periods, physical appearance is of importance to most. Individuals are more satisfied as they meet the idealized standards of attractiveness.[712] In order to assess appearance-related body image, it is necessary to define the yardstick against which physical attractiveness is judged and the ramifications of meeting or failing to meet the level of physical appearance deemed 'ideal.'

## 10.6 Physical Appearance

Spring et al.[713] proposed that across all societies, the most valued body shape is that which is associated with health and prosperity. While the lean physique is considered ideal in western societies, to ready themselves for marriage, young Nigerian females from affluent families spend up to 2 years in "fattening huts" in order to achieve the desired endomorphic physique. Likewise, men from Cameroon enter fattening huts to emerge appearing fat and prosperous, demonstrating prestige.[714] In general, the body type considered physically attractive depends on gender, social status, and sociocultural context. Western society lauds physical attractiveness, and having the "perfect" body symbolizes self-control, mastery, and acceptance.[684] Modern society goes to extreme lengths to strive for physical perfection, and to reward those thought to embody the ideal.[715] Attainment of the physical ideal is based on the belief that the body is malleable with the aid of diet and exercise.[683] The value placed on physical attractiveness is very evident in the fashion, fitness, diet, and cosmetic industries.[715] In a less obvious way, the value placed on physical attractiveness is reflected in body-image disturbances and the related pathogenic weight-control practices.[662,716]

As a self-concept construct, body image is greatly influenced by an individual's perception of physical attractiveness. Numerous studies have shown that perceptions of physical attractiveness are positively correlated with an individual's self-concept, self-esteem, personal judgment, depression, and emotional disturbance.[717,718] An individual's objective level of physical attractiveness can influence psychological experiences and development. While the cumulative effects of unattractiveness can negatively influence mental health, an individual's self-perceptions of physical appearance can differ considerably from reliable objective perceptions of physical attractiveness.[719] Thus, self-perceptions can have more salient implications for mental health than objective evaluations. These findings have important implications for the necessary support of obese children and adolescents. There is clearly the need to address the seriousness of the level of adiposity with reinforcement of one's self-concept and body image.

## 10.7 The Ideal Body Shape

All cultures value the body shape that is associated with health and prosperity, but the shape differs in relation to a society's degree of industrialization.[713] In affluent cultures characterized by an abundance of processed foods and convenient lifestyles, it is easy and unhealthy to become overweight and difficult to remain thin. Thus, it could be argued that in industrialized societies where the dominant causes of morbidity and mortality are chronic diseases associated with obesity, the ideal body type for both sexes is one that is predominantly lean mass.

The body shape considered ideal is not necessarily the one that is biologically determined, and for many is not biologically attainable.[720] Attitudes toward what constitutes a socially desirable body shape are learned early in life.[666] What is not learned, however, is that due to biological differences very few individuals will meet societal expectations. If body size and weight are normally distributed, only a minority of individuals can be expected to match "naturally" the ectomorphic, almost prepubertal female ideal,[715] or the male body ideal of "muscular mesomorphy."[721]

As the average weight of many populations is increasing, the real–ideal difference is also increasing. Fallon and Rozin concluded that a woman's perception of the ideal female body shape is a thin one, most likely thinner than the average weight of the population.[711] Studies of female adolescents reflect weight concerns comparable to those evidenced in women. Fisher et al.[722] reported that almost two thirds of the adolescent females tested described themselves as overweight, three quarters believed they were above the healthiest weight for age and height, and four fifths that they were above the weight deemed to make them most happy. Another study of adolescents found that whereas girls were more likely than boys to report a desire to be thinner (60.3 vs. 34.8%), boys were more likely to want to be taller (67.2 vs. 49.1%).[551]

## 10.8   Body Weight or Body Fatness — the Real Issue?

Body weight and fatness are fundamental elements by which people everywhere are judged.[713] The stigma attached to being overweight or obese in western cultures has implications for individuals of all ages. In western society the sexes appear to differ in the perception and appraisal of total body weight. The term "weight" appears to have a different meaning for males and females.[723] In contemporary society, weight is an issue of central importance to women; females are faced with the paradox of a hormone-induced increase in body fat at puberty and a socioculturally driven desire to be thin.[724] For females, the term "weight" may relate closely to perception of personal body size. Females may equate underweight with thinness, low adiposity, and an ectomorphic body type, all of which are viewed as favorable. In contrast, males may equate underweight as ectomorphy, and overweight as endomorphy, both of which are viewed as unfavorable.

Williamson devised a theoretical model, illustrated in Figure 10.1, that delineated how body-image distortion, preference for thinness, and body-size dissatisfaction interact with fear of fatness to produce static and dynamic disturbance of appearance-related body image.[686] It is evident from the model that a multi-dimensional approach incorporating measurements of each component of body-image disturbance must be employed if a comprehensive assessment of appearance-related body image is to be achieved.

Due to the varied approaches to defining body image, the number of appearance-related body-image assessment procedures has proliferated, with the majority focusing on the perceptual and subjective components.[725] Figure 10.2 illustrates the categorization of these measurement procedures.

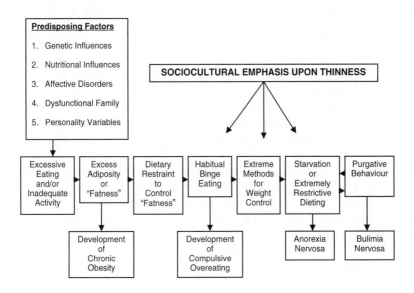

**FIGURE 10.1**
An etiological model for eating disorders. (Based on data from Ref. F31.)

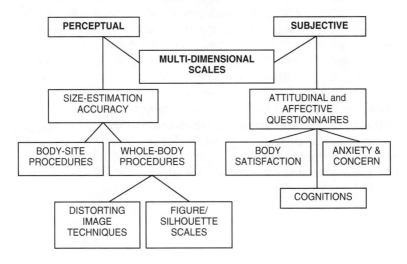

**FIGURE 10.2**
Categorization of appearance-related body image assessment measures. (Based on data from Ref. F32.)

## 10.9 Concluding Remarks

The intensity of body-image disturbances fluctuates widely even over short periods of time. When things are going well and a person with a body-image disturbance is in good spirits, he or she may not be troubled by the disability, although it may never be far from one's awareness. In contrast, in esteem-lowering experiences and a depressive mood state the unpleasant aspects of life may become focused on his or her obesity and the body becomes the explanation and symbol of unhappiness.

Despite such short-term fluctuations in intensity, body-image disturbances persist with remarkably little change over long periods of time and in concert with considerable variation in life circumstances. For example, weight reduction can have little influence for some individuals much to their surprise and dismay.

A number of factors may predispose an obese person to a disturbed body image. These include the age of onset of obesity, presence of emotional disturbances and negative evaluation of obesity by others during the formative years. Disturbances in adulthood are often commonplace in those who became obese during childhood or adolescence. While relative indifference to the condition may characterize much of childhood, adolescence is the most common period when a disturbed body image is likely to begin.

With the level of devaluation of obesity in society, it may appear redundant to mention negative evaluations as a cause. Obese individuals who have a body-image disturbance are often preoccupied with obesity, irrespective of their social status, intelligence, etc. Body weight is the overriding concern and the individual sees the world in terms of body weight. The individual may envy those who are thinner and feel contempt for those who are fatter.

Nevertheless, it is a mistake to assume that all obese individuals are psychologically or emotionally disturbed. There are no more anxious or depressed people among the obese than in the general population. Therefore, psychological problems do not occur in all obese individuals.

Irrespective of the mix of contributing factors to one's overweight or obese state, it is highly likely that psychosocial factors will be important in most cases. It may be argued that such factors are not considered as important as the physiological or metabolic, but do hold the key to treatment and management of the condition at all ages.

# 11

## Health Problems

The presence of obesity in childhood is associated with numerous medical problems related to physiological, metabolic, and structural changes.[63,181,726] Health problems in the obese include carbohydrate intolerance, coronary heart disease, diabetes mellitus, hyperlipidemia, increased total cholesterol (TC), and triglycerides (TG), along with decreased HDL-C and increased LDL-C, hyperinsulinemia, impaired heat tolerance, and decreased hormonal release. Additional problems include sleep apnea, osteoarthritis, respiratory infections, elevated blood pressure, gall bladder disease, and many others.

Nevertheless, it is important to recognize that obesity has not been conclusively earmarked as a primary independent risk factor for these problems. Adult obesity developed from childhood may be more problematic than adult-onset obesity due to an increased risk of the metabolic syndrome. Some authors suggest that irrespective of adult body mass, adolescent obesity is associated with elevated health risks and higher adult mortality.

Pediatricians and general practitioners perceive obesity in childhood as a serious problem that should be treated as early as possible since childhood obesity contributes to approximately 30% of adult obesity.[727,728]

Few longitudinal studies have considered the delayed, long-term effects of childhood obesity with respect to adult disease. Approximately one half of adolescents with more severe obesity, that is, a body mass index (BMI) at or above the 95th percentile, become obese adults.[182] Moreover, there is some evidence that obesity that develops during childhood and persists until adolescence can increase adult morbidity and mortality. As the severity of obesity can predict morbidity, the persistence of childhood obesity may be expected to account for a disproportionate share of the consequences in the adult years. In men who were obese during adolescence, all-cause mortality, and especially the mortality from cardiovascular diseases and colon cancer, were higher. In both genders, early obesity increased the prevalence of cardiovascular diseases and diabetes in adulthood. This may be related to the amount and distribution of fat. Various adverse psychosocial consequences were more frequent in females who were obese in childhood, and included completion of fewer years of education, higher rates of poverty, and lower rates of marriage and household income. The same result has not been found in males.[63,182]

A 50-year longitudinal study of a group of obese adolescents demonstrated that the mortality and morbidity from cardiovascular diseases were significantly increased compared with a group of subjects who were lean during adolescence. In addition, the influence of adolescent obesity on adult morbidity and mortality appeared independent of the effects of adolescent obesity on adult weight status. A more marked deposition of fat on the trunk starts to appear during adolescence.[18] Therefore, adolescent-onset obesity may be the forerunner to adult obesity as well as influencing mortality and morbidity in its own right.[51] This is one of the most important reasons why obesity should be managed as early as possible, at the latest, during adolescence.

Risk factors for coronary heart disease are present in obese adolescents, including an increased level of serum lipids with lower HDL-C, increased blood pressure, and a reduced fitness level.[557] These problems occur more frequently in children from families with an increased prevalence of these problems.[729] It is even more important to intervene when individuals are further handicapped by their family history.

## 11.1 Dyslipoproteinemia and Cardiovascular Risks

A 40-year weight history and adult morbidity and mortality were described in a cohort of Swedish subjects followed in Stockholm between 1921 and 1947.[730] The sample of overweight children remained overweight as adults. After the age of 55 years, BMI values started to decrease in both males and females. From postpuberty onward, female subjects were heavier than males. Subjects who died during the 40-year study and those reporting cardiovascular diseases were significantly heavier at puberty and adulthood than were subjects who remained healthy. There was a marked increase in the BMI between the postpubertal period and age 25 among those who subsequently died, those who developed cardiovascular disease, and particularly those who developed diabetes. In contrast, those reporting cancer had a lower BMI throughout. This study provides further evidence that overweight and obesity in adolescence may continue until adulthood and may be associated with serious health risks and increased morbidity and mortality later in life.[730]

The evaluation of long-term data on the health status of obese children showed that 28% had hyperlipidemia, 25% had an elevated blood pressure, 30% had asthma; 63% had an obese mother, 31% had an obese father and 50% had one or more obese siblings.[731]

Other studies revealed that overweight in adolescence can predict a broad range of adverse health effects that are independent of adult weight after 55 years of follow-up. Morbidity and mortality of obese adolescents aged 13 to 18 years, characterized by a BMI higher than the 75th percentile for age in a large national survey, were assessed in the Harvard Growth Study and compared to their lean peers (BMI 25th to 50th percentiles). Subjects who were still alive were interviewed about their medical history, weight, functional capacity, and risk factors. Cause of death was assessed from death certificates. The analysis revealed that obesity during adolescence was associated with an increased risk of mortality from all causes and disease-specific mortality among men, but not among women. The relative risks among men were 1.8 for mortality from all causes and 2.3 for mortality from coronary heart disease. The risk of morbidity from coronary heart disease and atherosclerosis was increased among men and women who had been overweight in adolescence. The risk of colorectal cancer and gout was increased among men and the risk of arthritis was increased among women who had been overweight during adolescence. Overweight during adolescence was a more powerful predictor of these risks than overweight in adulthood.[182,732]

The association between risk factors for coronary heart disease including obesity in 15- to 16-year-old schoolboys and adult mortality rates were examined in localities with a fourfold difference in adult mortality from coronary heart disease. Increased body fat, smoking, poor diet, and physical inactivity were greater among pupils from the school in the high-risk area compared with those in the low-risk area. Lipids, maximum oxygen uptake, and hypertension were similar in both schools. The risk of coronary heart disease seems to reflect the adult mortality rates in the area.[733] The reduction of obesity prevalence in childhood is therefore one of the important tools available to reduce coronary heart disease later in life.

Measurements in lean fit children showed lower total cholesterol (TC), low-density lipoprotein cholesterol (LDL-C), and triglyceride levels (TG), and higher high-density lipoprotein cholesterol (HDL-C) levels than in unfit children, which was not apparent after adjustment for body fat and/or abdominal fat. Unfit children appear to be at an increased risk of unhealthy levels of serum cholesterol due primarily to increased body fatness.

Cardiovascular risks were associated with leptin levels and nutrition in Korean girls aged $15.4 \pm 1.5$ years compared to normal-weight girls of a comparable age. Circulating leptin levels were significantly higher in obese girls and were significantly correlated not only with body weight and body fat, but also with systolic blood pressure, fasting blood sugar, TC, TG, and LDL-C. After correction for BMI, leptin was significantly correlated with percent body fat, TC, and LDL-C. Several cardiovascular risk factors were positively associated with circulating leptin that, in turn, was positively correlated with percent fat intake, and negatively with percent carbohydrate intake. These results show that a high-fat, low-carbohydrate diet was related to leptin levels.[526]

## 11.2  Blood Pressure

The results of the FRESH Study showed that in children aged 9 to 11 years, the level of physical fitness assessed using a treadmill test was usually higher in boys, and fatness and TG serum levels were higher in girls. Systolic blood pressure correlated positively with fatness in girls, but in boys there was only a trend toward a similar relationship. LDL-C in boys correlated positively with fatness and negatively with the level of physical fitness. Using multi-variate analysis, physical fitness was the primary correlate of total and LDL-C. In girls, fitness correlated positively with total and LDL-C, but this finding was reversed in boys. Fatness correlated negatively with HDL-C only in boys. Evidently, boys were more physically active, fitter, and carried less body fat. The level of physical fitness in boys was also positively associated with more favorable serum lipid levels. Along with other studies, these data suggest that consistent relationships among fitness, activity, fatness, blood pressure, and lipids are likely to emerge as children approach adolescence.[734]

In relation to risk factors for atherosclerosis in obese children, the following anthropometric parameters were suitable predictors: BMI in subjects below 9 years of age, BMI and waist circumference in males over 9 years, and BMI and waist/hip/height ratio in females aged above 9 years.[735]

Mathematical models have been fitted to individual semi-annual BMI values from 2 to 18 years of age and then at 2-year intervals from 18 to 25 years. Analyses showed that the higher the peak velocity and the BMI values at peak velocity and at maximum, the more likely adulthood obesity would develop. Birth weight also had an important role, the lower the birth weight the more likely the development of obesity in adulthood. The later the peak velocity and maximum BMI occurred, the higher the TG, the higher BMI at maximum velocity, and the lower the HDL-C.[736]

Results of studies from the National Heart, Lung, and Blood Institute (NHLBI) have confirmed that both obesity and high blood cholesterol levels in U.S. children are higher than optimal. The study suggested that the benefit of reducing the prevalence of these conditions in children and adolescents would be revealed later in life.[737] Research has focused on transition predictors to the obese state, the feasibility, efficacy, and safety of long-term dietary intervention during growth, and the effects of school-based programs that include various systems of positive interventions with respect to obesity.

Another study has confirmed some of the previous observations including that level of actual physical activity does not vary among obese and non-obese children. Correlations of physical activity and total cholesterol were low and not significant. However, both systolic and diastolic blood pressure and total cholesterol were higher in obese children. These observations indicate that obesity is associated with higher blood pressure and total cholesterol regardless of the present level of physical activity of children.[482]

Increased blood pressure is manifested in the obese under resting conditions and during physical activity. Comparisons of hypertensive obese and non-obese adolescents before and during a treadmill test revealed no differences under rest conditions, but during moderate exercise (stage II Bruce test), the differences became significant. The same was found during maximal exercise. Heart rate response to exercise was also greater in normotensive obese than in non-obese adolescents. These data show that obese hypertensive adolescents have higher blood pressure during exercise than lean, non-obese hypertensive adolescents. During testing of moderate intensity on a treadmill, it is possible to identify hypertensive individuals during adolescence and also to disclose mechanisms different from those at rest, which induce blood pressure elevation during exercise.[738] Under these conditions, an increased percentage of stored fat is a functional as well as a health handicap. Another study of 14- to 15-year-old obese boys and girls showed two or more risk factors for cardiovascular diseases in 25% of subjects, especially increased values of TC and a lower score of cardiorespiratory fitness.[739]

In a 3-year longitudinal study of anthropometric parameters and blood pressure in adolescents, there was a relatively greater proportion of female to male students who were overfat as seniors. Overweight trends for each of the four groups (that is, black and white boys and girls) were stable over the study period. A sharp increase in obesity occurred among black females. A significant association was found between percent of ideal weight, skinfold thickness, BMI, and blood pressure among females of both ethnic groups. These observations add support to the hypothesis that the early onset of obesity is an indicator of obesity in the later years of adolescence with many of the accompanying health risks including hypertension.[486]

Measurements in obese Czech children aged 9 to 16 years admitted to a sanatorium for the treatment of obesity showed a percentage of body fat from 29 to 44% (derived from skinfold measurements using regression equations for Czech children). Fat distribution was evaluated by the waist-to-hip ratio. In addition, blood pressure, lipoproteins and apolipoproteins, OGIT, and IRI were also evaluated. The level of physical fitness was assessed during a treadmill test. Paired tests and multiple regression analyses showed that fatness, diastolic blood pressure, and TG are independent factors for metabolic syndrome in obese children. These results provide further evidence that in the age range of 9 to 16 years, body fatness is related to risk factors for cardiovascular disease and diabetes.[568]

## 11.3 Insulin Resistance and Diabetes Mellitus

A study in Finland revealed that obesity is also associated with an increased risk of insulin-dependent diabetes mellitus (IDDM) in children. The prevalence of childhood obesity in children affected by IDDM was on average twofold from the age of 2 years onward compared to control children. In logistic regression analysis, the development of obesity 1 to 4 years before the diagnosis of IDDM was associated with an increased risk of disease in boys as well as in girls. This also held true after adjustment for maternal education and place of residence.[740]

Insulinemia of the mother can also influence the body fat of her children. A follow-up study in women with past gestational diabetes showed that the incidence of obesity in their offspring might have been reduced by antenatal insulin therapy. However, prenatal exposure to the metabolic effects of mild, diet-treated gestational diabetes mellitus (GDM) does not increase the risk of childhood obesity. Obesity prevalence in the offspring of mothers either with or without GDM showed a slightly higher prevalence in the offspring of mothers without GDM. There was also no difference in mean BMI adjusted for age and gender in these two groups of offspring.[741] Offspring of the mothers with uncompensated diabetes mellitus had significantly larger skinfolds at birth when compared to the offspring of normal, healthy mothers.[18,55]

The relative weight and 2-hr fasting plasma glucose were the variables most predictive of NIDDM in Pima Indians aged 5 to 19 years, participants in a longitudinal population-based study, and who were characterized by normal glucose tolerance. Fasting insulin was a significant predictor of diabetes but did not add to the predictive value of relative weight. Against a background of parental diabetes, high fasting-insulin concentrations predict diabetes, which is compatible with the hypothesis that insulin resistance is an early metabolic abnormality leading to NIDDM. But in this particular study, its predictive value did not add significantly to that of relative weight which is also an indicator of body adiposity, and with which fasting insulin is correlated.[742]

Insulin resistance with respect to glucose metabolism has been shown in obese adolescents; however, urinary sodium excretion and the pressor system remain insulin-sensitive. The sensitivity of the sodium-retaining action to hyperinsulinemia was higher in obese subjects when compared to non-obese subjects. For this reason, when compensatory endogenous hyperinsulinemia is raised by insulin resistance, these factors may result in chronic sodium retention and pressor system stimulation following hypertension in the obese.[743]

---

## 11.4   Multi-Metabolic Syndrome (MMS)

The prevalence of multi-metabolic syndrome (MMS) documented in obese adults has been examined in obese children aged 12.3 ± 2.2 years,[744] from the point of view of hypertension, hyperinsulinemia, hypercholesterolemia, hypertriglyceridemia, low HDL-C, and impaired glucose tolerance. In a subgroup, physical fitness and fat-soluble natural antioxidants were also studied. MMS was documented in 16 to 20% of obese children. Resting tachycardia, low physical fitness, and reduced α-tocopherol plasma concentration were also part of MMS in obese children.[744] Evaluation of exercise tolerance (exercise duration, $PWC_{170}$, and $VO_2$ max) in obese children with MMS showed a low level of fitness in children with multiple cardiovascular risk factors.

The relationship between morbidity and extreme values of BMI was evaluated in a group of Israeli adolescents at the age of 17 years. Functional limitations prevailed at both extremes of BMI distribution. Overweight was associated with hypertension and joint disorders in the hip, knee, and ankle.[745]

## 11.5  Hepatic Problems

In obese children and adolescents, hyperinsulinemia is an important contributor to the development of a fatty liver, apparently more so than overweight and increased fatness, blood glucose, or serum lipids. This was revealed in a study of Japanese children where the prevalence of fatty liver was 24.1%.[746] The results of a study of Italian children aged 4.3 to 20 years confirmed the importance of hepatic damage due to obesity during the period of growth and its relationship with metabolic alterations. Steatosis was found in 55.4%, hyperaminotransferasemia in 20.3%, and both these conditions together in 15.4% of children. In patients with an ultra-sonographic pattern of steatosis of the liver, there were significantly higher levels of liver enzymes (ALT, AST, gGT), triglycerides, and insulinemia. The degree of insulinemia correlated significantly with the presence or absence of steatosis.[747]

## 11.6  Respiratory Diseases

Respiratory symptoms were reported as worse in the obese during growth as the result of measurements in 7800 English and Scottish children aged 5 to 11 years. Positive associations were found between weight for height and the prevalence of bronchitis, "chest being wheezy" and "colds usually going to the chest" These data indicate that some respiratory illnesses can be reduced by preventing overweight or obesity in children.[748] For further information, see Chapter 6.

## 11.7  Sexual Development

Parents frequently consult a pediatrician when they believe the sexual development of a child may be abnormal, a particularly common occurrence in obese boys. The genitals are often so immersed in superfluous fat that despite adequate development, they appear to be retarded. Therefore it is recommended that children and parents with such concerns consult a medical practitioner. When this approach is taken, there is an increased chance that the problem of obesity will be treated.

Obese adolescent girls (aged 17.1 ± 1.4 years) often have menstrual disorders (oligomenorrhea, amenorrhoea, or irregular menses) and hirsutism. Polycystic ovary syndrome (PCOS) may begin at the perimenarcheal age, therefore the relationship between hyperandrogenemia and obesity in girls was analyzed. Subjects with any ovarial pathology were excluded. LH, FSH, testosterone (T), SDHEA, and insulin (Is) were measured in the follicular phase or after 6 months of amenorrhoea. BMI ranged from 18.3 to 34.5 and waist-to-hip ratio from 0.66 to 0.94. No correlation between the above-mentioned hormones and adiposity was found. Waist-to-hip ratio correlated significantly with T level, but not with Is. A significant positive correlation between BMI and T level was also found. These results suggest that in girls with menstrual irregularities, overweight is associated with hyperinsulinemia (as shown for other studies) and also with enhanced androgen production which may be a risk factor for PCOS.[566]

With respect to hormonal problems, the relationships may be double-sided. That is, some hormonal abnormality can result in obesity, and vice versa, obesity can significantly deteriorate hormonal activities in the developing organism. However, clinical cases of obesity caused by hormonal dysfunction in children are quite rare, and the majority of cases have other pathologies, most commonly resulting from an energy imbalance. But up to the present time, individual studies have not provided a satisfactory elucidation of the origins of obesity in all children. Much more research is necessary in this regard.

## 11.8  Orthopedic Problems

The structural consequences of obesity include the orthopedic conditions of Blount's disease, Legge-Calve-Perthes disease, genu valgum, flat footedness, and sub-talar pronation. Obesity has frequently been associated with the infantile form of Blount's disease (tibia vara). The increased stress on young bone resulting from excess weight may act on an underlying varus deformity and result in changes that are characteristic of Blount's disease. Dietz et al.[749] reported a similar incidence of the disease in obese children, for example, a slipped capital femoral epiphysis.

Numerous aspects of growth, development, and maintenance of body tissues are mechanically related. Inappropriate loading of the skeletal framework, particularly in areas of epiphyseal growth activity, can alter the pattern of growth in these critical regions. An increase in compression on one side of an epiphyseal plate may alter growth on that side, while normal proliferation occurs on the opposite side.[750] The end result of such unequal loading is a distortion in the normal angle of the epiphyseal plate. This may lead to unequal loading being experienced elsewhere and the direction of normal growth altered.[751,752]

Genu varus (bow leg) or genu valgum (knock knee) often produces additional lower extremity exacerbations that include compensatory pronation, talar adduction, and a degree of in-toeing. In addition to the abnormal loading forces mentioned, there is a predisposition to the early onset of osteoarthritis.[750]

Both cross-sectional and longitudinal studies corroborate obesity, or as yet unknown factors associated with obesity, as causing knee osteoarthritis.[753] The biological explanation for the link is unclear but obesity may initiate cartilage breakdown or promote joint destruction after the incipient lesion. It is evident that osteoarthritis does not remit but possibly either remains stable or progresses with time.

This has important implications for preventive measures early in life to avoid the disease. The role of weight loss in the alleviation of symptoms remains unanswered. One untested hypothesis advanced by Felson et al.[753] suggests that the likely mechanism by which obesity causes osteoarthritis in the knee is the increased force per unit area in the knees of obese individuals.

The consequences of pronation may also result in a flattened foot and hypermobile forefoot. The minimization of foot stability in these conditions requires greater muscle activity for normal-weight acceptance and transfer. Alterations in leg musculature, specifically the triceps surae and tibialis anterior muscles, tend to exaggerate the existing pronation.[754–756]

Body posture in obese children is also a common problem. However, some deviations of the vertebral column and the position of the scapulae are less noticeable as they are covered by a larger thickness of subcutaneous fat. Very often, the muscles of the abdominal wall are also flabby. Therefore, the prominent belly of the obese child is not only the result of fat deposition, but also of muscle weakness. Inadequate body posture combines to cause a hyperlordosis. The level of the shoulders is often uneven, and the head and neck are in a wrong position predisposing the individual to a poke neck. Obese children are also subject to the same range of postural deviations as normalweight children. As the development of musculature in the obese children is mainly sound, the deterioration of body posture can be rectified by appropriate instruction and exercises. Generally, obese children and adolescents are less fit than non-obese individuals of the same age which is a major concern for the musculoskeletal system, particularly overloaded joints.[757] A number of studies by Hills have demonstrated improvements in gait characteristics as a result of successful diet and exercise interventions in prepubertal children.[342,758–760]

## 11.9  Dental Caries

The relationship between dental caries and eating habits (24-hr recall and food frequency recall) has been studied in Brazilian children aged 1 to 12 years. Forty-two percent of children were born with an adequate birth weight and most of them had a mixed diet before 6 months of age. The main food provided after weaning was cows' milk in 40% of cases. The frequency of food intake was five times per day in 45% of the children. Thirteen percent of children studied were obese, and most of those ate white sugar and candies at least once a day. The prevalence of caries was 75%. These results indicate that children ingested more energy than needed. The data were insufficient to relate obesity to dental caries but the high intake of sugar indicates that this might be a factor in the increased prevalence of dental caries in children. However, other factors such as regular dental hygiene may be involved.

## 11.10  Immune Function

Obesity during growth can also alter the immune function.[761] Excess adiposity can be associated with impairments in host defense mechanisms, as shown by studies of the immune function in obese subjects. Total salivary IgA, serum C3 complement (C3c), and immunoglobulin A (IgA) were assessed in obese children aged 6 to 13 years. Comparisons with laboratory reference values for normal healthy children revealed that the data distribution showed higher frequencies near the zone of the highest reference values for serum IgA and C3c. When results of IgA in the saliva were expressed as a percentage of the normal value, 49.5% of the study population presented data lower than 76%. These results show a compromised secretory immune system without the incidence of clinical symptoms and infection, whereas humoral immunity might not be affected.[762]

## 11.11  Experimental Model Studies

Studies on the effect of increased fatness on health parameters using laboratory animals have been undertaken mainly in adult genetically obese animals. Rarely has the development of obesity been followed in normal animals from the early periods of life, except for those made obese with the help of an increased dietary intake such as cafeteria diet and hypokinesia.[18]

An experiment by Plagemann et al.[763] confirmed that the pathological effects of excess fatness developed as a consequence of early postnatal overfeeding in Wistar male rats from small (3 to 4 pups, overnutrition) as compared to normal sized (12 pups, normonutrition) and large (20 to 24 pups, undernutrition) litters. Serum insulin levels were significantly increased in overnourished pups from the smallest litters as compared to the other groups at the age of 15 days. These hyperinsulinemic rats had greater food intake and weight gains during the suckling period until adult age. The degree of overweight and obesity correlated significantly with basal hyperinsulinemia and increased blood pressure in small-litter adults. In addition, the early overnourished animals developed an increased type 1-like diabetes susceptibility to a sub-diabetogenic dose of streptomycin in adulthood. These results indicate the essential importance of food intake very early in life and predisposition to obesity, increased diabetes susceptibility, and increased cardiovascular risk in later life.

These conclusions are in agreement with the results of experiments following a reverse situation. Rats kept marginally malnourished from lactation until puberty and later realimented showed a range of different characteristics. Animals grew more slowly, showed a higher level of spontaneous physical activity (running in rotation cages), and were subsequently leaner in adulthood. However, they had the same sized vital organs (heart, adrenals, etc.) and were more resistant to experimental cardiac necrosis induced by isoprenaline in adulthood (lower spontaneous mortality, less damage of the heart muscle). In other experiments, the percentage of fat correlated with cardiac damage induced by isoprenaline as related to the level of physical activity (exercise and/or restriction of activity).[18,61,68]

## 11.12 Developmental and Nutritional Characteristics of Long-Living Populations

A long-living population in Abkhasia (living at a mean altitude of 600 m above sea level) was studied by Russian and U.S. scientists in the 1960s and 1970s. Children were never forced to eat more than they chose to spontaneously. Children grew more slowly and had smaller skinfolds, and overeating was considered unacceptable. These subjects were highly active from childhood to old age, had lower body weight, less fat in adulthood along with favorable serum lipid profiles, and a more positive health status. The population achieved a higher age (higher ratio of nonagenarians) as compared with a genetically identical population living in bigger cities nearby with quite a different lifestyle and nutrition. This involved eating more than was needed, with a food intake of undesirable composition, and with a restriction of physical activity.[764,765]

# Part II

# Treatment and Management Principles

# 12

## Effects of Different Reduction Therapies

Due to the multi-dimensional nature of obesity, the condition is often described as complex and particularly resistant to treatment. This may be due to the failure, in most situations, to provide the necessary multi-disciplinary support. Similarly, the longer an individual is obese, the more difficult it may be to change diet and exercise behaviors and therefore less likely that the condition will resolve spontaneously.

Effective long-term treatment options for overweight youngsters are critical for a successful reduction in the prevalence of adult obesity and its associated co-morbidities. The involvement of a team of health professionals using a range of behavior management techniques increases the chance of a successful outcome, that is, the maintenance of a desirable body weight and composition.

It has been recommended that in a multi-disciplinary approach to weight management, diet, exercise, and psychological support should be the three key components.[18,68,158] These components should be provided together as they are interrelated, interdependent, and have mutually supportive features. In most cases, weight control programs for obese children should focus on weight maintenance strategies as opposed to weight loss.[409] The particular features of these individual approaches, as well as any combined approach, depend on the degree and duration of obesity and the age of commencement of the condition. The child's past and present health and fitness levels and the family background are also important.[189,316,457] Further, consideration of the child's whole environment during the treatment period plays an essential role. Wherever possible, the overweight child should maintain a similar weight while growing at the expected rate, provided that the degree of obesity is not so severe that more intensive treatment is required. A severely restricted or crash diet has the potential to jeopardize normal growth and development of both muscle tissue and bone.[766,767]

In addition to the potential physical concerns as a function of inappropriate weight loss, the effects of a failure to lose weight should not be underestimated. There have been parallels identified between unsuccessful weight loss attempts and psychological problems, including a predisposition to eating.[768–770] A common problem in self-managed weight-loss attempts in young people who are poorly informed is the use of unhealthy eating practices and inappropriate exercise. Therefore, there is an important need for specific assistance from relevant health professionals. For dietary issues, a nutritionist or dietitian should be involved and an exercise physiologist should be responsible for the prescription of physical activity and exercise. Ideally, the management of obesity during growth and development requires mobilization of a team of health professionals from medical, pedagogic, psychological, nutrition, and exercise backgrounds.

A study comparing obese adolescents and their parents during behavioral treatment over 6, 60, and 120 months showed weight maintenance in adolescents, but a failure to maintain weight loss in parents.[771] Logistic regression analyses showed that children were more likely than their parents at each point in time to have percent overweight decreases greater than 20%, with over 20% of the children and less than 1% of the parents showing changes this large.

The effect of a weight loss intervention can be very different in individuals due to the degree of obesity and its duration. In addition, hormonal, biochemical, and functional parameters, plus family history and genetic predisposition play a role. During recent years, these issues have been the focus of attention of groups such as the European Childhood Obesity Group.[321,621,637] The specifics of the treatment and prevention of obesity in childhood have also been discussed in many meetings.[772] The individual approach to the treatment of obese individuals of any age, gender, and environmental background has been stressed in adults.[773] Particular effort must be made during the growing years to reduce excess weight and fatness.[18,30,51,63,182,183,774–776]

Attitudes toward obesity and its treatment may be biased and thus cause problems with respect to the management of obese individuals during growth and development. Dispelling the myths about children's obesity may represent a critical step in both the prevention and treatment of obese children.[777] Believing that all obese individuals overeat, eat too much junk food, and do not move enough suggests that the obese are social deviants, helping to justify the intense discrimination against them. Another myth is the inability to treat obesity. This notion has the potential to remove health-care professionals from the responsibility of understanding and caring adequately for obese children.

An understanding of the problems associated with childhood obesity is still lacking and needs to be improved and expanded. It is still poorly understood why in a family, one child is obese and the other not, in spite of the same environment and similar genetic background. The starting point for rectifying the problem is to use all the available knowledge on the mechanisms of obesity development and implement this knowledge as early as possible in life. The process must respect individual peculiarities. Therefore, any intervention must be the result of a careful and detailed profile of each particular child, including the history, degree and duration of obesity, health and fitness status, and psychological status.

## 12.1 Assessment of the Obese Child

The following list of assessment items is often referenced as important in providing an authoritative understanding of the status of each child or adolescent.

Physical growth history: an historical overview of size and shape during the growing years, comparisons with siblings, and patterns of growth of parents.

Anthropometric and body composition profile: height, weight, circumferences, limb lengths, skinfold measurements (NOTE: skinfold measurements may be unreliable in some overweight and obese individuals.).

Nutritional profile: assessment of energy intake, eating practices, and food preferences and aversions. An understanding of family eating practices is particularly useful at this stage.

Fitness assessment: indication of response to exercise through an assessment of health-related components of fitness.

Family interview: group meeting and discussion with all family members. This should be followed by the administration of psychological questionnaires including body image and body satisfaction instruments.

The authors use this approach in a clinical setting. The influence of the family should never be underestimated, from both an historical and a treatment perspective. Therefore, family members are potential key players during the assessment and subsequent treatment and management phases. Due to the wide variability in individual differences, each program, while following the same central themes in assessment, must be individualized. Variability must also extend to the respective families of obese children. The ability of practitioners to gain family involvement and support during the treatment and management phases may be one of the most influential factors in the likelihood of a successful outcome in the longer term.

### 12.1.1   Treatment Strategies and Markers of Success

As indicated previously, it is often extremely difficult to compare the results of studies in this area. Unfortunately, many studies are not homogeneous with respect to age, degree of obesity, health and fitness level of the obese subjects, duration and type of treatment approach, and all other approaches in the management of the child's obesity.

In the management of most individuals, the essential initial element is modification of the diet. This management component is addressed later in this chapter in more detail. Individual studies often fail to report the true nature of energy intake in the obese, as the consumption of food and drink is commonly under-reported in this population. The opposite is true for physical activity. It is customary for the obese to overestimate energy expenditure when self-reporting physical activity participation. Further, it is unusual for health professionals to know the full details of the historical nature of the health, nutritional, and physical activity status of the obese patient or subject.

The most important goals in the management of childhood obesity are the prevention of an increase in fat mass and the minimization or prevention of any immediate and long-term adverse consequences. When the degree of obesity is mild in infants and children, a desirable outcome of management is to keep body weight constant while body height increases. However, when fat mass is excessive and weight loss is considered mandatory in growing individuals, it is still critical to understand that from a growth and development perspective, the natural trend is for the young individual to increase and not to reduce total body weight.

The cornerstones of obesity management during growth are the modification of eating and activity behaviors, the combination of which results in a more active and healthy lifestyle. Any proposed change in lifestyle during the growing years must be cognizant of the individual's peculiarities, such as his or her period of growth, gender, plus environmental, social, economic, and psychological factors. In obese infants and school-age children, parent participation in the weight management process is indispensable. With adolescents who may be more motivated and have greater potential for self-management of their condition, parental support and encouragement are also of great importance but should act to mainly foster self-control in the individual.[339,778]

Less severe obesity can be managed by a reduction of energy intake and appropriate adjustments in the composition of the diet. However, in more severe cases, a very low energy diet may be implemented. Irrespective of the level of obesity, increased energy output is essential for long-term success. The promotion of physical activity followed by an individualized prescription of exercise must be incorporated wherever possible. With very large young people, a degree of caution should be used in relation to activity, ideally provided by an exercise physiologist with the joint supervision of a medical practitioner.

The response of children to a standardized treatment approach is variable.[779] Nuutinen and Knip considered the characteristics of children who had various degrees of success after reduction treatment.[768,769] Weight, body composition, and insulin levels were the main outcome variables and those who were successful after 1 year of treatment had greater weight loss, lower loss of lean body mass, and lower fasting serum insulin levels. Predictors of better success in weight loss at 2 years were the decrease in basal metabolism index (BMI) of the mother and documented energy intake over the first year.

Retrospective review and comparison of subgroups defined by age and frequency of visits to an obesity treatment center were conducted to determine if the timing and frequency of interventions influenced the outcome of treatment in obese children aged 1 to 10 years.[780] Children were seen within 1 year, with one or more subsequent visits in the next year at a nutrition evaluation clinic and an outpatient clinic in a metropolitan hospital. At the time of the initial visit, a comprehensive history, physical examination by a physician, and discussions with a registered dietitian and social worker were undertaken. A sound diet and exercise plan was suggested. A subsequent visit occurred after 1 month, with later intervals tailored according to individual need. A comparison of the outcomes of treatment in four groups subdivided according to age and frequency of visits showed that the most successful treatment of preadolescent obesity may be possible in the preschool years with frequent visits to the clinic or center. Therefore, to treat early and often may be the best method.

A multi-disciplinary intervention program was most successful in long-term weight maintenance for children who were only mildly obese at the beginning of the treatment program.[781] More than 70% of boys and 40% of girls grew out of their obesity if they could self-monitor their lifestyle on a permanent basis with a simple checklist. This was also revealed in a study of Japanese children involved in a multi-disciplinary program. This approach can potentially be used in a number of settings including with various medical practitioners and without the need for special facilities.[782]

Analyses of changes in obesity prevalence as well as experiences with different treatment modalities mean that it is possible to provide recommendations for both treatment and the prevention of obesity during growth. A study by Flanery and Kirschenbaum examined the effect of four classes of variables associated with weight reduction programs.[783] These included self-control techniques, degree of social support, attribution style, and self-reinforcement style in obese children. The results of this study conducted at two localities suggested that obese children who terminated ineffective problem-solving efforts quickly and who had more adaptive weight reduction attribution might be more likely to succeed in long-term weight reduction. Differential results in the two samples suggest that variables investigated in this study may play a greater role in weight maintenance rather than in initial behavioral change.

For an intervention to be effective, it is important to know the reliable predictors of treatment and the likely reaction of the obese individual. In a study of prepubertal American and Caucasian boys aged 9 to 11 years, total energy expenditure (TEE) by doubly labelled water (DLW), resting metabolic rate (RMR), the thermic effect of food (TEF), and substrate oxidation after the meal was assessed.[414] The primary endpoint was a 2-year change in the percentage of body fat measured by DXA. The best predictor of weight gain after 2 years was a high protein oxidation, followed by low energy expenditure and high RQ during the TEF. It was possible to conclude that energy expenditure, resting metabolic rate, and components of substrate oxidation are predictors of an increase in body weight and fat mass during late childhood. With this information, it may be possible to select individuals with an increased risk of remaining overweight.

The level of hyperinsulinemia is also considered a marker of success in the treatment of obesity.[784] Groups of obese children aged 5 to 16 years were assessed longitudinally and screened for insulinemia and glycemia after an oral glucose tolerance test, plasma levels of total cholesterol, HDL-C, and triglycerides. The sample was divided into subgroups on the basis of insulinemia and was similar according to all variables tested, except for weight loss and plasma triglyceride levels. The hyperinsulinemic group had a lower percentage reduction in excess weight and the results in this group were not dependent on the duration of treatment. This did not apply to the normo-insulinemic group of obese children.

As mentioned previously, various approaches are used in an attempt to encourage weight loss in children and adolescents, so results have not always been comparable or similarly successful. Reported results are as variable as the studies are different. Comparisons of study outcomes must include consideration of the changes in body weight, BMI, body composition, and other outcome measures. For example, an educational strategy to improve diet may have positive results in childhood obesity, as was the case in a Milano (Italy) population with young people (aged 3 to 18 years) in which mean prevalence of obesity was 13.4%.[178]

Current knowledge and understanding of various approaches in the treatment of pediatric obesity have been reviewed by a number of authors, most recently by Epstein et al.[33] Generally, the most effective combined therapy of the principles of energy balance improvement by diet and exercise and behavioral modification are recommended for children and youth.[18] This approach is also the most effective for adults. However, weight management treatment in obese growing subjects requires special approaches tailored to individuals in this age period.

Recommendations for improving childhood obesity treatment programs reported in the literature include the application of behavioral choice theory, improving knowledge of response extinction, and recovery with regard to behavioral relapse. These are some of the greatest problems of obesity treatment in children and adults. The individualization of the treatment and integration of basic scientific information with clinical research outcomes are additional recommended components of therapeutic procedures for obese children.[33]

The maintenance of a successful outcome in reduction treatment is a significant challenge in adults and the same applies to children, even when weight loss is often achieved more easily.[18,30,32,33,50,51,56,63,182,183,421,785–788] A study of obese children aged 6 to 16 years indicated that weight loss of at least 10% of the initial value after 2 years of treatment was the criterion of a 'successful loser.' Approximately half of the children succeeded in meeting this criterion. In children who were successful, body weight decreased by 24.7%, along with a significant decrease in total cholesterol (TC), triglycerides, and insulin, an increase of serum level HDL-C, and an increased ratio of HDL-C/TC. These positive results were maintained after 5 years of the study period. In normal-weight children, serum lipids and insulin remained stable during this period.[768,769] Similarly, an effective weight reduction program using a family-oriented approach and/or group approach had the best results.[789] In addition, a group provided with resources such as a manual on dietary change and overall lifestyle improvement including exercise did better than the group which only received written information. This program was included in "Cuidando El Corazon," a weight reduction intervention for Mexican-American subjects.

Findings of another study suggest that if aerobic conditioning is used to modify the heath risks of atherosclerosis, it is likely to be accompanied by a reduction of body weight.[561] Importantly, without a reduction of excess fat, health cannot be effectively promoted. A counterargument when considering the best approaches to obesity management in children incorporates the numerous negative examples regarding fear of obesity and an exaggerated reaction to it by excessively reduced diet and high levels of exercise. These phenomena may be a more common occurrence in adolescent girls with the potential for the development of symptoms similar to anorexia nervosa. A case of a girl aged 7 years showed an excessive reduction of food intake and elimination of carbohydrates and an excessive involvement in exercise.[790] Height velocity for this individual reduced from 6.0 to 4.1 cm.year$^{-1}$, compared to the values in control girls of the same age of $5.5 \pm 0.74$ cm.year$^{-1}$. The individual's eating behavior was finally normalized without specific psychotherapy. Such situations must be prevented because of possible longer lasting health, functional, and psychological consequences. These problems may be considered comparable or even more serious than problems resulting from obesity. Concerns regarding the treatment of childhood obesity were raised for these and related reasons in the earlier work of Woolley and Woolley.[791]

Young people are also exposed to a wide range of inappropriate health messages through the various forms of mass media. For example, one of the more common trends in recent years has been the societal tendency to glamorize thinness.[49,652] When a characteristic feature of the human race is diversity in body size and shape, this message is potentially problematic. A strategy to assist young people to cope with a wide range of potentially misleading messages is to provide them with the skills to critically appraise advertising. There is a wonderful opportunity for society to profit in a positive fashion through advertising to promote healthy eating and physical activity behaviors to counteract the widespread prevalence of poor or inappropriate lifestyle practices.

## 12.1.2 The Role of Family Support

The family of an obese child must play a lead role in the treatment process if the individual is to maximize the opportunity of a successful outcome. In families where obesity is more pronounced, Kalker et al. found that children were able to reduce their weight more than the average during treatment but regained the weight during the subsequent 3 to 5 years.[792] The highest levels of overweight were recorded after that time. The obesity level of the other members of the family, whether the individual was an only child, or the gender of the obese children did not influence the initial decision to stop or continue with the treatment. Boys were more successful in weight reduction than girls based on mean scores after both 3 to 6 months and after 5 years. However, this difference was not significant. Children without a family history of obesity were significantly less overweight at the beginning compared with those with a familial obesity, and similarly, they showed the best short- and medium-term results. Thus, in spite of good short-term results, obese children of obese parents should be regarded as those at greatest risk of weight regain and therefore should be checked and treated on a regular basis over a long period during the growing years.

Many claim that it is too difficult, even impossible, to achieve permanent change using standard procedures of obesity treatment. Therefore, the potential effect of the family must not be underestimated, especially for younger obese children. The prevention of obesity in such children can be most successful if initiated with the simultaneous prevention and treatment of obesity of a parent and/or older siblings. An early start is the best guarantee of an adequate result in the longer term. Epstein et al.[793] have suggested that in relation to weight loss in weight management programs, outcomes are related to the weight of parents and the present status of the obese child.

Epstein has also suggested that a family-based intervention program should be introduced to rectify energy imbalance in slightly older obese prepubertal children (approximately 8 to 12 years of age).[794] The involvement of at least one parent as an active participant in the weight reduction process can improve both short- and long-term effects of weight regulation. There is a dual benefit when family and friends support a child in behavior change, as those providing a supporting role also benefit.

Other positive changes have been reported in parent-directed weight reduction programs with young children. For example, the degree of compliance was significantly correlated with the change in percentage overweight of Taipei children.[795] A number of longitudinal studies over 1, 5, and up to 10 years have also illustrated the importance of parents.[771,786] The results after 1 year showed that the amount of relative weight change was related to the initial treatment success, the number of children in the family, and the gender of the child. Children who were initially more successful had fewer siblings and were female. These results suggest that family size may interact with the treatment to determine weight change.[786] When non-obese siblings are present in the family, the adherence of only one family member is very difficult to achieve.

Multi-variate regression analyses of changes in relative weight and fitness after 5 years of treatment in obese children showed two factors independently related to fitness change: maintenance of weight loss from the end of 6 months of treatment to the 5-year follow-up, and the initial level of physical fitness. Children with the lowest levels of fitness at the beginning of the treatment who were able to maintain weight loss for up to 5 years showed the largest improvement.[796] Another family-based behavioral treatment study conducted across a 5-year period with obese children aged 6 to 12 years provided the following results.[786] Treatments with conjoint targeting and reinforcement of both child and parent behavior, plus reciprocal targeting and reinforcement of children and parents were associated with the best outcomes for the child. Predictors of the child's success included self-monitoring, changing eating behavior, praise, and change in percent overweight of parents. Predictors for successful parental outcomes were self-monitoring of weight, baseline parent percent overweight, and participation in fewer subsequent weight control programs. Similar conclusions were gained in a 10-year longitudinal study. Long-term change in children depends on the mode of treatment; evidence converges on the importance of the family and other sources of support to a change to adequate eating and physical activity.[771]

Wadden et al.[797] considered the effect of a 16-week program on obese adolescent girls who were treated with different levels of parental participation. The greater number of sessions attended by the girl's mother, the greater the weight loss of the girl. Weight loss was associated with significant improvements in body composition, serum TC, and psychological status. Other studies by Epstein et al.[771,798] have demonstrated the essential role of an active approach by mothers and fathers in helping their obese children.

Parents should be active participants in all aspects of the treatment and management of their obese child to maximize the impact of both diet and exercise. Epstein has suggested that the motivational structure within the family that supports or discourages behavior change may be just as important as the specific behaviors that the weight management process is attempting to modify.[32] As might be expected, when parents and children are treated together, better results are gained than when children are targeted alone.

In a recent study by Golan et al.[770] the role of parents in the treatment of obese children aged 6 to 11 years was assessed. With the experimental group of children, parents were agents of change whereas in a comparable group, a conventional approach was used. Anthropometric and biochemical measurements and questionnaires to assess sociodemographic characteristics, diet, and physical activity in the family were completed at the beginning and the end of the study. Mean percentile weight reduction was significantly higher in children in the experimental group (14.6%) than in the control group (8.1%). This study provides further substantiation of the essential role of parents in rectifying obesity during growth.

In obese children treated on an outpatient basis, best results in a reduction program were obtained in subjects aged 4 to 14 years with two or more siblings plus an adequate adherence to the prescribed diet and good family support. In this study, the gender, level of obesity of other family members, initial age, and previous food and exercise behaviors did not have a significant effect.[799]

### 12.1.3    Individual vs. Group Approaches to Obesity Treatment

The results of treatment can vary according to whether treatment is provided on an individual or group basis. In a 1-year treatment program, it was found that both groups had a similar weight reduction, linear growth, and lean body mass development. Similarly, the serum level of HDL-C and HDL-C/total cholesterol (TC) increased and TG decreased significantly in both groups. However, fasting insulin levels only decreased significantly in the group treated as individuals.[768,769]

In Singapore where a high prevalence of obesity has been reported, three subgroups of obese preschoolers (with mild, moderate, and severe overweight) were studied.[144] The latter group was referred to dietitians for management while nursing staff using pre-planned counselling sessions managed the other two groups. There were differences among groups with respect to family history of obesity and hypertension. After 1 year of the intervention program, 40.4% of the children improved their obesity status and 20.2% reached normal-weight status. All groups significantly improved their health status.

Suttapreyasri et al.[800] studied the response of obese children in Bangkok using several training methods. After 3 months of training, knowledge about obesity increased significantly using each model; weight reduction was significant in the group provided lectures and rewards to decrease body fatness. After 6 months, each group showed similar increases in height and weight, but the group mentioned above had the lowest increase in weight.

In very severe cases of obesity in adolescents, a closely monitored program such as an inpatient approach must be considered the same as for similar cases in adults. The results of a follow-up lasting 33.3 months, with a mean duration of inpatient treatment of 6.8 months, showed that long-term inpatient treatment had a positive effect on weight change. Successful outcomes were induced using a permanent change in lifestyle brought about by a combination of nutritional therapy, psychotherapy, and exercise.[801] However, inpatient treatment of subjects who are obese but without co-morbidities is particularly difficult, especially due to the facilities required and the expense of such treatment.

## 12.2   The Effects of Diet

Considerable attention has been paid to the factors that determine food habits during the early years of life. Further consideration has been given to the possibility of influencing food preferences and eating patterns in a desirable way to achieve health promotion. The prevention or delay of adult-onset diseases may be facilitated by interventions in early childhood. Numerous common chronic diseases fit into this category and include ischemic heart disease, cerebrovascular accidents, hypertension, malignancies, and also obesity.[802]

The importance of the diet during early life is of central significance as this period is assumed to be the most critical and sensitive. Food intake and its composition during this period of growth can influence metabolic development and predetermine some future metabolic processes.[68,189,803] However, while the importance or significance of the potential benefits for young children may be undisputed, there are still some shortcomings in research in the area.

## 12.2.1 Dietary Allowances for Obese Children

The definition of food intake including energy and macro- and micro-components of RDAs for obese children and adolescents is a unique problem. Along with the reduction of stored fat, fat-free mass and functional capacity should increase to attain optimal health status.[804] A 2-decade study spanning the period from birth to 21 years revealed that 41% of children who were fat at 1 year of age were still fat in adulthood.[380] It was also revealed that one can be obese without being hyperphagic (at least during the period when children were followed-up). Therefore, the definition of a reduction diet must be qualified and an individualized approach used whenever possible. The evaluation of BMI is suitable; however, periodic check-ups of body composition status aimed at the provision of information, changes in fat-free mass, or a marked slowdown in height are recommended.

A monitored reduction in food intake is acceptable in obese children as it is in adults. However, the appropriate definition of the actual allowance for an obese child is quite difficult to quantify. Total food consumption should be less than before but should still include all the necessary items required for the adequate growth and development of lean body mass. Again, this may vary in different periods of growth and depends on the initial degree of obesity and health status of the individual. The preparation of meals on a daily basis can also be a very difficult task for families who are not specialists in nutrition. In addition, for families in which not all members are obese, it can be a problem to prepare separate meals for individuals, especially children. The effect of inadequate diets may not manifest immediately, but may be delayed to a point when rectification of the child's status could be more difficult.

Numerous dietary regimes have been developed but only the basic characteristics of the approach are generally reported. A reduction diet for a child is not simply a scaled-down version of food usually consumed by youth and adults. The diet must consist of reductions in the amount of high-risk items, for example, saturated fats, sweets, and highly processed food that is often high in fat and sugar. At the same time, adequate amounts of essential vitamins, minerals, fiber, and polyunsaturated fatty acids should be included to meet the recommended dietary allowances for the age and gender of the individual.

Caution should be exercised when any form of dietary modification is used and height velocity should be monitored during periods of weight management, as changes in velocity are more likely in growing individuals who lose, maintain, or increase weight more slowly than average. The same rule should apply to the health status, functional capacity, physical performance, and psychological status. Greater attention needs to be given to the identification of the optimal diet to support linear growth during weight loss. Dietz has suggested that a safe approach to employ in dietary restriction is to limit the amount of high fat food in the diet.[805] This may result in a reduction in total caloric intake by approximately one third. Attention should also be given to reducing the consumption of snack foods such as ice cream, potato chips, and soft drinks.[767]

A study of Japanese 4th and 5th graders showed a significant decline in obesity levels after 3 months of therapy using a low-carbohydrate, high-protein diet, and exercise.[806] After the educational program, dietary intake decreased, especially due to decreased carbohydrate intake. Nutrient intakes were in the appropriate range for boys, but energy and iron intakes were lower than the recommended dietary allowances for girls while protein intake increased. This diet and exercise treatment program was very effective as evidenced by the decrease in obesity level from 30% and above to 10.4% for boys and 7.5% in girls.

Children's eating patterns should be addressed with other components of a total weight management program that include parental involvement, reduction in energy intake, and increased physical activity and exercise.[33,51,339,341,522,786,788,793,794] Family eating and exercise patterns play a significant role in the etiology, treatment, and management of childhood and adolescent obesity. Eating is often considered an important indicator of the emotional state of family members and of interactions between parent(s) and child(ren). Optimal nutrition depends on the development of a positive relationship between parent(s) and the child(ren). The eating practices of children are enhanced when parents recognize and respond appropriately to the needs of the child.[807]

For some parents, concerns about overfeeding and causing obesity in their children are pervasive. While an appropriate awareness of food consumption in both type and quantity is necessary, being so concerned that food is withheld and hunger in children not satisfied can be problematic. This practice may be more prevalent if parents are anxious or concerned about their own eating practices. There is a real need for sensitivity on the parents' part to the child's likes and dislikes and feeding cues. The promotion of a positive feeding environment in the home that discourages rigidity and inflexibility regarding eating practices and behavior should be a central focus.

## 12.2.2   The Effect of Low Energy Diets

The aim of weight reduction in obese children is to achieve a loss of excess fat and preserve adequate growth in height and lean body mass. However, when the degree of obesity is already severe or morbid, a greater restriction of energy is necessary. A special protein-sparing, low-energy diet was used for severely obese adolescents, e.g., at the Hospital for Sick Children in Toronto.[808] The regime provided 2.0 to 2.5 g of protein per kilogram of ideal body weight, plus adequate fluid and nutrient supplements. The amount of meat, poultry, and fish that supplies this allowance of protein was determined using a protein equivalence system developed for the diet. The system allows both dietitians and patients to plan meals that minimize energy intake while maintaining protein adequacy and diet variety. When this diet is prolonged beyond the recommended 3 to 6 months, limited carbohydrate may be added in the form of selected vegetables. This type of diet must be properly supervised but its safety and efficacy have been demonstrated in adolescents.

In obese youth, the protein-sparing, modified fast diet produced significantly greater changes in percent overweight at 10 weeks (−30% vs. −14%) and at 6 months (−32% vs. −18%). At 10 weeks, a significant loss of adipose tissue with preservation of lean body mass occurred in the protein-sparing, modified fast group. A transient slowing of growth velocity was seen at 6 months in both dietary groups compared with the values at 14.5 months. Growth velocity approached normal levels at 14.5 months compared with standards for North American children. When dietary groups were combined, blood pressure decreased significantly at all points of the study. The initial average values of serum TC also significantly decreased and no biochemical or clinical complications were observed. The results indicate that it is possible to use hypocaloric diets without negative consequences for growth, but such diets should not be used without careful medical supervision.[809] Another longitudinal study also confirmed that moderate dietary restriction in overweight children with adequate dietary guidance does not have a negative long-term effect on children's growth.[798]

A study by Stallings et al.[810] considered the treatment of obese adolescents with the protein-sparing modified diet (PSMF) (880 kcal.kg$^{-1}$.day$^{-1}$ and 2.5 g protein.kg ideal body weight$^{-1}$.day$^{-1}$) for 3 months. Approximately three quarters of the subjects were followed up after 1 year and 48% had sustained weight loss, with the ideal body weight-for-height percentage decreasing from 154 to 125 over this period. Total body potassium (K) decreased 13% and total body nitrogen (N) decreased 14.3% over the year of study. The protein-sparing diet did not prevent some loss of K and N during this treatment; however, the decrease did not exceed their normal predicted values.

Figueroa-Colon et al.[811] used a clinic-based hypocaloric diet intervention in children aged 8.8 to 13.4 years in New Orleans. During the first weeks, super-obese children were placed on a 2520 to 3360 kJ (600 to 800 kcal) protein-sparing modified fast diet. Subsequently, the diets of all children were increased in a 3-month period by 420 kJ (100 kcal) every 2 weeks until a 5040 kJ (1200 kcal)-per-day balanced diet was attained. At 6 months, the super-obese dieters on the protein-sparing modified fast diet had a significant weight loss from baseline (−5.6 ± 7.1 kg) with a positive growth-velocity Z-score. Blood pressure and serum lipids decreased and no complications were observed. The diet was effective for the super-obese children in the medically managed clinic program implemented in a school setting. The effort of committed clinic staff, school officials, peers, and family involvement was crucial to the success of this intervention program over a period of 6 months.

Obese children have also been successfully treated using a classical hypocaloric diet.[812] At the beginning of the follow-up, energy intake of obese children was 98 ± 24% of RDAs, with 38.4 ± 4.2% of lipids, 47.8 ± 4.5% of carbohydrates, and 13.8 ± 2.5% of protein. The food consumed by the obese children contained a small amount of fiber and total water. The reduction diet included 1200 to 1800 kcal.day$^{-1}$, or about 65% of RDAs, with 20% protein, 30% lipids, and a total water volume > 1.5 ml.kcal$^{-1}$. After at least 6 months, the children exhibited a decrease in their excess P50 BMI from 155 ± 22% to 133 ± 16%. An evaluation of dietary intake after treatment showed a significant improvement. Total energy intake was lowered to 75% of RDAs, the percentage of lipids to 33.5 ± 5.3%, and total water was 1.28 ± 0.37 ml.kcal$^{-1}$. The percentage of proteins increased while the percentage of carbohydrates remained unchanged. This study revealed that the classical hypocaloric balanced diet had a significant effect on obese children, although the improvement of their nutrition did not accurately follow dietary recommendations for the particular age groups.[812]

Very low calorie diets (VLCDs) can be risky for the treatment of obesity in children, even when they contain a very high quality protein. This was shown in a study of a group of obese children monitored by frequent 24-hr Holter recordings for the appearance of cardiac arrythmias. After weight loss, cardiac arrhythmias appeared in some patients and can be potentially dangerous for the health of obese children.[813]

Concerns have been expressed about the marked reduction of food intake in obesity treatment. Zwiauer et al.[814] conducted a special study concerning cardiac function in another group of obese children with a daily intake of 500 kcal across a 3-week period. Electrocardiograph 24-hr recordings (Holter ECGs) were made and analyzed for a group of grossly obese children. Weight loss during these 3 weeks was 5.7 ± 1.6 kg. Average and minimal heart rate decreased constantly throughout the study period (Figure 12.1). During the second week, maximal heart rate increased significantly but returned to baseline values in the third week. Neither before nor during the period of therapy were any dysrhythmias monitored. These results indicate that a low calorie diet (500 to 700 kcal.day$^{-1}$) with a proper macro- and micro-component composition is a safe therapeutic approach for obese children and adolescents.

The composition of diets, i.e., diets with a low fat content, may be problematic in pediatric nutrition as already mentioned. The effect of obesity on the availability of essential and long-chain polyunsaturated fatty acids (LC-PUFAs) was followed up in a group of children. The results of the study

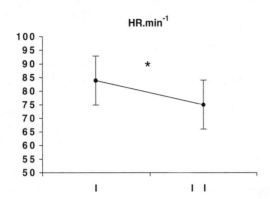

**FIGURE 12.1**

Changes in heart rate (HR) after a low calorie diet (I, LCD = 525 kcal.day$^{-1}$) and after weight loss (II, –5.7 ± 1.6 kg). * indicates (p < 0.05). (Based on data from Ref. F33.)

suggested that obese children do not require LC-PUFA supplementation to low fat diets during reduction treatment.[581]

An improvement in the diet of children can be achieved by reducing fat intake. For example, skim milk can be used instead of higher fat alternatives. This is an economical, single-food strategy that makes it possible to achieve contemporary RDAs of macro- and micronutrients and maintain nutritional adequacy. It is more of a challenge, for example, when replacing normal meat with entirely lean meat. In such cases, some slight deficiencies, i.e., vitamin E, may appear.[815] A concerted effort is needed to replace the present, common but unsuitable, high fat diet with healthy alternatives.[816]

An adequate dietary intake in terms of quantity and composition, modified according to the needs of the individual and program, is the most indispensable tool and most often used approach to rectify body weight and composition. Where inpatient support is not available, dietary counselling at schools or other institutions is highly advisable. However, some problems may appear when attempting to restrict food intake which might be inappropriate. These include the changes mentioned in relation to height velocity.[18,767]

There is some variability in studies that have considered slowing of growth after treatment for obesity using a restricted diet. For example, a study by Epstein et al.[788] showed that after 5 years of treatment (from 6 to 12 years), obese children still remained taller than the norm (65th percentile). A study of Russian children showed that dietetic management produced a different effect in obese children, which attests to the heterogeneity of the disease. Therefore, more detailed analyses of the causes of obesity and a more exact diagnosis should be used prior to involvement in such programs.[817]

This approach was used in a group of obese children during a 2-year period in a school health-care setting (group II), as compared with a group of severely obese children with intensive treatment (group I). The age range of the children was 6 to 16 years; they were treated over 1 year and observed for another year.

Food intake data were collected by a 4-day record method. At baseline, there were no differences in food consumption or nutrient intake between obese and normal-weight children. The group with intensive therapy (I) significantly decreased fat intake during treatment, which was permanently maintained throughout the observation period. Weight loss was 16.2% of the initial value, in contrast to group II in which no change was revealed. Body fat and relative weight were significantly correlated with the decrease in energy intake. Both the dietary counselling group in the school health care setting and the control group displayed no change in daily fat intake. The conventional approach for obesity treatment appeared to be far less effective as shown in group II.[818] In another study, dietary instruction lasting 13 weeks partially rectified the degree of obesity (as evaluated by Rohrer's Index) and some serum biochemical characteristics in Taiwanese children in the third to sixth grade.[819]

Body composition and resting energy expenditure (REE) in obese adolescents changed significantly following weight loss due to a low-energy, high-protein diet (800 kcal, 3349 kJ.day$^{-1}$). Total body potassium (TBK) and extracellular, intracellular, and total body water (ECW, ICW, TBW) did not change significantly after weight loss, indicating a preserved body composition. The REE decreased with weight loss; however, when expressed as kcal.kg$^{-1}$ body weight and/or fat-free mass, no significant changes were revealed.[820] The hypocaloric diet decreased RMR in obese adolescents after 6 months of mixed hypocaloric diet resulting from a weight loss of 5.4 ± 1.2 kg (Figure 12.2).[392]

Nitrogen (N) balance was studied in a group of obese children after a liquid formula very low calorie diet containing 1339 kJ (44 g protein, 33 g carbohydrate, 0.9 g fat) was consumed, resulting in a weight loss of 15.3 ± 4.6%. There were no complaints of hunger or discomfort, and no serious side effects were observed. Half of the patients achieved N-balance during the second week and all but one in the third week. Great interindividual variance was found in the rate of N-loss during the course of the study. No significant correlation was revealed between cumulative N-balance and weight loss and initial body weight. Blood parameters remained unaffected except for blood glucose and urea, which slightly decreased. Uric acid concentrations increased slightly and in some patients increased more than 8 mg.day$^{-1}$ and was treated by allopurinol. Total serum protein decreased and serum albumin values did not change. This type of VLCD proved to be efficient from the point of view of rapid weight loss. A marked improvement of N-balance in 3 weeks could be achieved with the VLCD containing 1 g protein.kg ideal weight$^{-1}$.day$^{-1}$. This amount of protein seems to be indispensable for achieving a sparing effect in growing subjects during weight reduction by VLCD.[821]

The effect of a low-calorie balanced diet (LCBD) was assessed in Japanese children aged 3 to 15 years using bio-electrical impedance analysis (BIA);[487]

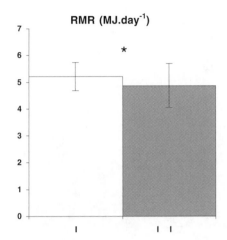

**FIGURE 12.2**
Changes in resting metabolic rate (RMR) before (I) and after (II) weight loss ($-5.4 \pm 1.2$ kg) during 6 months of a mixed hypocaloric diet. * indicates ($p < 0.05$). (Based on data from Ref. F11.)

41% of obese males and 13% of obese females increased their obesity index after temporary improvement of obesity status after 1 year. Fat and lean body mass did not change significantly, irrespective of the increment of obesity index. This was due to the increase of lean body mass during growth. These observations indicate the importance of a range of body composition measurements.

Maffeis, Schutz, and Pinelli indicated that the thermic response to a meal (TEM), which is lower in obese children than in controls, significantly increased after a slimming diet up to the values of controls, that is, to $73 \pm 30$ kJ.[538] These results support the hypothesis of a moderate thermogenic defect in some obese children, representing a consequence rather than an etiological factor of obesity during growth (Figure 12.3).

Total antioxidant capacity (TAC) and plasma levels of lipid soluble antioxidant vitamins ($\alpha$-tocopherol and $\beta$-carotene) are decreased in obese children. The effect of reduction treatment lasting 20 weeks on TAC was followed-up in obese children aged $16.7 \pm 1.2$ years. After a weight loss of $10.4 \pm 4.6$ kg, the plasma level of TAC normalized in contrast to those subjects who maintained or even increased their body weight during the same period.[580]

### 12.2.3 Administration of Supplementation in Reducing Diets

The use of supplements in conjunction with a weight reduction diet can help to reduce the energy content and promote satiety during meals and curb hunger between meals.[822] With respect to the prevention of obesity, it is recommended that fiber intake during growth be increased gradually up to the

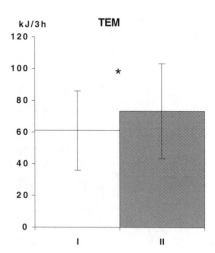

**FIGURE 12.3**
Changes in the thermic effect of mixed liquid meal (TEM) before (I) and after (II) weight loss by a hypocaloric balanced diet. * indicates ($p < 0.05$). (Based on data from Ref. F25.)

RDAs, and children be helped to adapt to eating sufficient fresh fruit and vegetables. A safe range of fiber dietary intake for children over age 5 years is up to 10 g per day. This range is considered safe even for children and adolescents with marginal intakes of some vitamins and minerals, and provides enough fiber for normal laxation. This is a difficult task for many people, especially considering the relative ease of availability of various types of junk food, which rarely include sufficient fiber and other healthy items. However, a diet too high in fiber is contraindicated during growth, although such a risk is limited given the nature of common diets available in industrially developed countries. The possible prevention of some chronic diseases including obesity can also be considered as due to an increased fiber intake.[823]

The effect of a diet with unprocessed wheat bran was studied in obese children. Blood glucose and immunoreactive insulin (IRI) concentrations using oral glucose alone, or combined with 15 g of unprocessed wheat bran, were measured during an oral glucose tolerance test. The latter combination significantly reduced body weight, blood glucose, and plasma IRI concentrations at 30 min of the tolerance test. These results support the inclusion of bran in the diet of obese children during reduction treatment.[824] Other results indicate the importance of an increased ratio of carbohydrates in children's diet, and a reduction in energy intake at the time of the main meals in the prevention of obesity.[210]

Vido et al. assessed the inclusion of glucomannan (1 g twice a day) in the diet of a group of children with an average age of 11.2 years and a placebo in the diet of the control group.[825] During the 2-month study period, all children followed a normo-caloric diet. At the beginning of the study, the drug and placebo groups were comparable. At the end of the study, the mean overweight of the drug group decreased from 49.5 to 41% and that of the placebo group from 43.9 to 41.7%. Decreases in both groups were significant. The only significant difference between groups was a reduction of some serum lipids. It was suggested that this metabolic alteration may derive from a primary decrease of α-lipoprotein, most likely because of inadequate water intake. Children on the placebo diet only displayed decreased triglycerides and Apo-b-lipoprotein.

### 12.2.4  Risks of Hypocaloric Diets

An uncontrolled restriction of food intake can cause deficiencies in obese children. This phenomenon was followed in a group of obese children and adolescents before and after a 13-week treatment with a hypocaloric balanced diet (HCBD) or a 10-week treatment with a protein-sparing modified fast diet (PSMF). The energy intake provided by HCBD and PSMF was calculated to be 60 and 25%, respectively, of the recommended dietary allowances (RDAs) for age and gender. No further supplementation was provided. The composition of the diet was assessed using a visual memory system for dietary intake recall before starting the weight-loss system. Both diets produced significant weight loss with a significant reduction in the arm muscle area of the PSMF group. After treatment, no significant changes were observed in serum Fe, ferritin, and transferrin in both groups, whereas erythrocyte zinc content increased significantly in both the HCBD and PSMF groups, along with an improvement in the erythrocyte index. A significant increase in plasma zinc was also observed in the PSMF group.[826]

### 12.2.5  The Effect of Hypocaloric Diets on Cardiovascular Parameters

Echocardiography was used to assess changes in cardiac characteristics in a group of obese adolescents.[827] The group lost a mean of 13.9 ± 4.3 kg, representing a decrease of 15.5 ± 5.0% of initial body weight. Serial measurements of intra-ventricular septal thickness (ST), left ventricular wall thickness (LVWT), and left ventricular volume assessed by standard m-mode echo cardiographic methods over 14 weeks, showed only slight insignificant changes (Figure 12.4).

In another study, surface electrocardiographic (ECG) parameters were followed in obese children aged 12.2 years, before and after a conventional low calorie diet containing an average of 525 ± 109 kcal.[828] The mean loss of body weight was 5.7 ± 1.6 kg. All electrocardiograms were within normal limits; however, a change in the ECG pattern was noted after weight loss. Heart rate and the QT interval decreased (Figure 12.5) and there was a tendency toward a rightward shift of the front plane QRS axis and a leftward shift of the horizontal plane QRS axis. Therefore, weight reduction in obese children and adolescents is associated with significant changes in ECG pattern.

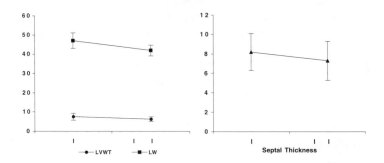

**FIGURE 12.4**

Changes of intraventricular septal thickness (ST, mm) before (I) and after (II) weight loss (–13.9 ± 4.3 kg) in obese adolescents after a 14-week diet (LVWT, left ventricular wall thickness; LVV, left ventricular volume). (Based on data from Ref. F34.)

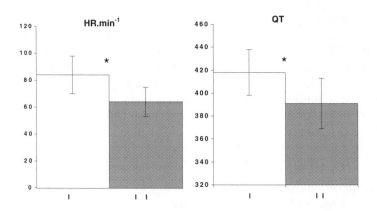

**FIGURE 12.5**

Effect of weight reduction (–5.7 ± 1.6 kg) on heart rate (HR) and surface electrocardiogram (QT interval, msec) of obese boys and girls (average age 12.2 ± 1.7 years), before (I) and after (II) reduction. * indicates ($p < 0.05$). (Based on data from Ref. 35.)

The effect of weight reduction on blood pressure using a hypocaloric diet has also been confirmed in obese children. Both systolic and diastolic blood pressure were significantly reduced. A long-term dietary intervention study of a group of obese adolescents showed a marked increase in erythrocyte sodium levels and maximal frusemide-sensitive sodium and potassium fluxes, but no changes in cell potassium or water and no effect on lithium-sodium counter-transport. These parameters are sensitive biochemical markers of human essential hypertension. A correlation between the decrease in percentage of body fat and the increase in cell sodium content suggests a link between the metabolic effects of reduced food intake and control of erythrocyte cation handling. Changes in body weight, especially weight loss, are important in studies of erythrocyte transport in spite of the fact that the mechanisms linking dietary energy restriction and changes in erythrocyte cation metabolism are unknown.[829]

The effect of sodium intake on the regulation of blood pressure in obese adolescents was followed after a 2-week period on a high-salt diet (greater than 250 mmol. Na.day[-1]) and a low-salt diet (less than 30 mmol.Na.day[-1]).[830] When the obese adolescents changed from the high-salt to low-salt diet, the obese group had a significantly greater mean change in arterial pressure (−12 ± 1 mm Hg) than did the non-obese group (+1 ± 2 mm Hg), (p < 0.001). The variables that best predicted the degree of sodium sensitivity were fasting plasma insulin level, the plasma aldosterone level while on the low-salt diet, plasma norepinephrine level while the high-salt diet was being given, and the percentage of body fat.

In this study by Rocchini et al.,[830] after 20 weeks of treatment, the subjects who lost more than 1 kg of body weight had a reduced sensitivity of blood pressure to sodium difference from the value during a high-salt diet to a low-salt diet. These results support the hypothesis that the blood pressure of obese adolescents is sensitive to dietary sodium intake and that this sensitivity may be due to the combined effects of hyperinsulinemia, hyperaldosteronism, and increased activity of the sympathetic nervous system.

## 12.6 Changes in Respiratory Parameters after Weight Reduction

As mentioned in Chapter 6, a number of respiratory parameters are changed in obese children and adolescents. A group of children and adolescents with medium to severe essential obesity was followed before and after a reduction diet lasting 6 months. More than one third of the subjects showed pathological values of peak expiratory flow (PEF) and/or forced expiratory volume (FEV) before dieting. All female subjects normalized their respiratory parameters after 6 months of the reduction (that is, forced vital capacity (FVC), and also PEF and FEV), while five of the seven males still had pathologic respiratory indices in spite of comparable weight loss.[831] These results indicate that obesity can cause a significant number of pathological changes in respiratory parameters in growing individuals. Improvements are not guaranteed when excess weight is reduced using a diet-only approach.

Morbidly obese children commonly suffer from sleep-associated breathing disorders that appear to be reversible after a reduction of weight. Hypopnea, obstructive sleep apnea, and the respiratory disturbance index improved significantly after a reduction of weight, but central sleep apnea did not.[832]

### 12.2.7 Changes in Biochemical and Hormonal Parameters after a Hypocaloric Diet

The positive effect of weight reduction on serum lipids has been repeatedly confirmed in numerous studies using various programs of obesity treatment. For example, family-based behavioral obesity treatment lasting 6 months showed greater weight reduction changes in obese children compared to a control group.[787] Simultaneously, a reduction of fasting serum triglycerides (TG) and TC levels, and an increase of HDL-C was found. After 5 years of follow-up of a small sample of children comprising the experimental group, improvement in relative weight and fitness from 6 months to 5 years was also associated with improvement in lipoprotein profiles.

A study of obese children aged 5.3 to 9.9 years of age in Spain showed increased serum lipid levels (total and lipoprotein cholesterol, triglycerides, apoprotein A1 and B).[569] After diet treatment lasting 6 months, the values of total body weight, BMI, and skinfolds (triceps and subscapular) decreased significantly. In subjects who responded well to this treatment, increased serum levels of HDL-C and Apoprotein A1 were found (Figure 12.6). The results indicate that prepubertal obese patients show alterations in lipid profiles; this is not correlated with anthropometric parameters, but a reduction in BMI and skinfold thicknesses also improved lipid profiles. Initial pathological serum lipid levels in subjects who responded well to the treatment were normalized, but in those who did not reduce weight, no positive changes in serum lipids were revealed.

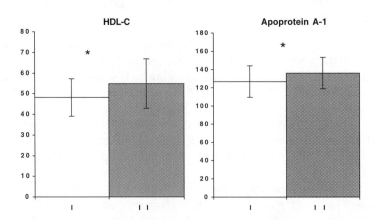

**FIGURE 12.6**

Changes in serum lipids (HDL-C, Apoprotein A-1) in obese boys aged 5.3 to 9.9 years, before (I) and after (II) reduction dietary treatment. * indicates ($p < 0.05$). (Based on data from Ref. F28.)

A longitudinal study of obese children with initially increased serum lipid levels and plasma insulin concentrations, but a lower HDL-C/TC ratio, showed a decrease in relative weight by 15.8% over the first year of reduction treatment, with a parallel decrease of TG and plasma insulin. HDL-C and HDL-C/TC ratio increased simultaneously. These changes remained stable over the second year of observations. At 5 years, the obese subjects still had a reduced weight (12.8% lower than initially) and a higher serum level of HDL-C.[833]

Similar results were gained in a study of the effect of a weight reduction regimen by diet in grossly obese children aged 15 years.[834] Mean weight loss was 9.6 ± 2.1% of the initial body weight. Highly significant decreases in TC, LDL-C, HDL-C, TG, HDL3, and Apolipoprotein B concentrations were also observed, while HDL2 concentrations remained almost constant. These observations showed that the decrease of HDL-C that occurs after weight loss due to treatment of obese adolescents with a hypocaloric diet does not result in a decrease in the anti-atherogenic HDL2 sub-fraction.

A special study of the effect of a reducing diet, either with or without enrichment by polyunsaturated fatty acids, was conducted across 8 weeks in children aged 12.5 ± 1.2 years.[835] The results showed a similar reduction in weight following both diets. TC, LDL-C, and Apo-B concentrations were also reduced after the diet enriched by polyunsaturated fatty acids, but there were no major changes in HDL-C levels.

As mentioned in Chapter 9, the GH-IGF axis is significantly altered in individuals with exogenous obesity. Most changes in the peripheral IGF system appear to be independent of GH secretion modifications. Results of a longitudinal study of prepubertal children with exogenous obesity before and after weight reduction on a calorie-restricted diet revealed that not all of the observed abnormalities were reversed with a significant reduction in the BMI SD score.[596]

In a study by Wabitsch et al.,[642,836] after 6 weeks of treatment by dietary restriction (1032 ± 125 kcal.day[-1]), obese girls lost 8.1 ± 2.0 kg, showed a significant increase in IGF-II and BP2, and a reduction of IGF-1, BP1, BP3, and IGF-I/IGF3. The ratio BP1/BP2 was ameliorated by caloric restriction. The decrease in IGF-I/BP3 ratio after weight loss, indicating a decrease in biologically active IGF-I, may contribute to the explanation of impaired growth velocity in obese children after reducing therapy with a restricted diet.[836]

In another study, obese girls aged 15.0 ± 1.1 years, with BMI 31.1 ± 3.8 kg.m[-2] had increased levels of IGF-I, IGFBP-I, IGFBP-2, and IGFB-3 and normal values of IGF-II.[836] After weight reduction by 8.1 ± 2.0 kg, IGF-II and IGFBP-2 increased, and IGF-I, IGFBP-1, IGFBP-3, and the ratio of IGF-I/IGFBP-3 decreased significantly. Fasting insulin levels were positively correlated with IGF-I, but inversely with IGFBP-1 and IGFBP-2. IGFBP-2 was associated with several metabolic parameters, namely, an inverse correlation with uric acid and triglyceride levels. The ratio IGFBP-2 to IGFBP-1 was inversely correlated with total cholesterol and LDL-C. In addition, IGFBP-2 was inversely correlated with the waist-to-hip ratio. The results indicate, too, that the decrease in IGF-I/IGFBP-3 after weight loss could be partially responsible for the impaired growth velocity revealed in obese growing subjects during treatment with restricted diets. Low values of IGFBP-2 and high IGFBP-1 levels are associated with an unfavorable atherogenic risk profile.[836]

Overweight children aged 12.5 ± 1.9 years placed on a short-term weight reduction in a camp setting showed decreased plasma leptin levels from 16.5 ± 9.8 ng.ml$^{-1}$ to 10.0 ± 8.6 ng.ml$^{-1}$ after a significant fall in BMI. Plasma ApoA-1 and HDL-C were independent predictors of leptin concentrations during weight loss. HDL-C transports a variable portion of leptin in circulation.[837]

The results of a hypocaloric diet were addressed in obese children in two visits to an outpatient department at intervals of 1.5 and 4 years. The group of children with a successful response to the hypocaloric diet treatment (a significant loss of weight) showed a decrease in the plasma levels of apoprotein A1 and B, triglycerides, non-esterified fatty acids (NEFA), and insulin together with an increase in the level of HDL-C. These changes were not significant in the group of obese children who did not lose weight. For obese children who had high levels of TC despite reduction treatment, the pathologic plasma profile did not show any change, while the group with a high level of insulin showed a significant increase of apoprotein A1 and B, and TC and HDL-C. The group in which insulin levels became normal after treatment showed a good development of the biochemistry parameters studied.[838] Weight loss due to a reduction diet decreased insulin resistance and increased insulin sensitivity in children aged 10.1 years.[839]

A significant reduction in serum triiodothyronine (T3) concentration in obese children, along with a REE decrease, was found after 6 weeks of a weight reduction program. The T3 concentration reduction, which was parallelled by FFM loss, could be responsible for RMR reduction.[578]

The effectiveness of a family-based, multi-disciplinary, behavior-modification program was also adapted for obese adolescents with insulin-dependent diabetes mellitus (IDDM). The measurement of skinfolds and glycated hemoglobin revealed positive results of reduction therapy, including an improvement of body image and self-esteem in these adolescents.[840]

As indicated by the above-mentioned results, there appears to be a certain bias when a restricted diet is used. There is a risk of a slow-down of growth in height and lean body mass and also changes in other parameters that are not always desirable. Therefore, another approach is preferred. That is, energy intake should not be drastically reduced but rather, an increase in total energy expenditure is preferred. A prescribed diet should certainly be introduced, but the intake checked and the composition of food monitored. Along with diet, a system of exercises plus an overall increase in physical activity level and modified lifestyle should be used.

## 12.2.8    Changes in Immunological Parameters after Hypocaloric Diet

Some of the changes in immunological parameters due to obesity were mentioned in Chapter 11. Kravets and Kniazev studied immunological parameters and serum lipids in obese children aged 3 to 14 years who were treated using a hypocaloric diet enriched by polyunsaturated fatty acids (PUSFA from non-purified oil, 0.5 to 1.0 g of weight as an additive to vegetable and meat salads, twice a week).[841] A statistically significant increase in the relative content of T-lymphocytes and theophylline-resistant lymphocytes with simultaneous reduction of null cell numbers was revealed in children with PUSFA. This might be associated with their stimulating effect on the differentiation of young precursor-lymphocytes, or with the release of T-lymphocyte receptors due to normalization of lipid metabolism, as found in other studies. This study showed the positive effect of a diet with PUSFA that acted as an immuno-stimulant on the general condition of children.

## 12.3    Exercise Management

The effect of exercise alone on obesity has less of an impact than low-calorie diets.[47] However, such diets are not always considered suitable for treating obesity during the growing years.[18,31,51,61]

The importance of physical activity to health, and specifically to weight management, is undisputed.[10,18] The increasing prevalence of overweight and obesity is always attributed to a number of factors, the most important of which is the decline in physical activity participation by children and adolescents with a concomitant increase in inactive behaviors. As mentioned in Chapters 1 and 2, inactive leisure pursuits such as television and video viewing and playing computer games are commonly coupled with the consumption of energy-dense snack foods high in fat and sugar. These practices combined with the use of cars or public transport instead of walking, plus an extensive array of labor-saving devices in the home and workplace, have resulted in reduced energy expenditure in daily tasks. These changes have had a significant impact on individuals of all ages.

The incorporation of exercise into weight control programs increases the chance of success (as determined by weight loss or weight maintenance) along with numerous additional benefits.[10,473,842] Individuals can increase their energy expenditure, protect against the loss of fat-free mass, improve cardiorespiratory fitness, muscular strength and endurance, and self-esteem through appropriate and regular physical activity.[10,18,846] Other positive benefits of regular physical activity may include appetite control, an increased likelihood of maintenance of weight loss, desirable changes in body composition, and potential changes in fat cell development.[843] Physical activity also has the capacity to improve lipoprotein profiles and normalize carbohydrate metabolism.[844] An increase in energy expenditure through physical activity is critical in view of the sedentary lifestyles pursued by many individuals and the documented reduction in metabolic rate coincident with diets low in energy.[845-847]

Exercise in isolation, or in combination with a reduction in energy intake, is recommended in the treatment of obesity, particularly in cases where an individual may benefit from improvements in energy efficiency.[848] Increased energy efficiency is characterized by a normal energy intake; therefore, it may be dangerous to attempt to modify the diet further and thereby potentially compromise an individual's health status.[849]

A more marked reduction in energy intake alone can cause the loss of lean tissue as well as fat.[31,51,61] There is also the potential for reduced basal metabolic rate (BMR), as tissues are broken down to provide energy. The loss in protein may be derived from muscle tissue and/or skeletal tissue.[850] There is some evidence to suggest that hypocaloric diets that contain a large proportion of carbohydrates might minimize the protein deficit.[851] However, both the sensitivity of different tissues to carbohydrate intake and also the degree of protein loss from all tissues are uncertain.

Exercise can contribute to maintenance and potential increase in lean body mass while maintaining a decrement in fat mass.[766] When diet alone is the focus of weight reduction, up to 25% of lean tissue may be lost.[852] This loss may be reduced to approximately 5% by adding exercise.[853]

Interestingly, there have been relatively few intervention studies that have considered the benefits of strength training in obese children. The best results for changes in BMI and body composition and also physical fitness, behavioral improvement, and psychological status were gained in summer camps where both diet and physical activity are monitored.[18,61,189,316] Treuth et al.[415] assessed fitness and energy expenditure following a school-based, low-volume strength training program. Obese prepubertal girls in this study demonstrated gains in strength but no significant increase in energy expenditure. The authors recognized that energy expenditure might be further enhanced with a more intensive strength-training program and/or in combination with aerobic training. In this study, more attention was given to the influence of the activity on energy expenditure, as measured by 24-hr calorimetry and doubly labelled water (DLW), although aerobic capacity was also assessed.

Bar-Or has suggested that resistance training in children is safe as long as they adhered to necessary safety precautions.[757] Importantly, an experienced adult should supervise such training. Weight-bearing exercise has also been considered alongside resistance training. The benefits of weight-bearing activities during the formative years have been well established, but less attention has been paid to the effects of such activity for those who are overweight or obese. There are numerous ways in which innovative activities that combine resistance with loading can be used with great effect. Examples of the types of tasks that can be employed with children are outlined in Chapter 13.

A range of studies have shown that exercise alone can reduce body weight, both in experimental animals and humans. Gradual reductions in weight are possible with modest modifications to activity patterns.[854–856] It may be postulated that an early exercise intervention with growing individuals may produce a greater opportunity for the enhancement of weight reduction and most importantly, exposure to the necessary skills and practices required to enjoy and sustain a long-term commitment to physical activity. Motivation to move plays an essential role in the introduction of an increased physical activity and exercise regime for an obese child unadapted to greater workloads.[857] Also, structured exercise using resistance training of various kinds can be applied in a multi-disciplinary outpatient treatment program for obese children and youth.[858]

Wilmore reviewed studies of exercise and obesity with physical activity as the sole focus and reported that loss of body weight was minimal.[855] There is general agreement that while weight loss is low, there are usually increases in lean body mass and reductions in body fat. While exercise may have a negligible impact on total energy expenditure when basal requirements account for a major proportion of energy utilization,[859] there is a contribution to prolonged post-exercise metabolic rate that may influence weight loss.[846,860]

A multiple regression model was used by Barbeau et al.[861] to analyze the results of the effect of 4 months' exercise training (4 days per week, 40 min per session, heart rate $157 \pm 7$ beats per min, energy expenditure $946 \pm 201$ kJ per session). Body fat decreased and bone mineral density increased, and most importantly, frequency of exercise and decrease in energy intake resulted in an increase in vigorous activity.

Increased physical activity can be augmented through an increase of common everyday activities such as more walking and stair climbing. In adults,[862] 30 to 40 min of activity, such as walking, working in the yard or at home can significantly reduce cardiovascular disease risks. Such modifications may be more effective than programmed exercise for long-term weight prognosis. Exercise programs should promote increased energy expenditure and the loss of body fat and the maintenance of lean body mass, and also lead to permanent increases in habitual physical activity. Greater benefits in both weight loss and adherence have been reported in studies that have used behavioral approaches to weight management.[846,863]

Weight control programs for children have traditionally been employed in a variety of settings with the involvement of health professionals and other adults.[473,864] Sole practitioners and various group approaches have included school personnel, such as physical and health educators, medical practitioners, exercise physiologists, nutritionists, dietitians, and parents. A team approach to weight management is generally superior to an ad hoc approach and is likely to help maximize potential long-term success for the patient.[473,865]

Physical activity and exercise are therefore considered important components of a weight-reduction program, mainly in combination with a diet.[10,18,409] However, in adulthood, the efficiency of physical activity alone as a means of significant weight reduction is doubted, especially with respect to its permanent effects.[189,399] Experience shows that even in the individuals who are very disciplined, resistance to fat loss generally occurs before body composition is comparable to that of normal-weight individuals.[866] However, even a small weight loss can reduce health risks resulting from obesity.

Evidence of the effect of exercise on obesity and its role in the prevention of excess fatness is still inconclusive. As mentioned previously (Chapters 4 to 6), some authors have not found a significant relationship between physical activity, energy expenditure, and overweight and obesity. In most cases, such studies of physical activity and energy expenditure were limited to a brief, short-term analysis rather than the more desirable longitudinal approach.

On the other hand, other studies have provided evidence of the positive outcomes of increased physical activity and exercise, especially in the treatment of the obese.[55,189,774] This has been best illustrated by longitudinal studies in the same growing individuals over longer periods of development.[18,316,450,452]

As mentioned in Chapter 1, there are numerous methodological problems and constraints concerning the measurement of physical activity levels during growth and development.[49,409,867] These problems may be magnified, for example, in young children where methods used are more appropriate to older individuals and if implemented in children, provide unreliable data. Therefore, evaluation of the effect of physical activity and exercise has the potential to be biased.

The growing organism is in a unique situation with respect to physiological control. A restricted energy intake is not recommended due to the potential negative effects on the growth and maturation processes. In contrast, an increase in the level of activity is easier to achieve in most children compared with obese adults. This is particularly the case when there is not an excess deposition of fat. In the case of severe or morbid obesity, the situation is more similar to that in older individuals. For such individuals, special restricted diets must be introduced along with a modified exercise program.

When defining an adequate physical activity and exercise regime for children, it is necessary to consider that spontaneous physical activity and the type of games preferred change during growth.[2] There are differences in children's play as a function of age, growth and developmental stage. It is very important to recognize the potential contribution of games and play to the maintenance of energy balance and a desirable body composition in young children. Three kinds of play physical activity with consecutive age peaks can be distinguished. The first, *rhythmic stereotypes*, peaks in infancy and is hypothesized to improve control of specific motor patterns. This is followed by *exercise play* that peaks in the preschool years and is related primarily to strength and endurance; the evidence for possible benefits for fat reduction and thermoregulation is less clear. Finally, *rough-and-tumble play* is characteristic of the childhood years and peaks in middle childhood. This type of play has a distinctive social component and primarily serves dominance functions.[868] The latter two forms of play are more prevalent in males.

The role of these types of children's activities in the maintenance of a desirable body composition warrants further analysis.

### 12.3.1 Relationships between Body Composition and Fitness during Growth

A parallel study of the development of aerobic fitness, blood pressure, and BMI revealed significant interrelationships, indicating the possible implications for the development of interventions directed to the primary prevention of hypertension.[869] A study of free-living children aged 5 years at baseline who were followed over a mean of 19.7 months was undertaken. Aerobic fitness was assessed during a treadmill test. Mean systolic blood pressure was 95.3 mm Hg (SD ± 8.38) and increased by 4.46 mm Hg per year. Mean diastolic pressure was 53.9 mm Hg (SD ± 5.81) at baseline and did not change significantly. Children in the highest quintile of increase in aerobic fitness had a significantly smaller increase in systolic blood pressure when compared to children in the lowest quintile (2.92 vs. 5.10 mm Hg.year$^{-1}$; $p < 0.03$). Children in the lowest quintile of increase in BMI did not differ significantly in the rate of increase in systolic blood pressure compared to children in the highest quintile (3.92 vs. 4.96 mm Hg.year$^{-1}$). In a multiple regression model including baseline systolic blood pressure, aerobic fitness, height, BMI, and other co-variates, a greater increase in fitness ($p < 0.01$) and a lesser increase in BMI were associated with lower rates of increases in systolic blood pressure. In a similar multi-variate analysis, an increase in fitness was also associated with a lower rate of increase in diastolic blood pressure ($p < 0.02$). These data indicate that development of an increased level of aerobic fitness, along with reduced adiposity, which is usually the result of an increased level of physical activity and exercise, can contribute to a reduced deposition of fat and a lower BMI, plus a reduced risk of hypertension.[869]

Trends in relation to the development of spontaneous physical activity and fatness, for example, during the preschool years, show a clear relationship in normal-weight children. The natural trend for changes in subcutaneous fat in children is as follows. When the level of spontaneous physical activity is high, there is maintenance of the same amount of subcutaneous fat in girls and a slight decrease in boys which precedes adiposity rebound.[61,201,255,293,299] The development of body composition and aerobic power runs parallel in growing boys indicating the peak of natural physical fitness and lowest deposition of fat during puberty.[18,56,68,522]

### 12.3.2 The Effect of Regular Exercise during Growth

The significant effect of physical activity from an early age was shown in the Framingham Children's Study in which children aged 3 to 5 years together with their parents were followed longitudinally.[870] Physical activity was monitored using an electronic motion sensor. On average, girls who had a higher than median activity level increased their triceps and subscapular skinfolds by 1.0 mm, while inactive girls gained 1.75 mm. Active boys lost an average of 0.75 mm in the triceps skinfold, while inactive boys gained 0.25 mm. When age, television viewing, energy intake, baseline triceps, and parent BMI were adjusted for, inactive preschoolers were 3.8 times as likely as active preschoolers to have an increasing triceps slope during follow-up. As predicted, a lower level of physical activity already had a considerable effect on fatness.

A number of studies have demonstrated the significant effect of increased physical activity in preschool children.[68,405] Children who were more spontaneously active tended to have a lower BMI, smaller deposition of fat, higher cardiorespiratory fitness, and significantly increased serum level of HDL-C (Figure 12.7).

In a study of French children aged 10 years, Deheeger et al. considered physical activity, body composition, and food intake.[871] A validated activity questionnaire covering the previous year, nutritional intake (dietary history method), and anthropometric measurements (including triceps and subscapular skinfolds) were assessed. BMI, arm muscle, and arm fat areas were calculated from these measurements. Anthropometric measurements and dietary intake were recorded for the same children at the age of 10 months and every 2 years from the age of 2 years. At the age of 10 years, more active children had a significantly higher energy intake due mostly to a higher energy intake at breakfast and in the afternoon. Greater energy intake was mainly due to a higher ingestion of carbohydrates. Intake of fat was similar in both active and less active children, as was protein. In spite of the higher energy intake in the active group, BMI values were the same in both active and less active children, but body composition indicators were different (Figure 12.8). Active children had less fat and a higher ratio of fat-free, arm mass. Adiposity rebound (AR) occurred later in active children. Body fatness was positively related to the time spent watching television and playing video games. The higher level of physical activity resulted in an improved growth pattern and a more desirable body composition with less fat, in spite of a higher intake of energy.

Previous longitudinal studies have followed the effect of increased exercise on the development of body composition in healthy adolescent boys aged 10.8 to 17.7 years with normal nutritional status. Subjects varied significantly with respect to the physical activity regime that was controlled and supervised. The most active group of boys was enrolled in regular sports training (track and field, basketball) for at least 6 hr per week. Training was supervised and boys achieved a high level of exercise intensity during the whole school year. In contrast, the least active group participated in physical education at school (as did more active boys) and less than 2 hr of unorganized physical activity per week. Under such circumstances, both groups of boys developed an almost identical BMI, but in the active group, the absolute and relative amounts of lean body mass were significantly larger than in the least active boys. Consistent with this result, the relative and absolute amounts of

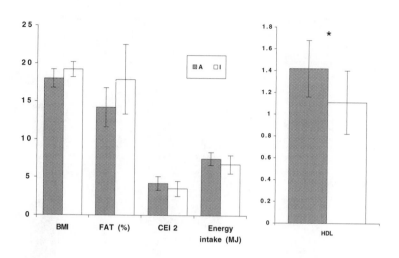

**FIGURE 12.7**

Body mass index (BMI), percentage of stored fat (% fat), cardiorespiratory efficiency (CEI 2), energy intake and serum HLD-C level (mmol/l) in active (A) and inactive (I) preschool children (CEI 2 = kpm/HRw – 10 × HRr; kpm = body weight × height of step × 150; HRwr = heart rate during 5 min mounting the 30-cm high step, and during 3-min recovery; HRr = heart rate at rest, 150 = 30 mounts/min × 5). * indicates ($p < 0.05$). (Based on data from Ref. F22.)

stored fat were also lower in the active boys (Figure 12.9). These differences were significant from the second and third year of the study. The most active boys also reported eating more than the least active boys.[18,334,872]

In summary, the active group was significantly leaner and the least active group was significantly fatter. These results were confirmed over a longer period of development with sustained differences in the physical activity pursuits of the different groups. It must be stressed that the differences in the level and intensity of exercise undertaken were marked. Aerobic power was also highest in the boys who performed the greatest amount of exercise.[875] This value did not decrease after puberty as in the least active boys. These results are evidence that the level of physical fitness of the less active children has already peaked and begun to decline in adolescence.[18,55,328,333,872–875] There are no comparable data available for similar long-lasting (8-year) studies involving the same adolescents with such different physical activity interventions during which body composition (using hydrodensitometry), VO$_2$ during a maximal workload on a treadmill, and physical performance were tracked.[18,875]

Numerous other studies have demonstrated the significant effect of organized, supervised, and sufficiently intensive exercise under the guidance of physical educators or trainers on body composition in normal-weight adolescents. Such changes are commonly paralleled by adjustments in aerobic power and functional capacity.[2,49,340,653,875,876] In motivated self-monitoring children and adolescents, sufficient activity may be achieved without any external

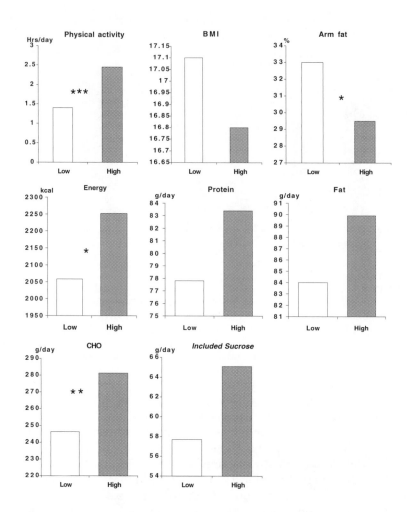

**FIGURE 12.8**

Differences in physical activity, anthropometric characteristics (BMI, arm fat), and intake of energy and macronutrients in 10-year-old boys with low and high physical activity level (hours per day). * indicates ($p < 0.05$), ** ($p < 0.01$), *** ($p < 0.001$). (Based on data from Ref. F36.)

support. However, during growth, this type of self-imposed discipline is rare and some assistance is preferable. For most children and adolescents, continued participation would only be sustained under proper professional supervision of physical educators and/or exercise physiologists. More research is needed to optimize the exercise prescription in children specific to the enhancement of improvements in body composition and functional capacity. Guidelines for exercise prescription along with suitable activities are provided in the following chapter.

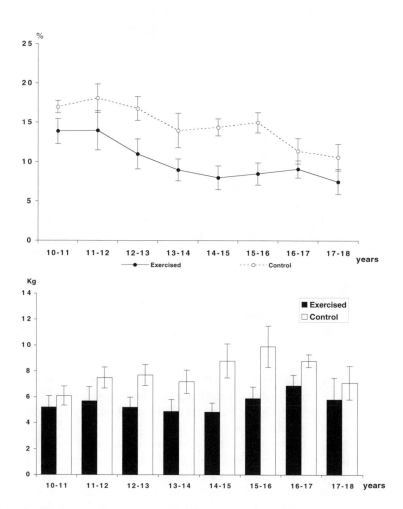

**FIGURE 12.9**

A longitudinal study of the development of stored fat: top (percentage); bottom (densitometry) in regularly exercised and control inactive boys. The differences between groups are significant from the 2nd until the 8th year. (Based on data from Refs. F6, F37–41.)

## 12.3.3 The Effect of Sports Participation

Studies of young athletes show that energy balance is maintained under conditions of higher energy output, for example, in gymnasts, hockey players, skiers, sprinters, divers, and runners.[877] Energy intake was consistently higher than the RDAs for normal youth of the same age with the exception of female gymnasts and sprinters. Protein intake in athletes was usually markedly higher. However, BMI was average (that is, around the 50th percentile) and there was a significant reduction of stored fat in the young athletes when compared to untrained individuals. Lean body mass in relative and absolute values was greater than in inactive peers of the same age. With respect to fatness and aerobic power, the best results were found in young athletes adapted to weight-bearing activities in dynamic (track and field, and running) and endurance sport disciplines.

A study of energy balance using heart rate monitors to register heart rate during the training day was conducted on male gymnasts who had a higher level of general fitness, including aerobic power. The experimental period lasted 1 week during a sport training camp in the mountains where the exercise intensity was even higher than during a normal school year and was supplemented by other activities such as hiking. Energy expenditure (EE) was derived using regression equations established for each individual on the basis of the relationship between heart rate and oxygen uptake during treadmill testing. Simultaneously, energy intake (EI) was measured using food diaries supplemented by interviews, and a computer program was used to provide detailed analyses of local foodstuffs. BMI was comparable to normal-weight boys of the same age. The energy balance during one week showed correspondingly increased values for both EI and EE. When EE is low, such a balance is more difficult to achieve, and commonly EI does not correspond to EE.[877]

This study illustrates that energy balance can be achieved without negative changes in body composition and BMI even with a higher energy intake compared to RDA. Despite an ability to balance energy values and an abundance of dietary intake, deficiencies in micronutrients and imbalances in macronutrients were found in some subjects.

Energy balance studies using the DLW technique have shown that the RDAs for young athletes may be too high for normally active children and adolescents living in affluent societies.[878] Commonly, the process of adaptation to an increased workload includes an increase in metabolic efficiency. Some measurements in adults have shown that energy intake does not always increase correspondingly to energy output without any negative consequences with respect to BMI, body composition, and level of performance. It is unusual for athletes in intensive training to have an inadequately high intake of energy. A higher intake of energy in an active, well-adapted athlete can be problematic if the intensity of training fluctuates.

A 5-year longitudinal study has shown the same increase in height, weight, and BMI in female gymnasts and a control group of untrained girls. The latter group showed a significant increase in the sum of 10 skinfolds. In the trained girls (Figure 12.10) the weight increment consisted of additional lean, fat-free body mass.[18,328]

Other observations in young female athletes aged 11 to 15 years have revealed a decreased body fat, lower levels of serum free fatty acids (FFA),

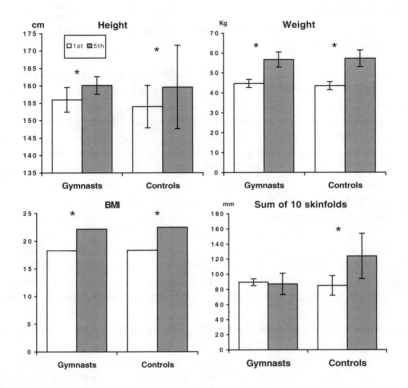

**FIGURE 12.10**
Differences in developmental height, weight, BMI, and sum of 10 skinfolds at the beginning and after 5 years of a longitudinal study in gymnasts with regular training and in control girls without training. Only sum of 10 skinfolds after 5 years is significantly higher in control girls without training compared to gymnasts. * indicates (p < 0.05). (Based on data from Ref. F6.)

and higher levels of HDL-C and Apo A-1.[879] Gymnasts are characterized by a low percentage of body fat and a lower percentage of stored fat. The most significant correlations were found between body composition and Apo A-1, and Apo A-1/Apo B in swimmers and control girls in whom the range of body fatness was much larger than in gymnasts. These examples show a beneficial effect of exercise, provided it is regular and sufficiently intensive. As yet, there has been no clear indication whether exercise training increases fat utilization in obese adult subjects at rest, or during exercise, or a 24-hr period. With regard to this problem under conditions of developed obesity, further studies are needed.[880] Aerobic training induced an increase in the response of plasma and subcutaneous adipose tissue concentrations of glycerol to β-adrenergic stimulation in adult obese subjects, in spite of the lack of changes in body weight and aerobic power.[881]

## 12.4 Studies of the Effect of Exercise on Experimental Animal Models

The classic study of Mayer et al.[882] showed that rats who exercised daily for up to 1-hr decreased food intake and body weight when compared to sedentary control rats. When the exercise duration increased beyond 1 hr, food intake was increased but only to the extent that body weight was maintained. At exhaustive levels of exercise (6 hr), both food intake and body weight decreased. Longitudinal physical conditioning studies in humans also show no change in caloric intake with mild to moderate intensity exercise training.[883] Evidence from a study of rats running voluntarily in rotation wheels showed an increase to 130% of energy intake as compared to sedentary rats. In contrast, when considered on a short-term basis, exercise suppressed food intake to prevent a potentially dangerous disruption of energy substrate homeostasis. Both exercise and food intake increased free fatty acids (FFA) and glucose in the blood of the laboratory animals. These changes, combined with the exercise-induced alteration in glucagon, corticotropin-releasing hormone (CRH), and body temperature, may contribute to the short-term anorexic effect of exercise.[884]

As shown in another experimental model, the effect of the adaptation to exercise, that is, increased energy output, was a decreased ratio of stored fat and an increased metabolic activity of the adipose tissue. The release of FFA *in vitro*, both spontaneously or after various doses of adrenaline added to the medium, was significantly higher from the adipose tissue of the animals adapted to daily exercise since weaning (daily running on a treadmill) (Figure 12.11). This was compared to control and/or hypokinetic animals (restricted to small cages). The intake of food was always highest in the exercised animals. The effect of exercise is relatively smaller, but that of reduced activity is relatively greater in growing animals. The reverse situation is apparent in adult or older animals; that is, a relatively greater effect of exercise and smaller or no effect of hypokinesia.[18,68] Restriction of activity has a more significant effect on metabolic activity of the adipose tissue in a developing organism during growth, resulting in an increased deposition.[18] This follows from the natural trends in physical activity during ontogeny. During growth, spontaneous activity is generally high and decreases with aging. Therefore, hypokinesia has a more marked effect during growth.[18]

The activity of lipoprotein lipase (LPL) was significantly higher in the heart and skeletal muscle of exercised animals. The inflow rate of applied FFA labelled with $^{14}C$ was spontaneously greater to the heart and skeletal muscle of the exercised animals but lower to their adipose tissue (Figure 12.12). In the control animals the situation was the reverse; that is, the highest inflow rate of labelled FFA was to the adipose tissue. Under the same conditions, i.e., after application of labelled FFA, the $^{14}CO_2$ expired by animals adapted to regular dynamic exercise was significantly greater (even under conditions of

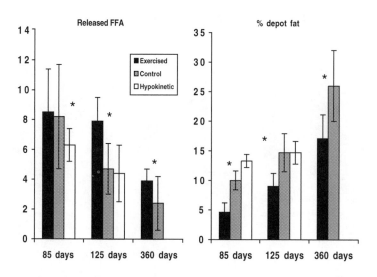

**FIGURE 12.11**

The comparison of released free fatty acids *in vitro* (incubation 60 min; FFA meq/1 ml medium/1/g adipose tissue) from the epididymal adipose tissue of exercised (daily run on a treadmill 2 h), control, and hypokinetic male rats (kept in small spaces 12 x 8 x 20 cm since weaning) aged 85, 125, and 360 days. * indicates ($p < 0.05$). (Based on the data from Ref. F5.)

anesthesia and complete physical rest) compared to control, inactive rats or to hypokinetic animals adapted to the restriction of activity. These data indicate a greater ability to utilize lipid metabolites, which results in a lower deposition of fat. The adaptation to regular exercise changes not only body composition and the ratio of stored fat, but also has more profound consequences with respect to the metabolic activity of tissues, especially the adipose and muscle tissues of experimental animals.[18] The results of some studies of trained and untrained adults are in agreement with the conclusions from this experimental model.

## 12.5 The Effect of an Interruption to Regular Exercise on Body Adiposity

The effect of exercise and sports training on the fluctuation of fat consumption with a change in the intensity of physical activity and training has been studied. A more detailed 5-year longitudinal follow-up of the female gymnasts mentioned above (Figure 12.13) revealed the following results. Girls were measured several times during the year (at the beginning of the

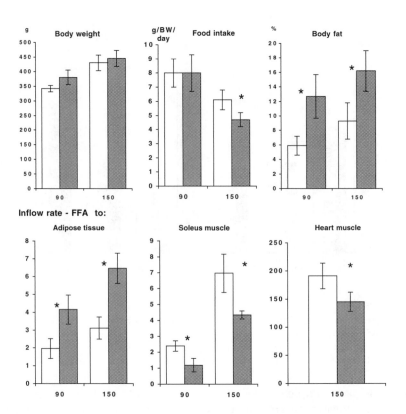

**FIGURE 12.12**

Comparison of body weight, food intake, percentage of body fat (%), and inflow rate of applied labelled fatty acids (14C; mmol.g$^{-1}$.min$^{-1}$) to adipose tissue, the soleus muscle, and the heart in exercised (clear) and control, inactive (shaded) male rats aged 90 and 150 days. * indicates (p < 0.05). (Based on data from Ref. F6.)

school year when the usual level of intensity of gymnastics was maintained, and before and after a summer camp in which training intensity was increased). The changes in body fat in response to a change in intensity of activity was rapid (Figure 12.14). Energy intake was also significantly higher during the period of intensive training when fat decreased, then declined significantly during the period of inactivity when fat increased.[18,885] The reduction in training intensity and energy expenditure was sufficient for an increased deposition of fat, in spite of a reduced energy intake. Girls in this study were not elite athletes but pupils of a sport school. Similar changes are even more apparent in some former athletes of any age who stop their exercise training.[873,886]

Corresponding changes are also seen following injury. A failure to maintain the usual level of sports training may result in an enhanced deposition of fat. When such a situation lasts for an extended period of time, development of obesity is a risk. For example, a longitudinal follow-up of an

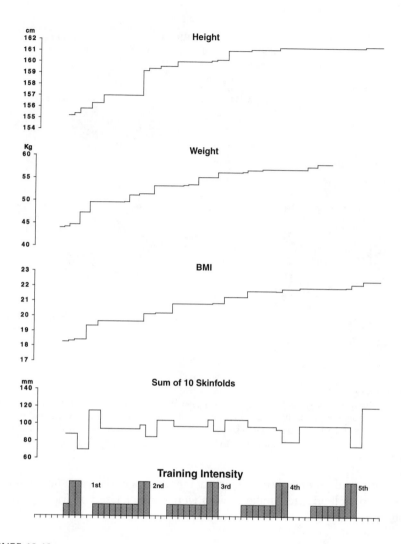

**FIGURE 12.13**
Development of height, weight, BMI, and sum of 10 skinfolds in female gymnasts assessed longitudinally over 5 years fluctuating training intensity. (Based on data from Ref. F6.)

adolescent football player who interrupted training because of a shoulder injury showed the development of obesity, a deterioration of aerobic fitness, and dyslipoproteinemia.[887]

Excess deposition of fat may occur in individuals who have adapted to an increased aerobic workload, had a permanently high energy output, and then decreased their activity level suddenly. An increase in body weight, BMI, and adipose tissue may result even when food intake decreases simultaneously.[18] The data of Jeszka et al.[888] have shown that young ballet dancers have lower proportions of fat and a high negative-energy balance. Food intake based on 24-hr recall data was lower than energy output (24-hr monitoring of heart

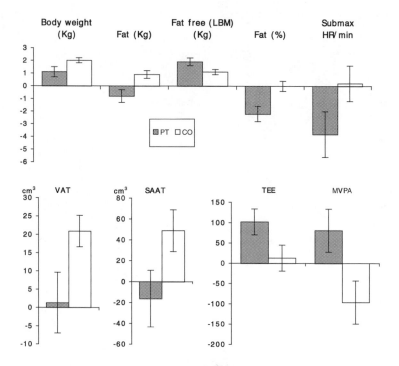

**FIGURE 12.14**

Effect of 4 months of physical training (PT) in obese children compared to control subjects (CO); changes in body weight, body composition, heart rate during submaximal work load (submax HR.min[-1]), visceral adipose tissue (VAT), subcutaneous abdominal adipose tissue (SAAT), total energy expenditure (TEE), and moderate to vigorous physical activity (MVPA) over 4 months. (Based on data from Ref. F42.)

rate) compared to control school girls of the same age. This situation was only possible in well-adapted subjects who were characterized by increased metabolic efficiency.[889]

## 12.6   The Effect of Exercise on Obese Children and Youth

The classical observations of Mayer showed that when lean and obese children claimed the same physical activity and exercise (as reported by questionnaire data) over the same time period, filming showed much less real motor activity and movement in the obese.[24] Even when exact measurements of the energy expenditure were conducted using the DLW technique, only information on the total amount of energy output per day, but not about the fluctuating intensity of workload during various periods of the day, could be determined.

A certain level of activity that achieves a well-defined threshold intensity for a sufficient duration and frequency during micro- and macrocycles can produce changes in body composition and aerobic power, or improvement of some motor skills and physical performance level.[18,406] These principles also apply to obese children. Stimuli that do not meet and exceed the necessary threshold values cannot cause significant physiological change. There appear to be contradictory conclusions on the effect of physical activity and exercise with respect to fatness and fitness with some studies confirming a positive effect while others do not.

Many obese individuals of all ages may be active, but generally for only very short periods of time and at an intensity that is too low. This level of effort does not increase the pulse rate above certain critical levels (which vary for different age groups). Importantly, such lower level activity does not significantly increase the intensity of workload and energy output of the organism over a certain period of time, which is a necessary stimulus for the development of systems involved in the improvement of functional capacity and physical fitness. When the fitness level of an individual is not improved, exercise remains a difficult and unpleasant task and the level of spontaneous physical activity and willingness to exercise remain low. As a consequence, any loss of fat mass may be minimal or non-existent.

The challenge in weight management programs is to encourage an increase in energy output in individuals whose previous experience of physical activity may not have been pleasant. Therefore, it is critical that particular care be taken to plan and implement an appropriate physical activity and exercise regime.[2,189] The prescription issue is considered in some detail in the following chapter. It is important to remember that much of the increased energy output in overweight subjects is due to higher energy costs of weight-bearing activities as a function of the higher load caused by excess body fat. The level of motor activity of an obese child during an average day is usually much lower than in normal-weight peers with a failure to achieve the necessary level of exercise in spite of an increased daily energy expenditure.[873,874]

Specificity in terms of the nature and intensity of exercise and training is essential for weight management.[10] A 5-month longitudinal study on the effect of a strength-training program on obese prepubertal girls showed a significant increase in muscular strength and $VO_2$ peak values ml.min$^{-1}$ (based on a treadmill test). However, this was not true when $VO_2$ was a co-variate for total and/or fat-free body mass. The same applied to resting metabolic rate (REE) measured by room respiration calorimetry. There were no changes in total energy expenditure (TEE), activity-related energy expenditure (AEE), and physical activity level (PAL), either unadjusted or adjusted for total and/or fat-free body mass. This long-term, school-based strength-training program favorably influenced muscle strength but did not increase the daily energy expenditure in obese girls.[415] These observations provide further justification for well-designed exercise programs conceived to improve body composition through a reduction in excess fat.

The effect of physical education on fourth and fifth grade elementary school students has been studied by Sallis et al.[890] Project SPARK compared the results of three different offerings of physical education: (1) usual physical education classes, (2) classes using classroom teachers, and/or (3) with physical education specialists. There were no significant group differences in triceps and calf skinfolds and/or in the sum of these skinfolds. However, there was a trend for higher skinfolds in group 1. After 2 years of intervention there was a tendency for lower levels of fat in groups 2 and 3, but the differences were not significant.[890] The intensity of exercise may not have been sufficiently different between groups.

A study of energy expenditure in preadolescent children over 4 years showed that the main determinants of change in fat mass adjusted for fat-free mass were gender (greater gain for girls), initial fatness, and parental fatness. None of the components of energy expenditure (total and physical activity-related energy expenditure measured by doubly labelled water) were inversely related to changes in fat mass. That is, reduced energy expenditure was not in this case the cause of the increased stored fat.[891]

There is widespread consensus that interventions to manage obesity should be implemented as early as possible. This approach has been employed in a number of studies in preschool children in various countries. As mentioned previously, the effect of a higher level of participation in physical activity is apparent in preschool age children. HDL-C serum level was significantly higher in active preschoolers compared to their inactive peers, along with a trend for a lower BMI, percentage of fat, and greater cardiorespiratory efficiency as assessed by a modified step test. Active preschoolers also have a higher energy intake.[61,68]

In Thailand, the effect of a school-based exercise program was tested in children in the kindergarten system (day care centers). Exercise consisted of a 15-min walk prior to morning classes and a 20-min aerobic dance session following the afternoon nap, three times per week, over 26 weeks. The prevalence of obesity at the end of the study decreased in both groups who exercised (from 12.2% at baseline to 8.8% of cut-off values for triceps based on National Center for Health Statistics guidelines) and control groups (from 11.7% to 9.7%). Differences between groups were not significant. Girls in the exercise group had a reduced likelihood of an increasing BMI slope than the control girls. The study concluded that exercise can prevent BMI increases in girls and prevent obesity in preschoolers.[892]

From a physiological perspective, the greater strain of participation in physical activity by the obese results in an increase in heart rate. A lower ventilatory threshold in the obese causes higher energy demands for the same activity compared to lean children. Further, this feature also contributes to obese individuals displaying more fatigue, greater stress, and heart rate increases during the same running workload. Each of these factors may contribute to a reduction in spontaneous physical activity and a preference for quieter and more sedentary activities for the majority of time.[215,241] This creates a vicious cycle and the chance of further decreases in activity levels that are already low.

Despite some pessimism with respect to the effect of exercise in the treatment of obese children, the role of physical activity and exercise has been stressed in many contexts as a suitable component in the management and treatment of the condition during childhood.[893,894] Data on dietary intake and activity regimes in children and adolescents have shown that the main lifestyle change in industrially developed countries has been a lower level of activity in all age categories, commencing with young children.[31,51,63,182,217,895] There is widespread acceptance of the link between activity and health as purported in the following statement: "America needs to exercise for health."[896]

In obese Chinese children, the exercise prescription deemed suitable to reduce weight and fatness has been defined according to the level of aerobic power development in local children. This equates with 50% of $VO_2$ max, 1 hr per day for 12 weeks with a frequency of 5 days per week. The exercise should be rhythmical and aerobic such as running and various endurance game-type activities, for example, football.[897]

Gutin has demonstrated the effect of exercise as a function of alternating periods of training and detraining.[264] After the initial 4 months of training, percent body fat decreased but increased after another 4 months of interruption in training. In the reverse situation, the group with no training during the initial four months maintained and/or slightly increased percent fat, but decreased after another 4 months of training. The Amsterdam Growth and Health Longitudinal Study (AGAHLS) showed a significant inverse relationship between the development of fat mass and the level of physical activity corrected for dietary intake.[459] Therefore, the level of fat mass provided was predictive of activity status. As is the case in childhood, the promotion of physical activity in adolescence appears to play a significant and effective role in the early prevention of obesity.

The effect of reinforcement on the behavior of obese children should not be underestimated. Following an individual choice between sedentary activities or movement-based physical activities, obese subjects were either positively reinforced for decreases in high-preference sedentary activity or were punished for high-preference sedentary activity, had access to high-preference sedentary activity restricted, or had no contingencies on activity (control group). Preference for sedentary activity decreased in the reinforced group, but increased in the restriction and/or control group.

### 12.6.1 Changes in Body Composition and Fitness after Exercise Intervention

Other studies have supported the significant effect of exercise on body composition in physically active children.[898] Black obese girls aged 7 to 11 years were subdivided according to physical activity and exercise regimes. Body composition, measured by DXA, skinfold thickness, circumference measurements, and the level of physical performance (evaluated during submaximal treadmill testing) showed a significant improvement. An increase in aerobic fitness and a 1.4% decrease of stored fat was reported after a period of organized aerobic training lasting 10 weeks with five sessions per week. The results were compared with a group that was engaged in weekly lifestyle discussion without formal physical training. The status of the latter group with respect to most fitness and body composition parameters measured remained unchanged.[898] This study demonstrated that it is possible to manage fat deposition and physical fitness through organized and controlled physical training in terms of intensity and frequency, even without diet intervention.

Another study showed that exercise results in a considerable weight loss with a normo-caloric diet. Weight management treatment was provided to a group of Cuban children who used a diet with energy content corresponding to the expected body weight-for-height. Growth and puberty occurred normally under these conditions of obesity management and lean body weight and muscle area of the mid-upper arm increased. A substantial loss of fat, as indicated by a reduction of fat weight, relative fatness, and fat areas of mid-upper arm was also achieved. Body weight-for-height shifted to lower percentile channels. These results underline the favorable effect of this obesity treatment approach which does not alter the normal course of development in obese children during the most rapid period of growth.[899] The potential bonus at this time is to profit from the reverse of the commonly observed decrease in fatness during this period of development.[18,61] This preadolescent period is one of the most preferable growth periods for obesity treatment because interest in spontaneous physical activity is still high and a decrease in lean body mass that often occurs when reduction therapy is applied later is absent.[18,56]

Body composition and heart rate also changed significantly in a group of obese children provided with physical training over a 4-month period compared with a control group with no training (Figure 12.15). A marked decrease in total and visceral adipose tissue was apparent after physical training.[876] The results of this and other studies using organized and sufficiently intensive exercise reveal the positive effect of an increased energy output in obese and also normal-weight children. The decrease in heart rate was most pronounced in subjects with the greatest weight loss.[876] Maximal and recovery heart rate also decreased following weight loss in obese children.[876]

Training for 4 months also increased bone density more than during the following 4 months without training. There were no differences in dietary intake during these periods.[900] The same period of training (4 months) did not result in significant changes in hemostatic factors (fibrinogen, plasminogen activator inhibitor 1, and d-dimer). Children with greater adiposity and concentration of hemostatic factors before the physical training period showed greater reduction in hemostatic variables after physical training than did children with lesser values.[901]

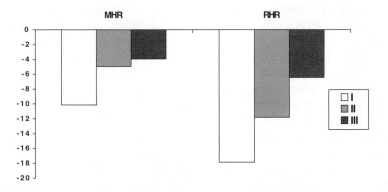

**FIGURE 12.15**

Effect of weight loss in obese children on the decrease of maximal (MHR) and recovery heart rate (RHR); (I) the change in children with greatest, (II) medium, and (III) least weight loss. (Based on data from Ref. F42.)

The physical activity regime provided for obese children's needs to be well planned and implemented in order to achieve maximum benefits regarding loss of fat mass and potential readjustment of BMI and functional capacity. The effect of an increase in exercise and a decrease in sedentary behaviors was followed in children aged 8 to 12 years.[66] After 4 months, significant differences in the reduction of the percentage overweight were observed between the sedentary and the exercise groups. After 1 year the sedentary group had a greater decrease in percentage overweight than the combined and the exercise groups and a greater decrease in percent body fat. All groups increased their fitness level. Children in the sedentary group increased their tolerance of high-intensity activity and reported lower food intake than did children in the exercise group. These results confirm that the reduction of time spent in sedentary activities without greater energy output can considerably increase weight loss during growth.

### 12.6.2 Hormonal, Circulatory, and Metabolic Changes after Exercise-Induced Weight and Fat Reduction

Participation in a light training program can improve the situation of obese children with respect to glucose homeostasis, insulin dynamics, and risk factors for coronary artery disease. A study of obese adolescents aged $13.3 \pm 1.4$ years before and after 15 weeks of supervised mild intensity exercise found that body weight, fatness, and $VO_2$ peak did not change when compared to the initial values. However, relative changes after training appeared in mean serum glucose and peptides, fasting glucose (–15%), total glucose response (–15%), peak insulin response (–51%), total insulin response (–46%), peak C-peptide response (+55%), and total C-peptide response (+53%). Systolic and diastolic blood pressure were also reduced as well as the serum level of LDL-C. Increases in hepatic insulin clearance (decreased insulin levels along with C-peptide levels) might also be the result of adaptation to an increased training load. While the intensity was low, the duration was sufficient to provide improvement. These results confirm that in obese children, health risks may be reduced by exercise even without more marked weight and fat loss.[902]

The failure to achieve weight loss might not be a sign of weakness in the management program but the result of changes in body composition. There was a simultaneous increase in lean body mass at the expense of fat. This result highlights the importance of testing other parameters, at least for the encouragement of the obese individuals. This finding also supports the rationale for weight stabilization in many children. If this is achieved with exercise and following metabolic changes, improvements are enhanced with the probable outcome being a significant improvement as the individual grows into his/her final height. Plasma leptin concentration changes in obese children are also related to exercise.[903]

### 12.6.3   The Effect of Exercise on Cardiovascular Parameters

Participation in an exercise-training program during a period of 1 year resulted in a significant decrease in body weight, degree of obesity, and resting heart rate in obese children. Left ventricular wall thickness did not change. The total voltage in SV1 + RV5 decreased after 3 months of training but returned to pre-training voltage after 1 year of training. There was no change after 2 years of training. In summary, these results indicate that after 1 year of exercise training, resting heart rate decreased while left ventricular end-diastolic dimension and left ventricular mass increased.[904]

The beat-to-beat variability in electrocardiogram intervals (heart-period variability) is a marker of cardiac autonomic activity that can predict arrythmias and mortality rate in animals and adults. This parameter was followed in obese children before and after a period of sports training over a 4-month period (5 days per week, 40 minutes per day) during which weight reduction occurred.[905] Cardiovascular fitness was assessed using sub-maximal heart rate during supine cycling. Resting heart-period variability was measured in the same position and body composition was evaluated by DXA. A pre-training to post-training change score was computed for each variable. A lower sub-maximal heart rate and percent body fat were found in the group who reduced weight and fat due to training compared to the group of obese children without training during the same period. All changes in the trained group indicated that physical training alters cardiac autonomic function favorably by reducing the ratio of sympathetic to parasympathetic activities.

In another study group of children treated by exercise, in addition to reductions in body weight and fat, multiple risks of coronary heart disease were lowered. This was not apparent in obese children treated only by diet and behavioral therapy.[729]

The effect of a regimented training program was followed in obese boys aged 10 to 11 years over 4 weeks with five 1-hr sessions of 45 min cycling per week at 50 to 60% of a predetermined maximal oxygen capacity ($VO_2$ max).[906] The aim of the study was to determine whether there would be an increase in the level of spontaneous physical activity of the obese subjects. No significant change in body weight, percentage of fat, sleeping metabolic rate, spontaneous activity (assessed by heart rate recording), and activity questionnaires was observed after 4 weeks. There was a 12% increase in average daily metabolic rate as measured by DLW, half of which can be explained by the energy cost of training and the rest by an increase in energy expenditure outside the training hour. These results indicate that training leads to considerable augmentation in the overall energy expenditure in obese children without a change in their level of spontaneous physical activity.

As indicated in an earlier section, many studies of obese children using hypocaloric diets have reported decreases in serum lipids along with weight and fat loss. A minimal decrease of fat-free, lean body mass is also often reported. Following the restriction of food intake, HDL-C commonly does not change or decrease, as is the case for TC, LDL-C, and TG. Changes were not found after a long-term supervised aerobic exercise program with obese children aged 11 years. The activity program was undertaken over 1 year during daily school life. The intensity of training consisted of running 20 min, seven times per week at a pace that corresponded to the blood lactate threshold. No dietary intervention was used in this study. After 1 year, the obesity index had decreased significantly. Weight loss was due only to stored fat reduction as confirmed by the simultaneous increase of lean, fat-free body mass. One of the most important results was a significant increase of HDL-C serum level in both boys and girls after the first year, an increase of 16 and 19%, respectively, with a slightly lower value in the second year. After 2 years, a significant decrease of TG was still found in obese girls. Serum TC was unchanged in both genders after 2 years. This study provides a clear indication of the benefits of a long-term supervised aerobic exercise program in obese children with respect to weight loss, positive body composition changes, and concomitant improvement of lipoprotein metabolism.[907]

## 12.7 The Results of Combined Treatment of Diet and Exercise

The combined approach of a comprehensive behavioral lifestyle program including increased exercise, a protein sparing modified fast, and a balanced hypocaloric diet has been suggested by numerous authors.[18,30,31,33,47,50,51,53,55,56,61,181,189,303,408,873,908,909] This multi-disciplinary approach is normally most effective in weight reduction of youth.[910] The physician and also the physical education specialist are essential in the treatment of obesity; in order to achieve long-standing control of overweight, a combination of the changes in eating and activity patterns using behavior modification techniques is recommended. A combined focus is also best for preventing obesity in the younger age groups.[47,473]

The combination of an increased energy output and controlled energy intake has been repeatedly recommended as the best means of obesity management during growth and development.[34,217,774,786,911–915] In adults, the same approach may be difficult to implement, particularly in the presence of co-morbidities. The implementation of a well-planned exercise and physical activity program can provide a significant benefit in relation to weight loss, improvement in fitness, motor skill, and posture.[10,12,339] This approach has been used to great effect in many countries.

In a study of Japanese children, more than 70% of boys and 40% of girls grew out of obesity if they could self-monitor their lifestyle on a permanent basis with a simple checklist. Instructions included eating meals three times per day on a regular basis with one snack per day. Children were advised to avoid extra dishes, juices, oily and greasy food additives, sugar and candies, but to consume in excess of 200 ml of milk per day. The energy density of the diet was not prescribed. Children were also instructed to play no more than 1 hr of video games alone at home per day. Each child (or family) was instructed to keep a checklist to evaluate (yes or no) if they observed the seven items (three meals and one snack a day, no night eating, video games, and housework duty) on a daily basis. The subjects visited the outpatient clinic at 3-month intervals for anthropometric measurements and reported on their checklist scores. Advice and instruction were provided to the family at each visit. The mean duration of the treatment was 526 days, with children being an average age of 8.95 years. This serves as a model for a combined mode of treatment and management commonly used within a pediatric department without special facilities.[782] Personal involvement plays an essential role in the outcomes of this process.

With regard to physiological acceptability during the period of growth and development, this combined method of treatment needs to be promoted. The decrease of weight, BMI, excess fat, serum lipids on the one hand, and an increase of aerobic power, physical fitness, and most often, HDL-C, were revealed after this treatment of obese children and adolescents. In another study of obese German children, physical training improved long-term weight control. In conjunction with such a program, it is important to assess the psychosocial background as a clue to lack of motivation in some children.[916]

A non-restrictive approach to diet is tolerated by many as it may establish more favorable conditions for the changes in lifestyle necessary for permanent improvement of the child's morphological and functional status. Such an approach can also be more easily applied under the conditions of outpatient treatment.[917] Some therapeutic procedures using a restricted diet alone have resulted in slightly reduced growth, especially with respect to body height. The advantages of treatment with a diet adequate for preservation of growth and maturation rates of children during early stages of obesity have also been demonstrated.[918]

Comparisons have been made between procedures comprised of diet, exercise and training, education and psychological support. The only difference between these approaches was the energy content of the diet. The first diet was restricted to 0.17 $MJ.kg^{-1}$ of expected body weight for stature, while, in the experimental group, the diet was fitted to the physiological requirements for age, gender, and physical activity (0.25 $MJ.kg^{-1}$). The results showed that the consumption of restricted diets for 6 months impaired the velocity of growth, maturation, and lean body mass accretion. The incidence of dropout was slightly higher in the restricted group with no relapses registered in the other groups. In the combined approach it was sufficient to reduce risky foodstuffs (fat, sugar, and delicacies) without marked restriction of food intake. This group used exercise of sufficient intensity over an extended period of time.

### 12.7.1 Changes in Body Composition and Fitness following Weight Reduction

The relative success of a combined diet and exercise therapy should be judged using stringent measurements of body composition. Some studies have shown that during weight loss, particularly in more severely obese children and during the later stages of puberty, lean, fat-free body mass may be lost in greater quantities.[18,56,189,328] These results may also be due to simultaneous loss of body water that can indicate a loss of not only fat but also fat-free tissue.

Rolland-Cachera et al.[255] considered the results of a 5-month weight reduction program on obese children. The program consisted of exercise and a low-calorie diet with either a high or moderate protein content. The protein content of the diet did not affect weight loss and change of BMI, which was reduced in both groups.[918]

Body composition measurements using DXA before and after a combined diet and exercise program for 12.8 ± 2.6 year-old children revealed that total weight and fat mass decreased, but fat-free body mass was maintained. The results were not dependent on age, race, gender, or stage of development.[919]

A comparison of the results of a study consisting of diet only, and/or diet combined with aerobic exercise (approximately 250 kcal per session) showed a greater decrease of overweight in the combined group after 4 months. This decrease was –25 ± 13.5% compared to –15.8 ± 10.8% in children treated by diet only. Treatment compliance was also better in the group using both exercise and diet.[470]

Aerobic power ($VO_2.min^{-1}.kg$ body weight$^{-1}$) increased significantly along with a decrease of BMI and percentage of body fat in adolescent boys after 7 weeks of treatment (Figure 12.16).[18] The program included a monitored diet (1700 $kcal.day^{-1}$) with sufficient liquids (unsweetened) and an all-day

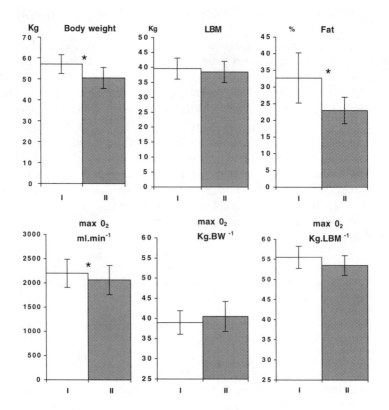

**FIGURE 12.16**

Changes in morphological characteristics (body weight, lean body mass (LBM), percentage of stored fat (%) and oxygen uptake in absolute and relative ($O_2$ ml.min.kg$^{-1}$ body weight, and/or kg lean (LBM), fat-free body mass during maximal workload on a treadmill in obese pre-pubertal boys and girls before (I) and after (II) reduction treatment by monitored diet and exercise in a summer camp. * indicates ($p < 0.05$). (Based on data from Refs. F6, F8, F43, F44.)

exercise program with sports activities suited to children with varying degrees of obesity.[18,68,189]

As a function of the intervention, improvements in functional capacity were found with respect to the economy of work during standard workload testing on a stationary bicycle. The economy of work and energy efficiency are lower in obese children compared to normal-weight children.[18,56,316] Following a reduction of weight and fat through exercise and diet in a summer camp, the energy cost of the same activity and workload was significantly decreased. The heart rate during the same workload was lower, oxygen uptake decreased, and a higher economy of work and mechanical efficiency was recorded (Figure 12.17). Vital capacity also increased significantly after a combined treatment program (Figure 12.18).[18,56,316,874,918,920] Similar results were gained during further follow-ups. The heart-rate responses during a standard workload on a bicycle ergometer test before and after weight reduction are

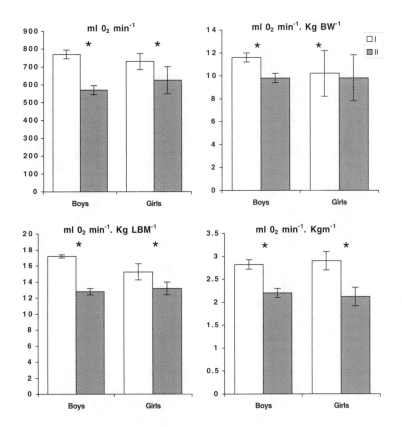

**FIGURE 12.17**

Changes in oxygen uptake in absolute and relative values ($O_2$ ml.min1.kg$^{-1}$ body weight, and/or lean body mass, LBM, and ml $O_2$.min$^{-1}$.kgm$^{-1}$ of performance) over a standard workload in obese pre-pubertal boys and girls before (I) and after (II) reduction treatment by monitored diet and exercise in a summer camp. * indicates ($p < 0.05$). (Based on data from Refs. F6, F9, F43.)

displayed in Figure 12.19. These results confirm that both peak performance and standard workloads (characteristic of tasks in everyday life) can be executed more favorably after reduction of excess fat.

Significant changes in functional parameters and body composition have been shown in relation to changes in the intensity of exercise in summer camps. The camps feature a combined diet and exercise program run each school year for 4 consecutive years. The combined effect of adequate intensity exercise on adiposity and fitness is displayed in Figure 12.20. During the earlier period of obesity treatment (11 to 12 years of age), there was a reduction in percentage of stored fat but lean FFM did not decrease. However, there was some reduction of lean body mass later. In spite of LBM being greater in obese than in normal-weight boys in a longitudinal study during the same growth period, it is preferable not to lose LBM. Therefore, it is more beneficial to start at a younger age during the initial phases of obesity. The

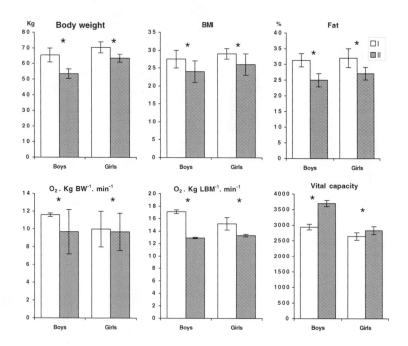

**FIGURE 12.18**

Changes in body weight, BMI, percent body fat, and oxygen uptake as related to total body weight and/or lean, fat-free body mass, and vital capacity over a standard workload in obese pre-pubertal boys and girls before (I) and after (II) reduction treatment by monitored diet and exercise in a summer camp. * indicates (p < 0.05). (Based on data from Refs. F6, F9, F43.)

changes in ventilation, oxygen uptake, and energy cost of the same standard workload were similar to results in other studies of obese children. Both the amount and distribution of fat changed after the treatment in summer camps.

The centrality index (subscapular/triceps ratio) was evaluated in obese girls and boys during a 3-year longitudinal study. The results of this index indicate that the reduction of fat was always relatively greater on the trunk than on the extremities of the obese girls (Figure 12.21).[53] Similar changes in the centrality index were observed in obese boys of the same age.

A 12-month reduction program that was comprised of individual nutritional counselling, guidance on physical activity, and supportive therapy found weight loss in the majority of children. $VO_2$ max.kg lean body mass$^{-1}$ (LBM) increased from 44.2 to 47.1 ml.min$^{-1}$.kg LBM$^{-1}$ (p < 0.025). There was no change in time allocated to physical activity during the weight reduction period but the children's participation in training teams of sports clubs increased. These data also indicate that obese children are less fit than children of normal weight, especially apparent with aerobic power. A loss of body fat improved the level of physical fitness significantly.[445]

The effects of diet-plus-behavior (DB) treatment and DB-plus-exercise treatment (EDB) were compared with respect to changes in basal metabolic

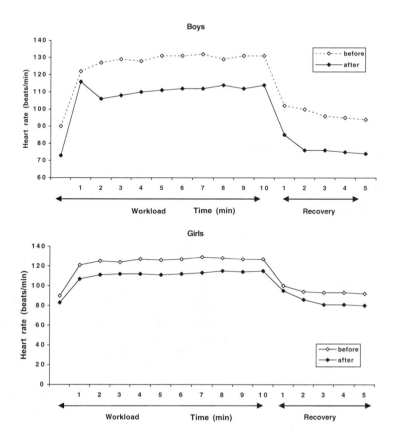

**FIGURE 12.19**
Changes in heart rate of obese boys and girls during standard, submaximal workload on a bicycle ergometer before and after weight reduction treatment by exercise and diet in a summer camp. (Based on data from Refs. F6, F8, F9.)

rate (open circuit spirometry) and body composition (hydrostatic weighing). Dietary management and restriction were based on the dietary exchange program and behavior management including record keeping, stimulus control, and reinforcement techniques. Aerobics 50 min per day, three times per week comprised the exercise component. Results revealed small but statistically significant improvements in body composition for both groups. However, no significant differences were found between groups. All control subjects gained a significant amount of body weight.[921] Following weight reduction, RMR and FFM decreased although no differences were found in RQ when comparing obese and control children.[392]

A weight loss program including exercise resulted in desirable improvements such as a decrease in resting systolic blood pressure and exercise diastolic and mean blood pressure.[922] In addition, obese adolescents showed structural changes in the forearm resistance vessels. These structural changes were reversed to a large extent in the weight loss program.

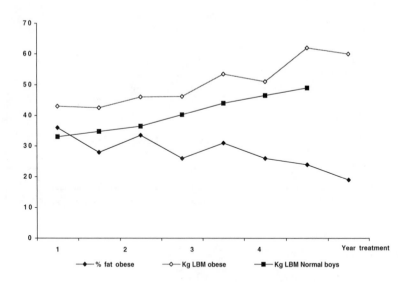

**FIGURE 12.20**

A 4-year longitudinal study of body composition changes (lean, fat-free body mass and % stored fat, measured by hydrodensitometry with simultaneous measurements of air in lungs and respiratory passages) after weight decreases in obese boys following four consecutive treatments through monitored diet and exercise programs in summer camps, and after weight increases during the school year (lean body mass kg in obese boys, lean body mass kg in normal-weight boys during the same growth period (longitudinal data), and percentage of stored fat in obese boys. (Based on data from Refs. F6, F44.)

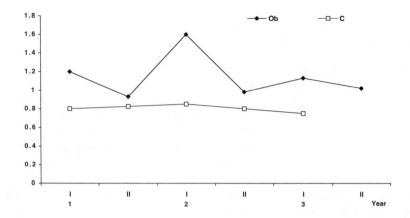

**FIGURE 12.21**

A longitudinal study (11 to 14 years) of centrality index changes (subscapular/triceps ratio) in obese girls over 3 years, before (I) and after (II) the reduction therapy by diet and exercise in a summer camp compared to values for normal-weight girls (C). (Based on data from Ref. F9.)

Blood pressure distribution in a group of obese adolescents was skewed 1 SD to the right of normal children (p < 0.01) after weight reduction due to a program of energy restriction and behavioral change alone, and/or combined with exercise. This distribution was no longer different from that in normal-weight adolescents.[922]

Other studies have shown that behavioral and public health models including dietary and exercise interventions can have long-term effects in obese juveniles. A modest effect on body weight, fatness, and blood lipids was found and the impact of the interventions endured the 5-year follow-up period.[923]

An evaluation of the effect of a multi-component and multi-disciplinary after-school intervention program in adolescent post-menarcheal girls showed successful results. This was especially the case with respect to reducing the rate of weight gain, reducing body weight by 11.5%, maintaining the pre-treatment amount of lean, fat-free mass, and improved eating and exercise behaviors. Changes in food habits included reduction of energy dense foods, reduction in frequency and amount of food ingested, and eating more slowly. Encouragement and praise from the group leaders played an essential role in weight control. The greatest obstacles to success were boredom, hunger, lack of family and peer support, and having food in sight.[924]

Similarly, positive experiences with a combined treatment and management approach were found in other populations, for example, in Brazilian obese adolescent females. Greater weight loss and a more favorable change in serum lipids and body composition were found in groups combining physical exercise and dietary education.[925]

The combined effect of diet and exercise was also studied in two groups of obese girls.[776] Treatment in the first group consisted of diet only and in the second group regular supervised exercise (walking or running 3 miles, three times per week). Both groups of girls significantly reduced percent overweight after 2 months of this treatment; however, after a further 4 months, girls who exercised still had a reduced percent overweight and improved their level of physical fitness. The percent overweight in girls in the diet-only group decreased during the first period from zero to 2 months but not from 2 to 6 months.

The effect of a weight reduction program on body composition in obese children and adolescents across the pubertal barrier has also been conducted (8.5 to 14.8 years). Lean body mass (LBM) was estimated from the resistance index (RI) and was obtained by bio-electrical impedance analysis (BIA) before and after the 3-week program of weight reduction. All individuals lost body fat during the treatment, whereas the change of lean body mass was heterogeneous. The individual change in body fat was inversely correlated with change in lean body mass. A number of subjects were reevaluated after 4 months. The regain in body weight during this period was inversely correlated with the change of LBM during the weight reduction period. These results indicate that changes in LBM during a weight reduction program can predict the short-term results in those children who manage to maintain or even increase LBM and lose weight only through a decline in stored fat. Changes in LBM during weight reduction seem to predict the long-term outcome; that is, loss of LBM is associated with greater regain of total body weight in the longer term.[926]

The effects of lifestyle modification and exercise in a 1-month YMCA program on body composition and serum lipids were studied in a group of obese sedentary children. The measurements at entry, after the intervention and subsequently, 1 and 4 months after completion, showed a non-significant decrease in body weight and sum of 2 skinfolds and a significant increase in the number of sit-ups and distance covered in a 9-min run. There was no change in flexibility and a non-significant decrease in TC.[927] A longer program would be necessary to consider the continuity of positive changes in morphological, motor, and serum lipid parameters.

Another combination of therapeutic approaches for obesity treatment was used in Cuban children. Children were divided into four groups (diet, exercise only, diet and exercise, and control group). In both genders there was a significant positive effect of exercise on body weight, efficacy index, and a significant interaction between fiber intake and exercise in girls, but not in boys. These results suggest a possible effect of fiber in the diet that may be accentuated by exercise.[928]

### 12.7.2  Serum Lipid Changes

A combined treatment was used in long-term observations of German children aged 9 to 12 years. Children who maintained the nutritional habits introduced during the program and who remained active in sports were able to maintain a desirable body weight.[929] Serum lipid profiles, along with morphological variables have also been best managed by combined strategies using physical activity and dietary management.[930] Whether short-term benefits gained in childhood will continue into adulthood and help to reduce the cardiovascular risks later in life needs to be assessed by further research. A combined reduction therapy using diet and exercise has a significant effect on serum lipids.

A group of obese boys was followed before and after 4 weeks of weight management. A hypo-energetic diet ($0.18$ MJ.kg$^{-1}$ expected body weight for age) and exercise reduced the values of relative fat body weight (calculated by regression equations for 5 skinfolds) and TC, TC/HDL-C ratio. TG decreased but did not reach significance; however, it had a better correlation with the reduction of adiposity (delta% body fat) than the two previously mentioned variables. The increase in lipolysis during the 4-week study is expressed in the significant increase of free fatty acids (FFA) and its correlation with delta% body fat ($r = -0.714$). There was a trend for an increase of HDL-C and a significant inverse correlation with delta% body fat ($r = -0.804$). This study also confirms the efficacy of the treatment by diet and exercise simultaneously to improve not only body weight and composition, but also serum lipid profile and therefore reduce health risks. Treatment efficacy and delta FFA were lower in subjects with lesser adiposity as related to muscle mass at the middle third of the upper arm (measured through energy/protein index).[931] These conclusions concur with other results from experimental models mentioned previously.[61,189,920]

Children treated by diet and moderate exercise during 15 days of hospitalization were assessed with the diet of one group supplemented with fiber. Weight loss was observed in both groups along with the reduction of TC and LDL-C. Triacylglycerols, VLDL-C, and HDL-C did not change in this short timeframe.[932]

The effect of a hypo-energetic diet (0.18 MJ.kg$^{-1}$ expected body weight for age) combined with physical exercise and psychological support was reported in another study of obese children aged 10 to 14 years. Significant changes in total body weight and composition (using skinfold measurements) occurred along with changes in serum lipids and physical fitness evaluated by the efficiency index (EI). Significant correlations were found between the EI values and changes in TC and TC/HDL-C ratio. Although the increase in HDL-C was not significant, the values were highly correlated with EI during the first and second assessments. Differences were found in the magnitude of increase in free, non-esterified fatty acids (delta FFA) which suggest that lipolytic mechanisms were not uniformly impaired. Treatment efficiency and delta FFA were lower in subjects with less adiposity as related to muscle mass at the middle third of the upper arm (measured via the energy/protein index).[933]

After 4 weeks of combined therapy (energy-restricted diet and exercise), the weight loss achieved in a group of obese children was 8.4% of the initial body weight.[933] The values for serum lipids were higher than in normal-weight control children before the reduction treatment and were significantly changed after the treatment. HDL-C was low before and unchanged after treatment. Serum apolipoprotein A-1 level was normal before treatment and significantly reduced after weight reduction (Figure 12.22). Serum apolipoprotein B level was significantly higher before treatment as compared to controls and decreased to the normal range after treatment. The ratio of apolipoprotein B to apolipoprotein A was significantly high at admission and decreased significantly after treatment. Serum apolipoprotein E level was normal but also decreased after treatment. The benefits of an improved serum lipid and apolipoprotein concentration are also important in reducing the risk of future development of atherosclerosis.

There is considerable support for the continued use of exercise in combination with diet for treatment and management of obesity in children and adolescents. However, the limited number of well-controlled studies indicates the need for more research in this area. The potential impact of exercise programs in the prevention and treatment of obesity during growth has been extensively reviewed.[72,935,936] Similarly, the role of the family has been highlighted in the combined treatment by diet and exercise. Future work must address the specifics of exercise prescription including the effect of the

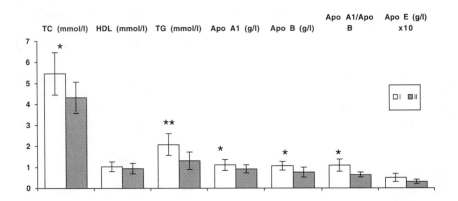

**FIGURE 12.22**

Effect of energy restriction over 4 weeks on total (TC) and HDL cholesterol (HDL-C), triglycerides (TG), apolipoprotein-A 1, B and E, before (I) and after (II) reduction treatment. * indicates (p < 0.05; ** (p < 0.01). (Based on data from Ref. F45.)

intensity, type, duration, and frequency of various exercises. Insufficient information on these factors makes it difficult or even impossible to compare and analyze the results of available studies.

### 12.7.3   Hormonal Changes as a Result of Diet and Exercise

Significant weight loss and decreases in serum leptin and fasting insulin concentrations occurred as a result of obesity treatment.[588,589] There was also a correlation between the reduction of relative body weight and serum leptin but not of fasting insulin. A significant reduction of IGFBP-3 and an increase of the IGF-1/IGFBP-3 molar ratio were also found after weight loss in obese children and adolescents.

Obese Czech children aged 9 to 16 years were admitted to a sanatorium for the treatment of obesity using both monitored diet and exercise suited to severe cases of obesity.[568] Serum leptin decreased significantly after the reduction of weight and BMI along with reduction in lipoproteins and apolipoproteins, systolic and diastolic blood pressure (Figure 12.23). Risk factors for cardiovascular disease and diabetes were therefore also reduced.

In a study involving systematic physical activity together with energy restriction in obese 14-year-old boys, Rychlewski et al.[937] determined immuno-reactive insulin (IRI), C-peptide, fructosamin, and binding of 1251-insulin. Management of exercise and diet resulted in a decrease in body weight, a reduction in stored fat, and an increase in physical efficiency. Insulinemia and insulin-resistance as measured by the amount of 1251-insulin-binding were also reduced by 20%. Over the 3-week period, the obese boys had a daily physical workload on a bicycle ergometer with a load of 1 watt.kg body weight$^{-1}$ lasting 30 min. Diet during this period equated with

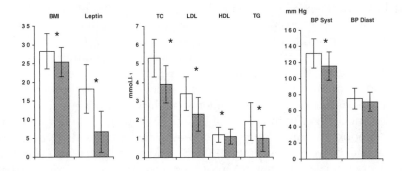

**FIGURE 12.23**

Changes of body mass index (BMI), serum leptin level, total (TC) and LDL-cholesterol (LDL), triglycerides (TG; mmol/l), systolic and diastolic blood pressure before (I) and after (II) 1 month of treatment in a spa, with a diet consisting of 5.217 MJ/day (protein 23%, fat 30%, carbohydrates 47% of energy). Energy expenditure (EE) elevated by 10 MJ/week by exercising 25 min/day at 70% of maximal heart rate. * indicates (p < 0.05). (Based on data from Ref. F46.)

1300 kcal.day$^{-1}$. Testing involved a bicycle ergometer protocol at an intensity of 75% VO$_2$ max.

Glucose-induced thermogenesis was tested in obese children aged 14.3 ± 0.3 years before and after 6 weeks of treatment by diet (5441 to 6279 kJ.day$^{-1}$) and aerobic exercise training (walking, jogging, calisthenics, and swimming) and compared to controls.[938] The thermic effect of 100 g glucose tolerance test (calculated as the area under the response curve for 3 hr in excess of resting metabolic rate) was similar in obese adolescents before treatment and controls. After treatment this value was lower in obese subjects. The area under the response curve for glucose was elevated in obese subjects before treatment compared to controls. Before treatment, the insulin response was similar in obese and controls but it decreased in the obese after treatment. The improvement in peripheral insulin sensitivity after 6 weeks of obesity treatment by exercise and diet and after weight loss was not accompanied by favorable changes in carbohydrate-induced thermogenesis in obese adolescents.

Plasma leptin, TC, and apolipoprotein (apo) A-1 and B were measured in obese children aged 12.5 ± 1.9 years before and after 3 weeks of weight reduction in a special camp.[939] Binding of endogenous and exogenous radiolabelled leptin to lipoproteins was studied by stepwise and continuous density gradient ultra-centrifugation. As in other groups, plasma leptin level was significantly higher in obese than in non-obese subjects and decreased from 16.5 ± 9.8 ng.ml$^{-1}$ to 10.0 ± 8.6 ng.ml$^{-1}$ after weight reduction (p < 0.001). In a multi-variate regression, relative BMI and apo A-1 were significant predictors of baseline leptin and accounted for 38% (p < 0.003) and 15% (p < 0.006) of the variance of baseline leptin concentrations in obese children. The change in plasma leptin associated with weight loss was independently predicted by a difference in plasma HDL-C explaining 29% of the variance of leptin changes (p < 0.0032). A substantial portion of both endogenous and exogenous labelled leptin was recovered with the HDL-C fraction. These results indicate that plasma leptin decreases in obese children undergoing weight reduction. Therefore, plasma apo A-1 and HDL-C, respectively, are independent predictors of leptin concentration during weight loss. HDL-C also transports a variable portion of leptin in the circulation.[837]

Important changes in the levels of insulin, cortisol, growth hormone, thyroxin, triiodothyronine, along with non-esterified fatty acids (NEFA), glucose, lactate, β-hydroxybutyrate (β-OHB), and triacylglycerols (TG) in the blood were followed-up in a group of boys aged 13.7 years during a period of weight reduction. Boys were examined initially (I), then after a 10-day stay in an inpatient department (II). The reduction treatment then continued in a spa. The initial assessment was performed with an 11 MJ diet (approximately 110 g of protein, 100 g of carbohydrate, and 80 g of fat). The energy was then decreased to 5.2 MJ (110 g of protein, 100 g of carbohydrate, 45 g of fat).

In addition to the diet, supervised low to moderate aerobic activity was performed 4 hr per day. A blood sample was obtained after 10 days (II), with the final sample after 52 days or at the end of the treatment in the spa (III). The changes in the above-mentioned indicators are provided in Table 12.1. All parameters except for the serum levels of NEFA and β-OHB decreased after the first 10 days of treatment when the daily weight loss was 300 g. After the next period, insulin did not change but a significant decrease throughout the period of treatment was observed for the concentration of cortisol, thyroxin, and triiodothyronin. The substrates showed a different pattern of change after the treatment, following an important modification of their levels during the first 10 days. An opposite trend followed so that the initial level was similar to that obtained on day 52. This was the case for glucose, with lactate presenting similar shifts but not significantly. The levels of NEFA and β-OHB displayed a mirror-like picture. The changes in growth hormone level were not significant.[567]

Another complex study of morphological, serum lipid, and hormonal changes before and after weight reduction in a 6-week diet and exercise program was conducted using overweight and obese adolescents.[597] Body weight, BMI, and fat percentage decreased significantly along with reduction of waist and hip circumferences, waist-to-hip ratio, and blood pressure (Figure 12.24). IGF-1, IGFBP, leptin, and insulin concentrations decreased during the program.

After weight loss due to energy restriction and an exercise program, plasma leptin concentrations decreased in severely obese French children from 21.2 ± 12.1 to 4.2 ± 4.0 ng.ml⁻¹ (p < 0.0001). After weight reduction the correlation of BMI and leptin plasma levels increased slightly to r = 0.89 (p < 0.004).[637]

Obese children were evaluated before and within 48 hr after the completion of a 5-month exercise training program (ETP, 3 aerobic sessions per

**TABLE 12.1**

Changes of Body Weight, Hormonal, and Biochemical Parameters in Adolescent Obese Children Aged 13.7 ± 1.3 Years during Three Periods of Reduction Treatment

| | I | | II | | III | |
|---|---|---|---|---|---|---|
| | X | SD | X | SD | X | SD |
| Body weight (kg) | 77.4 | 12.0 | 74.4 | 10.9 | 68.2 | 11.2 |
| Insulin (mU/l) | 15.4 | 5.6 | 12.7 | 5.0 | 13.0 | 7.4 |
| Cortisol (µmol/l) | 746.0 | 456.0 | 648.0 | 648.0 | 539.0 | 357.0 |
| Growth hormone (ng/l) | 8.2 | 12.2 | 2.1 | 1.2 | 15.7 | 21.2 |
| Thyroxin-T4 (nmol/l) | 108.0 | 33.0 | 107.0 | 36.0 | 94.0 | 29.0 |
| Triodothyronin-T3 (nmol/l) | 2.89 | 0.64 | 2.15 | 1.0 | 1.9 | 0.49 |
| Glucose (nmol/l) | 5.46 | 0.061 | 4.09 | 0.45 | 5.32 | 0.87 |
| Lactate (nmol/l) | 1.13 | 0.35 | 0.82 | 0.24 | 1.25 | 0.51 |
| NEFA (nmol/l) | 0.27 | 0.06 | 0.36 | 0.08 | 0.24 | 0.10 |
| β-OHB (nmol/l) | 0.65 | 0.28 | 4.48 | 2.06 | 0.49 | 0.25 |
| Triacylgycerols (nmol/l) | 1.35 | 0.81 | 0.78 | 0.24 | 0.81 | 0.81 |
| Protein (g/l) | 79.0 | 3.6 | 79.4 | 3.4 | 77.7 | 3.4 |

Based on data from Ref. T4.

week, each increasing the energy expenditure by approximately 300 kcal) and a moderate diet restriction. Weight gain after ETP was minimal, and improved insulin tolerance and an unexpected increase in the response of gastric inhibitory polypeptide (GIP) were revealed. Even after ETP, obese children continued to secrete more insulin than normal-weight children. Glucose tolerance, similar to pre-ETP for obese subjects and controls, did not change following ETP. An improvement in glucose utilization in obese children following ETP was associated with an increase in GIP secretion. This finding contrasted with reports that energy restriction would improve glucose utilization with decreased insulin and GIP secretion. This study demonstrated an uncoupling of GIP and insulin secretion and suggests shifts in peripheral tissue sensitivity to insulin-induced glucose uptake. These shifts may, in part, be influenced by GIP.[940]

Body weight correlates significantly with insulin levels and blood pressure in obese and non-obese adolescents. Following weight loss, a decrease in insulin levels and blood pressure was observed. The reduction of blood pressure during weight loss correlated significantly with the change in both insulin and body weight.[601]

The influence of physical training (PT) on components of insulin resistance syndrome (IRS) was examined in obese children aged 7 to 11 years. This was under two conditions of reduction therapy: (a) 4 months of PT followed by 4 months without PT, or (b) 4 months without PT followed by 4 months of PT. The results were analyzed using ANOVA. A significant interaction indicated that the changes over time were different for the two groups. During the 4 months of PT compared to the period without PT, there were significant decreases in the TC/HDL-C ratio, TG, insulin and percent body fat. Following periods without PT there were increases in insulin and percent body fat.

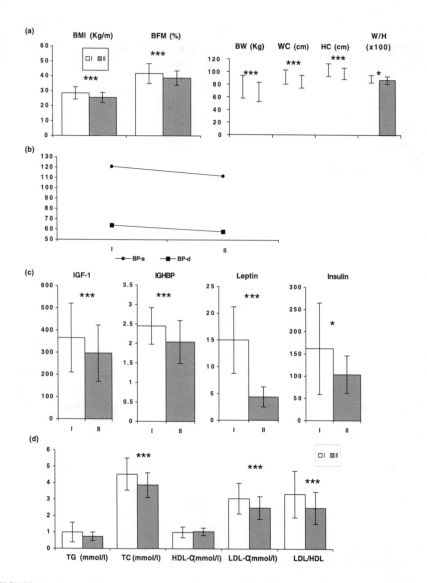

**FIGURE 12.24**

Changes of (a) anthropometric (body mass index (BMI), percentage stored fat (%), body weight (BW), waist (WC) and hip (HC) circumference and their ratio (WHR)); (b) blood pressure; (c) IGF-1, IGFHP, leptin, insulin; and (d) serum TG, TC, HDL-C, LDL-C, and LDL-C/HDL-C ratio in overweight and obese adolescents before (I) and after (II) weight reduction by 6 weeks of exercise and diet. * indicates ($p < 0.05$; *** ($p < 0.001$). (Based on data from Ref. F47.)

Thus, PT improved some components of IRS in obese children with some benefits being lost following its interruption.[941]

A further study confirmed higher fasting-plasma concentrations of IRI and C-peptide, and also a lower C-peptide to IRI molar ratio in obese children aged $11.4 \pm 2.5$ years compared to normal-weight children of the same age.[942]

Obese children also had reduced erythrocyte insulin binding over the physiological range of circulating insulin concentration. A negative correlation between insulin tracer binding and relative weight was revealed. This weight reduction program resulted in a decrease in mean relative weight score and, after treatment, obese children decreased fasting blood glucose levels. The same applied to IRI concentrations at 90 min following an oral glucose load when compared to the onset of therapy. No significant differences between the insulin binding characteristics at the beginning and at the end of the reducing therapy were found.

A lower body weight after reduction therapy is usually accompanied by a decline in serum insulin concentrations. In a study by Chalew et al.,[971] BMI decreased significantly from 39.1 to 34.7 $kg.m^{-2}$ after a low-calorie diet lasting 5 to 8 weeks. Insulin also decreased significantly, but these changes had little effect on the integrated concentrations of growth hormone (IC-GH). Factors other than circulating insulin levels are likely to play a major role in mediating the reduced levels of GH usually found in obese children.

In another study, French obese children were tested after the completion of a 3-month inpatient weight reduction program. The initial GH-U concentration in the urine (pmol/mmol creatinine) was 0.0256 on admission, and 0.0352 on discharge (p < 0.0001; normal values 0.031 ± 0.019). Using a two-level hierarchical model with adjustment for age, gender, and initial BMI, the increase in GH-U was facilitated by enhanced physical activity depending on the time spent by a child participating for more than 1 hr above the average.[943] After GH excretion, the restoration of its values was correlated with various anthropometric parameters to define which one could be a predictor for GH increase after weight reduction. GH restoration was significantly related to hip, not waist, circumference decrease. This suggests that subcutaneous fat is more important than visceral.[944]

The effect of an 8-week reduction treatment (1000 $kcal.day^{-1}$) on thyroid-stimulating hormone (TSH) and prolactin (PRL) responses to thyrotropin-releasing hormone (TRH) was followed in obese subjects aged 8.5 to 17.4 years, before and after reduction of weight. In females at baseline, fT4 serum levels were significantly higher than in control girls with normal weight and fell significantly following weight reduction with rT3 increasing following weight loss in the whole group. Other changes also appeared in the TSH and PRL peaks after TRH following weight loss in girls, as well as in other parameters in the whole group. However, the results of this study suggest that thyroid function is normal in obese adolescent subjects and not influenced by the restriction of energy intake even though a reduced hypothalamus dopaminergic tone on pituitary thyreotrophs and lactotrophs could cause subtle alterations on TSH and PRL release, partially influenced by gender and the level of sexual development.[945]

Weight loss due to reduction treatment also had an effect on adrenal androgens in obese boys who were followed-up before puberty (group I) and at the first stage of sexual maturation (group II). Pregnenolon and dehydroepiandrosteron plasma levels were significantly higher in both groups (I and II) of obese boys when compared to normal-weight controls. These values decreased to normal values following weight reduction, apart from pregnenolon in the prepubertal group I. Progesterone was significantly increased in both groups, and was normal following weight reduction. 17-OH-progesterone plasma levels showed no significant difference between obese and control groups. Androstenedione was higher in the prepubertal obese group I before the treatment, and then showed normal values after weight reduction. No significant difference was found in the other groups. Testosterone and estradiol showed normal values in the two groups both before and after weight reduction. Cortisol showed a similar pattern. It can be concluded that cortico-adrenal activity is increased in obese boys while the same was found in obese girls. The increased secretion of adrenal androgens might be due to an increased secretion of cortico-adrenal stimulating hormone, or to an enhanced adrenal sensitivity to the hypothetical hormone. These results could also explain the precocious menarche that often occurs in obese adolescent girls.[946]

Protein utilization was also influenced by an increased physical activity program that was used in children either alone (walking program 5 days per week, 2 to 3 miles per day), or in combination with diet. [15]N glycine was used to assess protein synthesis and breakdown as well as the net turnover (NET) and N flux. When only diet was used, NET decreased, protein synthesis decreased, and protein breakdown did not return to baseline levels.[947]

### 12.7.4　Changes in Cardiovascular Characteristics and Motor Performance

Weight and fat loss after 7 weeks of treatment by diet and exercise in a summer camp improved the level of cardiorespiratory fitness through an increased aerobic power. Similar results were found in repeated follow-ups before and after similar treatment in both boys and girls.[18,53,68]

Finnish children treated by diet and exercise over 2 years also showed a marked improvement in cardiorespiratory parameters following losses of excess weight and fat. The level of physical performance increased along with an improvement in serum lipid profile. The most active children, those who had ambulatory check-ups most frequently, achieved the best results from a morphological, functional, and biochemical point of view.[914]

In another study, preadolescent obese subjects were assessed before and after a 6-month behavioral weight control program. Significant improvements were found for both weight and fitness levels, which were also reflected by changes in heart rate during exercise and a recovery period. The most successful children decreased their maximal and recovery heart rates and the reverse was found for the least successful subjects. The severely obese subjects improved their fitness only when weight loss was substantial.[915]

An intervention study by Cohen et al.[927] showed a non-significant decrease in body weight and sum of 2 skinfolds, significant increases in the number of sit-ups (23 to 35), and distance covered in 9 min (1201 to 1419 yd). There was no change in flexibility and an insignificant decrease in TC (178 to 155 mg.dl$^{-1}$).

The effect of diet and exercise was assessed in an experimental group of obese children simultaneously with a control group without intervention. At the beginning, obese children were significantly inferior to normal-weight children in fitness items such as standing long jump, pull-ups, sit-ups, step-test and total fitness scores. No differences in lying trunk extension and standing trunk flexion for body flexibility were observed. Obese children were superior in static strength, that is, hand grip strength and back strength. Deterioration of physical fitness was due to enhanced deposition of fat rather than to increased body weight alone, which was more pronounced in boys than in girls. The results in the experimental group showed significant improvement in fitness of most items, especially in abdominal muscle endurance and aerobic capacity. This treatment did not limit growth velocity or reduce the development of lean body mass.[500] Similar results have been reported by other studies.[339–341,507]

### 12.7.5 Changes in Bone Mineral Density

Growth is usually accelerated in obese children. Bone mineral content (BMC, measured by DXA) was studied in obese children before and after a weight reduction program, including moderate energy restriction and exercise lasting 9.3 ± 3 months. Before weight loss, 25 OH vitamin D was below safety levels in some children. PTH, osteocalcine, and 1,25 OH vitamin D were normal in all subjects. However, bone density of the lumbar spine was lower. During weight loss, BMC increased and became similar in the subgroups supplemented and non-supplemented with the above mentioned vitamins. BMC was correlated with height increase, but not with plasma content or the increase of any biological parameters measured.[948] Gutin et al.[900] also found increased bone density after physical training.

## 12.8 Drug Therapy

Drug therapy in obese children has also been considered. Generally, the oral administration of appetite suppressors has been deemed inappropriate. Because of occasional poor results of other therapeutic approaches, especially under conditions of outpatient or school-based treatment, drug treatment for resistant, very severely obese cases, has been implemented. In São Paulo, Brazil, the results of diet and exercise therapy were compared to the results of the same therapy supplemented by 30 or 60 mg (according to age) of the racemic form of fenfluramine (D,L-fenfluramine) in two groups of obese youth. The groups did not differ in baseline mean age, BMI, percentage of ideal weight, and were followed-up over 1 year. Part of the exercise and diet (placebo) group was unwilling to continue in their therapeutic program. The subjects of the drug group lost significantly more weight, as expressed by the reduction of BMI values (29.2 ± 4.5 to 23.1 ± 3.9 kg.m$^{-2}$) as compared to the placebo-treated group (BMI 29.9 ± 4.3. to 28.6 ± 4.1 kg.m$^{-2}$). Dry mouth and drowsiness were the most common complaints, occurring in about 18% of the subjects during the first 2 weeks of therapy, and disappearing with a reduction of D,L-fenfluramine dosage.[949] However, few studies have been conducted using drugs for the treatment of childhood obesity. The use of fenfluramine showed undesirable side effects, for example, heart valve problems, and is no longer recommended or on the market, even for adults. In spite of problems not being reported in the study by Madeiros-Neto, the use of similar drugs is not recommended.[949]

A pilot study in obese adolescents has shown caffeine/ephedrine (Letigen) as a safe and effective component of the treatment of obese adolescents who lost significant amounts of weight and fat. This decrease was significantly greater than in the subjects treated by a placebo. Adverse effects were negligible and did not differ in the Letigen and placebo group.[950]

Leptin injections have resulted in the reduction of body weight in primates, although human clinical trials have not been reported until recently. No similar effect has been shown in the obese of all ages.[59]

## 12.9 Surgical Interventions

Gastric surgery has also been used in adolescents aged 11 to 19 years. Subjects were interviewed an average of 6 years postoperatively. The mean pre-operative BMI was 47 while at follow up, BMI averaged 32. Two thirds of the patients weighed within 9 kg of their lowest post-surgical weight at the time of follow-up and three patients had sought additional obesity surgery. Excellent psychosocial adjustment, improved self-esteem and social relationships, and more a satisfying appearance were reported by these patients, but compliance with exercise and dietary instructions was poor. Long-term patient monitoring and commitment are recommended, for example, prescribed multivitamin and calcium supplements were taken only by a limited number of subjects.[951]

Plastic surgery was suggested to improve the consequences of important weight loss (that is, more than 30 kg) in morbidly obese adolescents. Abdominal and mammary ptosis and adipose gynecomastia on the trunk, and wing-like arm deformities and lipomeria of the medial aspect of the thigh on the limbs, were observed. At the facial and neck level, no changes were usually found. Irritations with maceration and skin surinfection that can result in a sepsis were also revealed.[952] Psychological complications due to such a situation are commonplace so intervention with the help of plastic surgery has to be considered, especially in more serious cases. The procedures are almost the same as in adults with this complementary treatment being determined by close cooperation between pediatrician and plastic surgeon.[952]

## 12.10   Intragastric Balloon Therapy

This form of intervention was reported in five morbidly obese adolescents aged 11 to 17.7 years with a BMI between 30.3 to 52.7 kg.m$^{-2}$ who previously failed to lose weight with a conventional weight loss program. Gastric balloons filled with 4 to 600 ml saline solution were inserted during general anesthesia. Vomiting and abdominal distension lasted only 1 day. Weight loss after 3 months was between 3.5 and 14.5 kg; however, after another 6 months, all subjects had regained the initial weight lost, or gained more weight than before the treatment. The feeling of abdominal distension and early satiety lasted only 1 to 2 weeks. In two subjects, spontaneous deflation of the balloon occurred with a spontaneous loss per annum in one of them after 6 months. No further complications were observed after the removal of the balloons at 6 to 7 months, but the results showed that gastric balloons had only a transitory effect on weight loss in morbidly obese adolescents, and that other approaches should be used.[953]

## 12.11   Alternative Approaches

In addition to the combination of diet and exercise, auricular acupuncture was used in weight reduction treatment in obese Taiwanese subjects aged 16 to 70 years. The rate of effectiveness was 86.7% and weight rebound was only 6.7%. The effectiveness of weight reduction was significantly correlated with the compliance of participants with each therapeutic method and not with age. There were no side effects reported.[954]

The efficacy of acupuncture as a method for weight reduction was assessed in obese children. Electro-acupuncture had a beneficial effect on various pathogenic components in obese children. This was manifested by a cessation of subjective complaints, increased weight and fat loss, increased performance level and increased efficiency of the cardiovascular system, and a decrease in serum lipids to normal values. Therefore, the authors recommended this method in comprehensive treatment of children with constitutional exogenic obesity.[955]

# 13

## Practical Programs for Weight Management during the Growing Years

Interventions in early childhood may have a substantial effect on an individual's lifestyle behaviors, particularly with respect to dietary intake and physical activity or exercise. There are numerous opportunities for young people to learn good eating habits, for example, using computer games at school and profiting from the topical nature of this technology. The effect of such pro-active approaches can be substantial and can capitalize on a high interest factor for most children. The introduction of healthy food habits from a young age is particularly important for children who have had impaired food intake.[956] The importance of childhood diet in the prevention of adult obesity is essential and must start early, as is the case for a proper regime of physical activity.[950,957]

### 13.1 Arrangement of Weight Management Programs for Obese Children

As mentioned in the previous chapter, the combined approach of diet, exercise, and behavior modification in weight management programs gives the best and often permanent results.[10] It has also been demonstrated that for both diet and exercise regimes, it is essential to adhere to the monitored change on a permanent basis. This may be difficult in a situation where only one individual is attempting a lifestyle modification. The preference is for all family members to assist the child by following and benefiting from the same lifestyle changes.

As previously mentioned, an alternative approach is to employ an inpatient treatment program. This type of approach is rare given the cost and lack of suitable space, with institutions unwilling to commit the necessary resources. However, this approach is the most suitable for the treatment of morbidly obese children. Summer camps or health clubs offer similar possibilities for obese children, particularly where the necessary supervision for both diet and exercise can be guaranteed. The better possibility for most obese children is a supervised activity program as a distinct component of a school or university clinic setting. The school-based approach may be an after-school or holiday period opportunity. In the university-based clinic of one of the authors, a designated program called "PhysKids" provides an on-site opportunity for young people to be active in a fun group setting.

### 13.1.1 Ambulatory and Outpatient Programs

The combination of diet and sport has been used successfully as an ambulatory program for obese children; for example, an outpatient program attended by obese children aged 9 to 13 years over 1 year consisted of a diet of 1200 kcal.day[-1], exercise three times per week, and psychological support. The results of this therapy were an increased level of physical performance, improved coordination and endurance, and greater self-confidence. A reduction of approximately 20% of the initial weight was achieved but only in the age range of 12 to 13 years. In the younger children the level of reduction was smaller. During the initial period in this study HDL-C decreased but increased within 4 to 5 months to exceed pre-treatment levels. No vitamin deficiencies were reported.[34]

Primary (elementary) school-based programs have been well-defined as effective means of preventing obesity during childhood; for example, Sahota et al.[958] included dietary interventions with nutritional education incorporated in the curriculum. Policy changes included snacks consumed during breaks, "Fit is Fun" programs with improved playground facilities, the development of after-school physical activities along with activities such as cooking, health weeks, and competitions. The program was extremely popular with the participants and it was recommended that similar programs could be of great assistance in the prevention of obesity.

The effects of various levels of physical activity have also been reported in Italian children aged 9 to 14 years (Di.S.Co. project: experimental community project for preventing chronic-degenerative diseases). The program included nutritional habits and status, anthropometric parameters, and motor abilities. This study underlined the widespread trend of poor nutritional habits (including of those enrolled in regular sports activities) and a poor attitude toward voluntary physical activity. The school has a privileged opportunity to help in the promotion of healthy lifestyles and the correction of poor habits starting from an early growth period.[441]

Group programs that do not rely on the use of special diets and standardized training programs, but rather concentrate on changing food and physical activity habits can be very effective; for example, Vitolo et al.[959] used programmed monthly meetings of obese Brazilian children aged 13 to 15 years with pediatricians, nutritionists, physical educators, and psychologists. The result was a decline of BMI from 36.0 to 30.3 after approximately

9 months. The key to success in this approach was the management of children in a group setting with a sharing of experiences.

Outpatient programs should try to maintain a permanent increase in energy expenditure through participation in a mixture of organized (structured) and unstructured exercise. This should be over and above the non-negotiable everyday physical activity. Children should be stimulated and encouraged to undertake as much as possible the usual physical activities such as walking, climbing the steps, household tasks, working in the yard, etc. If this is achieved, it is possible to increase the level of functional capacity and physical fitness which then makes it possible to adhere to exercise and sport programs more readily and comfortably. In addition, enhancement of body awareness plays an important role in adherence to regular physical activity. Examples of body awareness activities for young children are provided later in this chapter.

Long-lasting changes in eating habits that result in weight and fat reduction may have a greater chance of success through individual consultations and regular check-ups of parameters such as BMI, skinfolds, serum lipids, and other biochemical parameters. Tracking of functional testing during standard and maximal workloads on a bicycle ergometer or treadmill is also particularly valuable and enables fine-tuning of the exercise prescription.

Consultations with staff should also include the parents to assure adequate cooperation of the family. Eating habits and food choices should be controlled with the help of interviews and the completion of diaries over a 3- to 10-day period. Because they lack experience, development and an inability to record, this approach is difficult in young children and may only be possible in adolescents. Discussion of results should occur with the child and at least one, but preferably, both parents. Greater success in modifying the nutritional habits of children is possible if parents have an adequate and well-balanced approach to their eating.

### 13.1.2 Treatment in Summer Camps

A combined approach to weight management using both diet and exercise can be implemented and controlled in healthy obese individuals most readily under conditions of inpatient treatment. However, the best and more natural option for children other than school-based programs is to participate in summer camps. Such camps have been run successfully in several countries in the past. For example, in former Czechoslovakia starting in the 1950s, camps were used, with satisfactory improvements in body composition and functional capacity of many participants.[18,55,316,568,960]

In the U.K., a 3-year follow-up of an 8-week diet and exercise program for children attending a weight-loss camp was completed by Gately et al.[961] A group of children entered the program in 1994, and returned in 1995, 1996, and 1997. Body weight and height were assessed during each program in which energy intake was restricted to 1600 kcal per day and the daily exercise prescription was five 1.5-hr sessions. This program was structured in the form of fun-type, skill-based activities which were used to give children the necessary motor abilities that enabled participation in physical activity with peers when they returned to their home environment. Educational information on nutrition, exercise, and lifestyle was also included. BMI decreased from 30.2 (pre-1994) to 25.5 (1997). Seventy-seven percent of subjects had reduced their BMI after the 3-year program. These results indicate that a program that concentrates on increasing skills and improving the motor habits necessary for participation in sport activities assists in producing successful lifestyle alterations. This program, initiated by the Leeds Metropolitan University, continues and was re-implemented using the same principles in the summer of 1999 for children aged 11 to 17 years.

The effectiveness of the complex treatment of obese children in a sanatorium-type camp was ascertained in Russian children.[962] The results of similar summer camps for obese children have also been reported from other countries and have involved 4-day stays with 4 hr daily spent learning and practicing eating and exercise skills conducive to weight loss.[963] In conjunction, parents of the obese children involved met weekly to discuss the program content and to explore their role in the management of their children's weight. A significant reduction of body weight, percent overweight, and skinfold thicknesses was achieved. Improvements were also shown in self-reported personal habits and participant's knowledge of weight management concepts. The results of this form of obesity management reveal that an intensive program of eating and exercise behavior instruction, practice, and monitoring can be particularly effective under conditions similar to a home setting, which may have special importance for children in this age period.[963]

A study by Jirapinyo et al.[964] reported on the impact of a 4-week camp on Thai children aged 8 to 13 years with moderate or severe obesity. Dietary restriction during the time at the camp and dietary self-control at home were incorporated. Various types of exercise including swimming and group therapy were incorporated into the program. Weekly sight-seeing trips outside the camp were included to interest and motivate the children and this feature was very attractive for all participants. After the program, children lost, on average, approximately 5% of their initial weight. Most of the weight loss was due to the reduction of stored fat and not of lean body mass. The character of the camp-based program did not cause any complications. These results provide further justification of this approach for the treatment of childhood obesity, especially during the initial periods.

Treatment in a summer camp using a group approach also resulted in a more marked and longer lasting weight loss in a group of obese Belgian children.[965] Similarly, a study of Polish obese adolescents treated in a 3-week-long summer camp using energy restriction (5.51 MJ.day$^{-1}$) and exercise resulted in a significant weight loss with positive changes in body composition. However, in this study, the results were gender dependent with better results for boys than girls.[888]

A number of pediatric weight-loss programs have also been reported in Taiwan. In a 'pediatric-obesity club,' four fundamental components, namely, diet, exercise, behavior modification, and the involvement of parents were included in a treatment program. In this family-based, parent-directed program, 11% of the participants showed a decrease in the degree of obesity after a 1-year follow-up, compared to 3% of a control group. In another individualized outpatient counselling clinic, the success rate was 59% after 1 year. Although continued long-term effectiveness of this approach cannot be determined, it seems that a realistic and culturally sensitive weight reduction program should be developed for each country. There is an urgent need in countries such as Taiwan and other Asian countries to develop such programs as early as possible because the prevalence of obesity is increasing.[143]

### 13.1.3   School-Based Programs

Schools have the opportunity, mechanisms, and personnel to deliver nutrition education, to promote physical fitness, and in many cases, to provide a school food service capable of preparing an adequate diet suitable for preventing excess deposition of fat. A 2-year longitudinal study on the effect of an enhanced physical activity program and modified school-lunch program was conducted on elementary school children in Nebraska.[966] At year two, lunches had significantly less energy (9%), fat (25%), sodium (21%), and more fiber (17%). Physical activity in the classroom was 6% greater in the intervention groups, but physical activity outside school was approximately 16% less for the pupils comprising the intervention group compared to control pupils without intervention. No significant differences were found for body weight, stored fat, cholesterol, insulin, and glucose; however, HDL-C was significantly greater and TC/HDL-C was significantly less for the intervened pupils compared to controls. This finding indicates that the total volume and especially intensity and mode of exercise during selected periods might significantly influence at least some parameters, in spite of the lack of differences in the total amount of activity. A regular intervention in the management of physical activity programs is necessary in order to make them more efficient on a broader scale.

Bar-Or et al.[47] has rightly suggested that the school is in a strong position to encourage and provide physical activity opportunities for all children but particularly for the overweight and obese. Logically, staff with the necessary expertise, whether physical and health educators, school nurses, or sports coaches, are well placed to provide innovative and targeted assistance. Furthermore, most schools have a range of physical facilities and equipment onsite without the need to consider a move to other venues. Most schools are also underutilized, certainly outside of school hours.

There are also great opportunities to use break times for physical activity during the school day plus before and after school and in timeslots on weekends. The school academic year is also very short with long holiday periods dotted throughout. Such times are prime opportunities during which activity programs should be provided.

One of the contributing factors to the increase in overweight and obesity in the pediatric years has been the demise of physical education. Very few children are provided with quality experiences of physical activity at school during their formative years.[2]

School physical education, if used effectively, is a major avenue for the promotion of physical activity among children. During childhood years (approximately 5 to 7 years of age), the young start to make comparisons between their physical performance and that of their peers. Children are conscious of the potential rewards associated with success in physical activity, such as feelings of competency and mastery, improvements in self-esteem, and the accolades of others. It is important that children's perceptions and considerations of the value of participating in physical activity are recognized. These include fun and enjoyment, health and fitness, desire to learn new skills, the chance to achieve, friendship, and cooperation.

## 13.2   Principles of Weight Reduction Diets for Obese Children

In the treatment and prevention of childhood obesity, adequate, monitored food intake is essential. According to the physiological situation of a child during growth, dietary treatment should be aimed mainly toward an improvement in the composition of the diet. This includes the recommended ratio of the main macronutrients, an adherence to RDAs, and monitoring of the energy content of ingested meals. As mentioned in Chapter 7, in more severe cases of childhood obesity, hypocaloric diets or special protein-sparing diets restricted in energy have a place in obesity management.

Every child has a unique personality and this relates to and includes nutritional and motor components. The term 'nutritional individuality' was coined by Widdowson and reflects the individual variability that exists in dietary intake, absorption, metabolism, and utilization of nutrients.[967] The more that is known about the child and his/her eating habits, the greater the chance of having an impact in rectifying the child's health problems, including obesity. Sound knowledge and understanding also minimize the chance of making fundamental errors of judgment that may be critical to the success of the treatment process.

General guidelines for treatment should reflect the combined needs of a compatible reduction of excess fat and preservation or increase of lean body mass, with a continued increase in height. These features, along with an improvement in functional capacity, should be the major goals. Another important treatment principle is to respect food and physical activity preferences. For example, no child should be forced to eat meals and foodstuffs he/she dislikes because an adult deems them to be appropriate. It is far more preferable, although potentially difficult, to structure a diet according to the child's preferences. It may be necessary to patiently experiment in order to find what is the most acceptable to the child. If this is achieved, there is greater hope of the individual adhering to the modified diet and the result might be a long-lasting or permanent change in eating behavior.

The suggested procedure for defining an adequate diet is as follows:

1. One of the most important principles is the use of an individual approach according to the child's health status, physical fitness, and psychological traits. Consequently, a medical examination by a pediatrician, plus consultations with a nutritionist and other specialists are necessary. There should also be a concurrent consideration of physical activity habits and exercise recommendations. Co-morbidities also need to be identified, and where necessary, treated simultaneously.

2. A comprehensive analysis of food intake history including the individual's dietary habits should be undertaken prior to prescribing a recommended diet. There is a range of options available. The most suitable and feasible option would be the inventory methods using daily diaries over 1 week, preferably during at least 3 weekdays and 1 weekend day. The food frequency method can also be used. These assessments should be representative of the usual dietary regime of the child. When necessary, more sophisticated and demanding approaches may need to be implemented.

3. On the basis of such analyses, an individualized dietary intake should be defined for each child. The composition of the diet should correspond to the RDAs of WHO, EU, and the U.S. Academy of Science, all of which recommend 12 to 13% of total energy intake from protein, up to 30% from fat and 50 to 60% from carbohydrates.[274] Proteins should comprise 50% from animal and 50% from plant origin. Also, the composition of fat should include one third saturated, one third mono-unsaturated, and the rest polyunsaturated fats. Carbohydrates should be mostly complex polysaccharides (dark bread, cereals, and so on), and only up to 10% of the energy intake should be sugar.[274]

   Depending on previous practices, some food items may need to be reduced, especially if they used to be ingested in excessive quantities. According to numerous authors, this mainly concerns fats (especially saturated fats) and simple sugars. The combination of these items in sweets is a significant risk for the deposition of excess fat. Thus the energy content and composition of the diet for each individual can be assured. Such foods should be replaced by other items such as fruits and vegetables. An individual approach considering the age, gender, degree and duration of obesity, and energy output is also necessary.

4. Vitamin and mineral content in the diet should always correspond to the RDAs for the particular age and gender of the child. In the case of a more markedly reduced food intake which provides a certain risk of some deficiencies, these items may need to be supplemented.

5. The frequency, timing, and regularity of meals and consumption of the necessary major nutrients during the day are very important. For example, skipping breakfast and ingesting the majority of energy during the second half of the day, particularly having a large meal for dinner, may provide a higher risk for obesity in some individuals. A regular intake of meals, which may be at least five smaller meals during the day with an adequate breakfast and a light evening meal, should be the goal. Better control over the time of eating may be just as important for many children as any individual component of the prescribed diet. For example, discouraging eating prior to going to bed when there is little further potential for increasing energy expenditure until the following day is an important goal. Similarly, limiting the size of bites and also eating speed are important eating behaviors to change if applicable.[968]

6. The consumption of regular snacks, particularly those high in energy such as chips, corn, and sweets must be progressively reduced. This is also the case for all delicacies and foodstuffs high in saturated fats. These foods must be limited and/or eventually eliminated. The same applies to the consumption of soft drinks that commonly contain a high amount of sucrose. These habits should be replaced by eating more fruit which is not too sweet (apples, grapefruit, oranges, strawberries) and vegetables (tomatoes, raw cucumbers, cabbage). These changes may be difficult, as children are not adapted to eat such food items because they are 'addicted' to various widely advertised energy-dense snacks.

7. Drinking an adequate amount of fresh water (when available), or club soda with lemon juice, or a small amount of non-sweetened fruit juice is also a priority. Obese children need to be properly hydrated, but, at the same time, preventing increased intake of energy from inadequate beverages is necessary. The same principle applies for normal-weight children, especially in parts of the world where water losses from the body are increased due to the climate. An adequate intake of liquids is critical.

8. The general principle for the use of reduction diets for obese children is to make only the necessary reduction in energy intake on the basis of the energy needs of each particular child. When the degree of obesity, overall health, and functional status is well defined, energy intake should be lower than for a child with normal weight. In special cases of severe or morbid obesity, a protein-sparing, very low-energy diet or classical hypocaloric diet

is warranted. On the basis of a number of studies, the use of such an approach over a short period of time does not have negative consequences. The implementation of such restricted diets is mainly recommended if another health problem exists concurrently with obesity. Restricted diets must only be used under strict medical supervision, preferably in a controlled environment, such as an inpatient department in a hospital or children's clinic. Under normal family or school conditions, severe dietary restrictions should be avoided.

The purpose of this volume is not to provide a list of special recipes for individual meals, but rather to define and specify the main guidelines. Fundamentally, it is necessary to appreciate that a detailed and unified approach common for all children who need to reduce excess fat cannot be prepared. To ensure the successful impact of a diet, the nutritional and physical individuality of each child or adolescent must be respected. This includes the conditions and dynamics of the obese individual's family and the broader environment. For example, it is counterproductive to insist that a child ingest a foodstuff that he/she has hated since early childhood. The choice of meals, especially at the beginning of treatment and management, should be adjusted for each obese individual.

Similarly, a diet to reduce body fat in a younger child with a moderate degree of obesity would be quite different and much easier to define than a diet for an older individual with more developed, longer-lasting obesity. The avoidance of difficult cases of prolonged obesity in children and adolescents is another argument for the effective prevention of obesity during growth.

9. The role of the family and appreciation, knowledge, and understanding of the whole environment are essential. As mentioned on numerous occasions throughout this volume, there may be a much greater challenge to treatment and management when only one child in the family is obese and other members are of normal weight. The role of the mother or responsible adult who is preparing the meals is a pivotal and often difficult role. From the commencement of management, at least as a start, meals should be the same or similar for the whole family so as not to make the child feel segregated and mistreated. When all members of the family, especially siblings who are not obese, have some solidarity and accept the fact that they should eat similar meals to their obese brother or sister, the process of management may have more chance of success. The diet should serve as a good model for all members of the family as their food habits may have been sub-optimal. They, too, may be at risk of obesity in the longer term if poor dietary practices continue. There is always the possibility of supplementing the energy intake of other family members as necessary when

the obese child is not present. After a period of time, the obese child may more readily accept his/her special position and be happy to eat a different meal than others if this is necessary. This degree of acceptance and attitude is more likely when the child is supported and treated appropriately from a psychological perspective and most importantly, self-identifies with the necessary regime of nutrition and physical activity.

It should not be necessary to add that proper adjustment of the family diet to prevent obesity or to assist in the treatment of a mild degree of obesity in a young child by appropriate and smaller dietary modifications is preferable. In summary, the consideration of energy balance and turnover is critical. A modest reduction in the energy intake and a substantial increase in energy output through physical activity and exercise are preferable. This lifestyle approach provides the best guarantee against obesity development.

Behavior therapy has been identified as an important part of the treatment and dietary management equation, including that of the obese child's family. The utilization of behavior management may well have an important place in the process, but does require the understanding of the techniques involved and must be seen as a component rather than the stand-alone option or answer. Successful behavior management requires a combined approach, cognizant of the complexity of the condition and its multi-factorial etiology. A comprehensive approach is necessary as the human mind cannot simply be sub-divided into various parts in which different types of treatment and management are used. Behavioral therapy has an important place in management but may be more effective when considered in the broader context.[969]

## 13.3  How to Define General Principles of Physical Activity and Exercise for the Obese Child

Increased energy output through physical activity and exercise is an essential component of the weight management process. The choice of activities must reflect the physical capabilities of each individual but be dominated by dynamic, weight-bearing aerobic exercise of well-defined intensity, duration, and frequency. This type of activity increases aerobic power and enhances the increased mobilization and utilization of lipid metabolites.

A dynamic, weight-bearing workload is possible in growing individuals with a mild degree of obesity. In cases where obesity is more advanced, beginning activities may be limited to exercises in the swimming pool that allow the individual to profit from the Archimedes principle. After some initial success in weight reduction and improvement in the level of fitness in the aquatic activities, the larger individual would benefit from a progressive introduction of specific exercises in a lying or sitting posture. Depending on the age and interest of the individual, this may include work on a bicycle or rowing ergometer, or resistance-training exercises supplemented by some weight-bearing activities. As soon as appropriate for the individual, but usually following further improvement in body composition and functional capacity, it is possible to include a proportion of mainstream exercises and sport activities that would be prescribed for normal-weight children. This approach also serves to assist in maintaining results achieved during the earlier phases of the weight management program.

Given the differences in the initial levels of health, functional capacity, and physical performance, plus the different levels of adaptation to a workload, the prescription for individual children is quite variable. Some obese children have very good levels of motor and physical performance but many have an insufficient, low level of fitness.[2,507] Because of individual variability in health and fitness, it may be appropriate for children considered as candidates for weight management to be examined by a team of health professionals (pediatrician, physical educator, exercise physiologist, and psychologist). With the help of the child or adolescent, an appropriate exercise prescription can be defined. Inadequate and unrealistic workload demands on an obese child at the commencement of treatment and management can completely discourage the individual and jeopardize the potential for a positive outcome of the weight management process.

Weight reduction during growth and development is not a natural trend for a young person. It is necessary to be very conscious of this and guard against any compromise to the normal development of height, lean, fat-free body mass including all individual systems. This also has implications for physical fitness and performance that usually improve following weight loss. The aim in the weight management process should be to optimize these functions, which is possible when using the right factors. The most important goal should not be forgotten. The aim of a weight management program should not, in the first instance, be only to decrease body weight and fat, but rather to improve functional, motor, psychological, and behavioral abilities.

### 13.3.1  Aims of Physical Activity and Exercise Interventions

The primary aims of intervention for children and adolescents should be to promote confidence and enjoyment in physical activity and enhance the physical well-being of an individual with the attainment of a desirable body composition. During growth, such an approach is of primary importance as it is necessary to influence the child to self-identify with all aspects of the weight management process.

The objectives for improved opportunities in physical activity may be encompassed in the characteristic needs of children:

- The need for vigorous activity to promote optimal growth and development.

- The need to maintain a desirable body weight and composition.
- The need for regular physical activity along with a nutritious and well-balanced diet.
- The need for physical and motor skill development to enable enjoyable participation in physical activity.
- The need for involvement in group activities with peers of a similar size and shape to provide support and the opportunity for social interaction.

The overweight or obese youngster should be mainstreamed into activity settings at school and in the wider community at the earliest possible opportunity.

### 13.3.2    Attitudes of the Child

The expected outcomes for overweight and obese children who participate in a quality activity program can also be summarized on the basis of relevant attitudes, knowledge, and skills.

A psychological focus should be incorporated in any intervention so the child achieves:

- An appreciation of one's own body as unique and desirable.
- An understanding of the health benefits of a nutritious diet combined with regular physical activity.
- An improvement in self-esteem and body image.
- A tolerance and understanding of the capabilities and interests of others.

### 13.3.3    Knowledge

The child should have the necessary knowledge and understanding of the weight management process in conjunction with the same information being provided for all family members. Information may be provided from a physical educator, teacher, parent, family member, or a friend. Knowledge and understanding should encompass:

- An understanding of a range of physical activities that suit the individual's interests and capabilities.
- An understanding of one's body, its growth, development, and physical limitations.
- A comprehension of the importance of regular physical activity.

### 13.3.4   Skills

Achievement of an adequate level of motor and related skills is indispensable for maintaining a consistent and meaningful involvement in physical activity. An allied goal is to develop and maintain a reasonable level of health-related fitness represented by cardiorespiratory endurance, flexibility, desirable body composition, and muscular strength and endurance.

- Acquire motor skills: balance, agility, coordination, and speed.
- Develop social skills: ability to accept oneself, tolerate and cooperate with others.
- Develop a range of related sport and physical activity skills.

In order to maximize the opportunity for individual and group success in the activity setting, the following guidelines are essential:

- Work hard to construct and maintain an appropriate psychological climate.
- Appropriate design and delivery of activity sessions are of central importance.
- The grouping of participants must be sensitive to individual needs.
- Recognition of good performance and measurement of personal improvement on an individual rather than a collective or comparative basis.
- Evaluate sessions taking special note of activities that are more or less popular.
- A key to the receptiveness of participants is their perceived readiness to be involved and attempt particular types of activities.
- Opportunities for success in the physical activity setting are related to an emphasis on short-term goals and attempts to maximize motor skill development and learning.
- Motivation in children can be enhanced if individuals are evaluated for improvement and effort rather than solely performance and loss of weight.

Of overriding importance for the child are enjoyment and fun which relates to one's perception of competence and accomplishment. The attractiveness of the activities and the nature of the activity setting have a major influence on children's fun and enjoyment. The interest taken by the teacher or responsible adult, and their empathy for each individual are further influencing factors.

A major aim is to have children make a commitment to physical activity and value the physical activity choices they make. If innovative opportunities are provided to enhance activity and sessions are social experiences, in the longer term, there might be less of a reliance on clinic initiatives. The more a home-based activity is attempted and maintained, the more likely self-responsibility will be maximized.

Responsible adults need to capitalize on the basic interest of children in physical movement and this should be started from a very young age. The focus of this interest should be the enhancement of fundamental motor skills. In time, when these skills are well developed, these basic skills can be extended progressively to sports-specific skills.

To a large extent, particular aspects of the physical activity program should be well understood by the individual child; for example,

- The expectation of increased energy expenditure and the degree of tiredness and fatigue one might experience.
- The purpose of the activity program.
- The importance of being provided with feedback.
- There is a graded increase in health and fitness expected, but children should be aware that they should not experience excessive discomfort.

Aerobic exercise should be a specific focus of group activity programs and individual home-based programs, with as much variety incorporated as possible. Examples of core activities include swimming, cycling, riding stationary bicycles, walking and jogging, treadmill walking and running, stair-climbing, and a wide range of active games. Water-based activities, particularly for those who are comfortable with the aquatic environment, can be particularly valuable. The benefits provided by enhanced buoyancy mean that even non-swimmers can be provided with a meaningful activity session. Aerobic work should be combined with a cross-section of games, skill work, gymnastics, dance, and movement activities that are enjoyable.

Benefits cannot be maximized without careful planning and the design and implementation of a quality program. A high priority should be given to developing appropriate attitudes toward physical activity and associated health benefits.

The overweight child is at a distinct disadvantage when participating in most physical activity, particularly when relocating the total body weight. Difficulties in participation tend to be the reason why obese individuals withdraw from vigorous activity. This, in turn, perpetuates low levels of physical fitness and reduced motor skill development. Therefore, activities in a program need to focus on increased levels of participation in conjunction with opportunities to enhance motor skills.

### 13.3.5 Factors to Enhance Program Design and Implementation

A number of factors may enhance program design and implementation:

- There should be a gradual progression from activities that promote a low level of energy expenditure to those at a higher level, and should provide for and encourage maximum participation by every child.
- Caution must be taken to prevent injury in the activity setting. This consideration is important throughout the program but critical in the early stages.
- Exercise must be vigorous enough to cause a training load on the cardiorespiratory system. Therefore, the intensity of exercise must be closely monitored in aerobic activity.
- Every attempt should be made to make activities enjoyable and as a consequence, self-motivating.
- Overweight and obese individuals often recount poor experiences with physical activity, particularly where non-obese children have been present. While a major goal should always be to provide the necessary skills to facilitate the mainstreaming of the obese child in physical activity settings, initial success is enhanced when groups of overweight individuals work together.
- Water intake should never be restricted as this could result in dehydration.

### 13.3.6 Exercise Prescription

The current guidelines for exercise prescription for weight management are general in nature; therefore, much work is still to be done to identify more specifically the amount, type, and intensity of exercise necessary to produce weight loss while maximizing desirable metabolic adaptations.[10]

Exercise prescription or exercise dose generally involves four integral components. The *mode* or type of exercise is reflected as cardiorespiratory (aerobic) training or resistance weight training. The *frequency* of exercise or how often one exercises, is usually represented by how many days per week or number of sessions per day. The *duration* of exercise or period of time is also represented as total energy expended (kJ) or total energy (kJ.kg body weight$^{-1}$). *Intensity*, or how hard one works is quantified as% $VO_2$ max,% maximum heart rate,% heart rate reserve, rating of perceived exertion (RPE), lactate threshold, and metabolic equivalent (MET).[10]

The goal for all overweight and obese children should be to increase their energy expenditure in an adequate way, that is, with achievement of the necessary threshold intensity tolerable by the child. For those who have been largely inactive, a short dose of activity may be all that they are able to tolerate in the short term. The aim is to progressively increase the volume of exercise that can be managed and ideally to sustain it over an increasingly longer period of time. Depending on the physical condition of the individual, a start may be made with as little as one or two brief sessions of 10 to 15 min per week.

### 13.3.6.1 Medical Examination and Pre-Participation Screening

Prior to undertaking an exercise program, all prospective participants should obtain a medical certificate or referral from their medical practitioner. One of the most important factors is gaining the interest of the child and his/her motivation and self-monitoring in the recommended exercise program.

As is the case for dietary intake of an individual, it is not possible to provide a unique and homogeneous recipe for exercises that will result in an improvement in body composition. It is possible to provide a general overview and instructions for use by a trained adult or parent to introduce an appropriate mode of exercise. Generally, guidelines and recommendations are superficial, for example, aerobic exercise at a certain ratio of aerobic power with no further details.

### 13.3.6.2 Mode of Exercise

Exercise should have a significant cardiorespiratory element. Potential dynamic activities include walking, jogging, treadmill walking and running, swimming, stair-climbing, bench stepping, and skipping. Children should be encouraged to start with brief sessions and gradually increase the length of sessions over time. A longer-term goal is the encouragement of increased habitual physical activity with additional activities as often as possible, ideally every day. The choice of activities should be based on the likes and dislikes of individuals, enjoyment, and the provision of an appropriate challenge. Activities that foster a combined improvement in motor skill are favored.

There is no selective effect of training mode on body composition changes if total work output is equivalent. However, individual variability in overweight and obese individuals means that there are differences in the suitability of exercises.

Walking is one of the most effective modalities for children, adolescents, and adults, particularly in the early stages of a program. There are numerous advantages of this modality, including the following: lower risk of musculoskeletal injury than running, convenience, ability to produce a training effect if used appropriately, and it requires no particular skill. While skill level may appear to be unimportant, the efficiency with which one walks is very much associated with ability and management of the extra load to be carried.[274,391] Particularly with the immature child, extra care and attention may need to be provided in order to maximize the value from a relatively simple locomotor task.[760,759]

Exercise performed in water has the advantage of the buoyancy effect and a reduced loading on joints. This enables a more rapid progression in terms of total volume of exercise and less risk of injury.[10] Additional water-based activities (other than swimming) are kickboard exercises, aqua-aerobics, and deep-water running.

Resistance training is recognized as an essential element of weight management programs for people of all ages. Growth and maintenance of metabolically active tissue are critical and integrally linked to regular involvement in physical activity.

### 13.3.6.3   Frequency of Exercise

Ideal initial frequency of exercise would be three to four times per week but additional benefits may be gained by exercising more frequently, even daily where possible. As mentioned above, it is important not to be overzealous in commencing regular physical activity. Individuals too often commence a program full of enthusiasm and with the best of intentions but stop soon after due to soreness, injury, or tiredness.

### 13.3.6.4   Duration of Exercise

Any increase in activity beyond the level of commitment prior to commencing a program is a good start. For many children, particularly those who have not been completely inactive, approximately 20 to 30 min of sustained activity per day is a good starting point if the aim is to improve cardiovascular fitness. This timeframe assumes that one is active for the full time period with the heart rate elevated to an appropriate training level. If the child has been extremely inactive, a shorter timeframe may be needed initially.

### 13.3.6.5   Intensity of Exercise

A substantial training effect can be accomplished by exercising in an appropriate heart rate range. As fitness improves, the heart rate response lowers for a given workload or activity. As for other components of the exercise prescription, there needs to be a progressive increment in work output to provide cardiorespiratory system overload to gain an improvement.

Intensity of exercise is by far the most difficult to quantify and is a particular challenge in young people. The better approaches for determining intensity of exercise are heart rate monitoring and rating of perceived exertion.[10] Ideally, one might suggest that an allied goal of activity participation is to understand the physiological response of one's body. Young people, particularly those in late childhood and adolescence, can be trained to measure heart rate with a reasonable degree of accuracy but this ability is a challenge for some. The use of heart rate monitors is a logical alternative but this technology may only be available in a clinic setting. The Borg RPE scale has also been used to determine exercise intensity in obese children but its widespread use is also cost prohibitive.[473]

The challenge is to work with children to increase their knowledge and understanding of physical responses to exercise. Knowing one's own body provides enormous benefits when prescribing exercise. Too often we are reliant upon others for advice and this is certainly the case for young people. We need to balance the adult prescription mentality with objective indications of intensity from children. This includes the opportunity for children to make decisions about how hard they work. In this way, adult imposition that may include greater expectations of work output than are desirable could be minimized.

In a simplistic sense, exercise intensity for weight loss may involve exercising at an intensity as high as possible for the available time period. This may suit some young people but may be fraught with problems for others, including cardiovascular and musculoskeletal risk and adherence to activity.

Exercise prescription for weight management may be described as a conundrum. The total volume of energy expended will determine the amount of weight loss, along with the composition of the exercise.[10] For all obese individuals, but particularly children and adolescents, the real challenge is to individualize the exercise program wherever possible knowing that this will influence the individual's tolerance, interest, and adherence to physical activity in the longer term.

## 13.4  Exercise Program

The exercise program for obese children consists of the following considerations:

- A physical fitness or conditioning component.
- Participation in appropriate physical activities, sports skills, and recreational pursuits.
- Guidance in lifestyle habits that encompass exercise and diet.

### 13.4.1  Conditioning Program

The capacity for exercise varies widely between individuals. This is even the case with individuals of a similar age and physical status. For this reason, it is important to structure activities based on each individual's response to exercise. Activity sessions may include the following sequence of activities:

- Preparatory warm-up activities.
- A set of stretching exercises.

- A cardiorespiratory conditioning period.
- Muscular strength and endurance activities.
- Dance, gymnastics, or other motor skill activities.
- Games and sports skills incorporating a cool-down.

### 13.4.1.1   Warm-Up Period

The focus during this period should be on low intensity activities involving large muscle groups. This period serves to elevate the heart rate in preparation for more vigorous activity to follow.

### 13.4.1.2   Stretching Activities

An extension of the warm-up in which a core of stretching exercises are completed and others chosen according to the specific focus of the main section of the activity session to follow.

### 13.4.1.3   Cardiorespiratory Endurance and Strength Activities

These activities form the bulk of the exercise program and are designed to improve the efficiency of the heart, lungs, and associated blood vessels. A range of strength tasks is incorporated using a combination of partner resistance and gym equipment.

### 13.4.1.4   Dance, Gymnastics, and Other Motor Skill Activities

Obese individuals should be exposed to a wide cross-section of experiences in these areas on a rotating basis. Dance is often a good choice since it is very attractive for children and adolescents even when they claim to be "too tired" from other exercises. The various forms of dancing to popular music can be quite energy demanding and are particularly suitable for an increased energy expenditure. Exposure to simple gymnastic activities and more structured classical gymnastic exercise can be especially helpful for the training of individual muscle groups and also improve body posture. Activities in these areas can be planned to suit obese individuals of various ages.

### 13.4.1.5   Sports and Recreational Skills

Activity opportunities should include a diversity of skills designed to improve a child's or adolescent's involvement in individual and team physical activity tasks. Obese children should be encouraged to swim, since the excess body fat of the individual enhances buoyancy, facilitates this sort of activity, and can involve all major body parts. This form of exercise can be undertaken year round if one has access to an indoor swimming pool, and is particularly suitable for a growing child. A wide variety of exercises can be conducted in the water with or without equipment, including deep-water running.[10]

Bicycle ergometer work can supplement the exercise program at the beginning of the program prior to the use of resistance-training exercises. Road cycling is a good alternative but only if safety is not compromised. Cycling as an exercise may be problematic for some individuals if the position of the chest is cramped and does not permit adequate breathing and the development of the chest muscles. In all activity tasks, the development of optimal breathing is one of the main aims of an exercise program for the obese.

Genu valgum and varum, a common condition in obese children, may be exacerbated, particularly during activities such as skating. This type of activity is not recommended under such circumstances or until weight loss and the adoption of the necessary skills. The careful introduction of cross-country skiing may also be a goal as the young person gains some success in the program. All weight-bearing activities such as running, jumping, and other track-and-field events can be gradually implemented. Various games are also an excellent choice depending on the individual's enjoyment of this form of exercise. Enjoyment of particular activities helps to maximize adherence to such a program.

## 13.5  Lifestyle Habits

The conscious modification of a number of key habits can help to reduce the tendency toward inactivity. Following is a short list of suggestions for adjustment:

- Use stairs instead of escalators and elevators.
- Walk children to school or to stores instead of driving. This may be a rotating responsibility of parents who may help supervise a group of children living in an area walk to and from school if safety is an issue.
- Take a brisk walk whenever convenient during the day.
- Walk everywhere!
- Encourage and support the young person in anything that incorporates an increase in physical activity.
- Attempt to practice and reinforce activity skills that have been introduced.

Some of the suggested activities may be unrealistic and therefore compromised due to safety concerns, especially in larger urban areas. This need not be a drawback but rather a challenge. Activity that is organized and supervised by appropriate adults is often a more suitable choice.

## 13.6  General Guidelines for Exercise Participation

### 13.6.1  Clothing

Clothing is important for a variety of reasons, not only from the point of view of suitability for exercise activities. Clothing can also play a role in adding to the attractiveness of the activity. This may be a strong factor in the pleasure gained by a young person in a range of settings, either in the gym, sports hall, or playground. This may be more of an issue for the participant than other instructions and advice he/she may receive.

Clothing should be attractive to the child as mentioned above, but of paramount importance is that items are comfortable and loose fitting. A concern for many overweight and obese individuals is self-consciousness. Empathy for this concern and doing everything possible to allay fears related to clothing, or lack of it, such as at the swimming pool, should be a high priority. Choose clothing with pleasant colors and with a style that is fashionable if this can help improve the likelihood of continued participation and enjoyment.

Children and adolescents should be discouraged from wearing any plastic or rubberized clothing while exercising. This practice is potentially dangerous, as the normal heat regulation of the body can be impaired. Resultant problems could include sharp increases in body temperature, dehydration, and possible heat exhaustion.[47] Only synthetic materials specially developed for champion atheletes would be acceptable.

### 13.6.2  Exercise Surface

While the chosen activity will be the major determining factor with respect to exercise surface, every attempt should be made to avoid repetitive exercises on hard surfaces. Excessive loading and jarring on such surfaces, particularly if combined with poor footwear, can predispose one to injury. Where possible, preventative strategies could include working on a grassed area to avoid the risk of jarring injuries.

### 13.6.3  Appropriate Time to Exercise

This is a very individual issue. Participation is the most important issue, not when exercise is to occur. Time of day to exercise is very much determined by adult preference rather than the child and when the chosen activity session or program may be offered, for example, during or after school, evenings, and holiday times. Avoid exercising in extreme weather conditions, particularly periods of high temperature and/or humidity. However, it is recommended that individuals exercise as often as possible under any suitable conditions.

### 13.6.4  Possible Complications Resulting from Exercise

There is always a possibility, especially in a more obese, clumsy child with too much enthusiasm at the beginning of a new regime, for illness or injury to occur. Physical activity should be modified, reduced, or eliminated according to ability and/or the severity of injury or sickness. Always consult a medical practitioner when in doubt. When an injury occurs, look for opportunities to maintain fitness by completing alternative modes of activity. For example, if an individual is unable to bear weight and run because of an injury to a lower limb, swimming or cycling may be a good alternative.

## 13.7  Motivation

Too often, exercise programs are started with the very best of intentions only to fail due to a lack of interest on the part of the individual. There are many things that can be done to help maintain one's motivation for activity. The fundamental starting point is to determine the likes and dislikes of the child. Capitalize on the activities the child likes and identifies as important, and use opportunities to attempt such tasks as stepping stones to new experiences. Commitment to activity is likely to be much greater, along with the chance to downplay the common excuses for inactivity: "too hard," "too boring," or "too embarrassing:"[47]

- Choose realistic and achievable short-term goals that are not performance based. This may relate to total activity time and type(s) of activity.
- Exercise at a regular time of the day and make this part of the child's daily routine.
- Exercise with a partner, in a small group of similar peers, or with the family.
- Monitor the body's changes; for instance, have participants write down how they feel and record any obvious physical changes they notice.
- Consider a system of reward for improvements in behavior. For example, improvements may include reductions in particular inactive behaviors such as television viewing, attaining a goal of being

active on a pre-determined number of occasions across successive weeks, or completing a given distance in aerobic activities.[47,875]

- Avoid a preoccupation with weight. Do not equate the loss of a certain amount of weight with success, or think of losing weight quickly as the only desirable outcome. For many children, weight loss may not be a sensible goal. Depending on the age and stage of physical maturation, most children and many adolescents may have considerable potential for further growth. Any minimization in potential for growth in height and FFM, a potential risk on a restrictive diet, should be avoided at all costs. If weight loss is a viable and necessary option, a logical approach is to remember that if weight has accumulated over a period of time one should consider any reduction in excess over a similar period of time.

- Payment of a deposit or bond that is repaid to the individual on the successful attainment of a goal or set of goals that was accepted at the commencement of a program. This approach or other forms of contract can be detrimental if too much emphasis is placed on the reward at the expense of any meaningful change in behavior. Nevertheless, young children and older individuals alike enjoy having their achievements acknowledged. Simple rewards in recognition of the individual's efforts and achievements such as T-shirts and movie tickets, or an educational item like a book can be powerful motivators.

- Behavior modification techniques need to be prominent in all work with children. Counselling should include techniques that will assist in behavior modifications that are desirable in relation to dietary and physical activity changes.

## 13.8 Self-Monitoring

A point system to reward time spent in physical activity may be one way to encourage modifications in behavior as a step toward self-monitoring. Role models also have an important place in the growth and development of children and adolescents. Useful modeling of behavior may be provided by peers, siblings, parents, and significant others such as teachers and coaches.[47]

Children need to be provided with examples to encourage both participation in activity and improvements in eating behavior. For example, if uncontrolled eating is a problem, identify then eliminate the troublesome cue or cues. Assistance from family members to help young people learn to avoid temptations is paramount. The avoidance of stores on the way home from school, excessive television viewing, consumption of foods low in nutritional value, discouraging poor eating habits and practices, such as the reliance upon the consumption of fast food, are all possible strategies.

Considerable attention has been given to the settings in which the greatest opportunity exists to help large numbers of children who are overweight or obese. University- or hospital-based clinics have a rather limited impact, even if these clinics also provide the opportunity for group activity programs to complement the individualized approach. Generally, such centers attract the more difficult individuals or the more obese children and adolescents. The limited number of centers providing a comprehensive and integrated program, along with the potential cost may also be a limitation to larger numbers of individuals accessing such facilities.

## 13.9 Home-Based Programs

Home-based programs provide numerous challenges. A desirable outcome is for the child or adolescent to take increased responsibility for his or her well-being. Very young people may have a limited capacity to take on such a role but nevertheless such responsibility should be fostered at an early age. The ability of individuals to self-manage their condition, preferably with the support of a program planned for them, is very much associated with their level of motivation and the support and encouragement they are given. Opportunities for support include parents, siblings, and/or health professionals who may take on the role of a personal trainer. As for clinic-based programs, the latter option while the most desirable, is not feasible except for a relatively small proportion of the population due mainly to the cost involved.

Home-based programs may work for some individuals but the number may be limited to those who have committed family members to assist as role models. Even with supportive family members individuals also need support through knowledge and understanding and appropriate educational materials. The authors have had some experience in this area and found that home-based activities can be a strategic component of a weight management program, particularly when running in tandem with a clinic or school program.[18,55,61,158,303,339,341,342,457,522,970] When parents have an integral role to play in such programs, their usefulness in the home setting can be maximized. With a written home program, parents can assist by providing supervision and assistance if instructed by other staff; for example, a physical educator or clinic staff member can verify work completed by children by signing off sheets as part of a contractual arrangement.

A good model for an integrated approach to a school or clinical setting complemented by home activities may be as follows:

- Initial screening, assessment, and support provided through an activity program in a university clinic or school setting.

- Personalized sessions with relevant health professionals depending on need; for example, medical practitioner, dietitian, exercise physiologist, and/or clinical psychologist. An individualized exercise prescription and dietary plan are required.
- Group activity program.
- Home-based program to complement the above.
- Educational material to support both settings. This should be resource material of particular benefit to all family members, in the form of a consolidated booklet or book with material specific to the individual provided. This may include completion exercises related to the program activities, providing complementary material to the theory and practice of nutrition and physical activity, diaries, questionnaires, growth charts, and a 'passport to health' that is the property of the individual child.[970]
- Educational seminar sessions on topical issues related to growth and development, body image, self-concept, self-esteem, nutrition, physical activity, and other relevant topics.

## 13.10 Recommendations for Leisure Time Activities

Video games and television programs have attracted considerable attention during recent years. They have been considered one of the main reasons for the progressive reduction in physical activity and exercise. A reduced level of sedentary activity of young people can result in an improvement in BMI, a loss of excess fat, and an improvement in the general health and functional status of obese children.

Especially in the early stages of treatment, it is recommended that the obese child becomes involved in some type of organized, regular physical activity. During such a monitored program, the time for activity is better utilized provided that adequate supervision and guidance from qualified staff are available. Unfortunately, there is a shortage of specialized staff available to provide the special approach that obese children require. Pedagogic experiences with normal-weight children are, of course, the basis of physical education for all children, but physical education is not readily available to all young children as it should be. Without the guarantee of a quality physical education program and the specific requirements for a special population such as the obese, increased demand is placed on the organization (school, clinic, hospital, and health and fitness center). Special programs are also more expensive but do provide a better guarantee of a safer and sustainable benefit.

Individual exercise and special sport activities implemented later must be chosen cautiously for obese children. Such children can be easily discouraged prematurely, for example, when they are unable to participate or are not achieving any noticeable results. Exercises must be selected according to the degree of obesity and its duration, and also to the age and gender of the child. As mentioned above, health status and initial functional capacity levels provide the necessary details to determine a starting point for the preparation of the well-planned exercise program.

Parents have a preference for supervised activities because many are afraid to let their children run freely without supervision in parks or playgrounds due to safety reasons. The possibility of long-term health benefits from a comprehensive weight management program with exercise as a central feature should also be a persuasive factor in encouraging the family to participate actively in management of the child's weight.

In more severe cases of childhood obesity, it is necessary to decide whether the individual should participate in usual physical education classes at school. Very obese children often have some additional health problems. Further, many obese individuals will try anything to avoid physical education with their normal-weight peers who can treat their obese schoolmates in a quite cruel and discouraging way. This is a major factor in the reduced interest in exercise.

The authors' experiences have shown that when children participated in physical education programs in summer camps where only obese children were present, their inhibitions disappeared. The children are able to achieve some level of physical performance and are competitive among themselves in sports activities along with weight lost over the duration of such a camp. Correspondence with parents is evidence of the acceptability of such camps to obese children, for example, "I feel very happy here and would like to stay here even longer." Camps lasting approximately 7 weeks resulted in a loss on average of 10% of initial weight and fat, improvement in performance, and increased self-esteem.[18,189] It is regrettable that this sort of weight management program is usually too expensive for the majority of families. Therefore, outpatient programs and participation in physical education classes for obese children during the school year are the most appropriate choices. However, even these opportunities are not very common in the majority of countries and especially in the bigger urban areas where they are most needed.

## 13.11 The Role of the Pedagogue and Physical Educator

The personalities of those who organize, supervise, and guide physical education and exercise for obese children are pivotal and must be similar to the role of the family. He/she should be patient, knowledgeable about all developmental aspects and problems of the obese child, kind and joyous, and sensitive to carefully reinforcing children even when errors occur. It is also very important to stress all successes, although they may be minimal in the eyes of others.

Adults who have had experiences with elite athletes of all ages are commonly not very suitable for the monitoring of exercise and physical education for obese individuals. Work and experiences with a select group of high achievers in the physical activity domain often means that such teachers and coaches do not have an empathy for the plight of the obese individual. Many often believe that "obesity is always the result of laziness and gluttony," and that it is necessary to be hard and tough with those who are obese. Such an approach may work in some cases, but for the majority of obese children, who are frequently shy and may have an inferiority complex, this attitude results in completely discouraging exercise. Nevertheless, it is possible to give some teachers the necessary skills to adapt their attitudes in order to work effectively with obese children.

## 13.12 Suggestions for a Balance between Physical Activity and Exercise

A sample program may include the following:

- Morning exercise for 10 to 15 min (may include stretching and muscular strength and endurance activities).
- Afternoon and/or evening (preferably both) of preparatory warm-up exercise lasting 15 to 30 min.
- A minimum of 2 hr of games, exercise, sport activities, walking, and running in the open air (each weekday).
- Twice a week, or whenever possible, participation in normal physical education classes that are modified to suit the obese.
- During weekends, at least 5 to 6 hr of physical activity of any sort including games, exercise, and sports. Whenever possible, this should occur in the open air and away from pollutants in large urban areas. Parents, siblings, friends, and peers, or anybody suitable who is willing to cooperate should participate.
- Exercise should involve all large muscle groups (including abdominal wall, chest, and back muscles mainly because of body posture).

At the beginning of a program, it is necessary to execute all movements slowly and in a controlled fashion. Movement that is correct and progressively becomes more economical and purposeful is the goal. Exercising in a setting where there are mirrors enables progressive improvement through the self-control of one's own performance. However, this might discourage some individuals, especially in the beginning of the intervention. Use of correct feedback, both visually and verbally, can also facilitate the progressive control of movement necessary to manage body posture and achieve a symmetric and stable gait. This work should not be exclusive to the obese but is also necessary for children of normal body weight. Any improvement in appearance is a bonus for an individual who may still have a long way to go in order to increase their interest in exercise.

## 13.13  Selected Exercises for Individual Parts of the Body

### 13.13.1  Body Posture

- The head is drawn up, with the chin and the neck at a right angle.
- Shoulders are spread and drawn back and down.
- Arms hang along the sides with elbows rotated out so the thumbs are directed forward.
- Abdominal muscles are drawn in and buttock muscles are contracted.
- The pelvis is reinforced and is mildly drawn backward flattening any exaggerated lordotic curve with protruding abdomen.
- When standing, the feet are oriented in such a way that body weight is evenly spread.
- The pronounced neck lordosis often found in obese individuals can be minimized by the contraction of muscles between scapulae and the vertebral column, especially between the 6th and 9th vertebrae.
- Simultaneously, the ribcage is lifted and the shoulders are drawn back and down. The position of the chest is improved which enables better breathing.

### 13.13.2  Breathing Exercises

Breathing exercises are only suitable when children have acquired an adequate body posture. During all exercises it is necessary to be aware of the airflow in and out of the lungs. Most children (not only those who are obese) breathe superficially, automatically, and without any conscious control.

Conscious breathing is best taught in a lying position. Attention must be paid to expiration, and various rhythms are used. During these exercises the abdomen should be drawn in, the pelvis tilted back, and the small of the back pushed toward the ground. Expiration should always last longer than inspiration since it has been shown that after a proper expiration, the lungs automatically inspire in a better manner. It is also recommended that the muscles of the ribs be exercised. The adoption of adequate breathing simultaneously improves body posture as well.

### 13.13.3 Other Exercises

For very obese children with a low level of fitness, it is best to prescribe exercise in an aquatic environment. Following some improvement in performance in an aquatic setting, it is recommended that exercise occur in a lying position, both on the back and abdomen. This can progress into sitting and kneeling positions. This progression reduces the load of one's own body weight that interferes with weight-bearing activities such as walking and running and also when exercising in a standing position. Again, it is important to start with a slow rhythm with a proper explanation of how to perform all exercises. Instruction should also include how the individual will benefit from such an exercise, and what should be avoided to execute all movements properly.

Coordination of exercise and breathing rhythm is essential. Relaxation after exercise when the muscles are mostly contracted is indispensable. Each exercise is performed four to six times at the beginning, later eight to ten times. A kind and empathetic approach at the beginning helps the obese children gain confidence. The creation of a nice and enjoyable ambience enables a better response from all involved.

All exercise can be executed in a right or wrong way. The latter not only results in limited benefits but could also cause some harm. Therefore, an experienced teacher or exercise physiologist should be responsible for exercise prescription for obese children, otherwise there may be some risk of injury if inappropriate procedures are introduced.

#### 13.13.3.1 Exercises for the Vertebral Column

Better functioning of the vertebral column involves strengthening of the muscles of the abdominal wall, and the relaxation and lengthening of the contracted muscles of the shoulders and back. One then needs to relax the hip joints and simultaneously strengthen the muscles around the joints. It is good to start in lying position. At the beginning, it is recommended that the supervisor assist the exercising child, for example, to help him/her get up from the lying position to the sitting position by pulling the child's hands. During all exercise, it is necessary to watch for free breathing, to consciously control and not hold breathing, and also not forget to concentrate on expiration.

A number of exercises for improvement of vertebral column posture in a lying position on the back and/or on the sides are available, involving various movements of the legs and arms. Other sets of exercises can be executed in a sitting, kneeling, or standing positions. Each exercise must be followed by appropriate relaxation.

### 13.13.3.2   Exercises for Upper and Lower Extremities

When exercising the lower extremities, strengthening of the thighs needs to be stressed. In spite of their large circumferences, thigh muscles are often too weak and flaccid in obese children. It is helpful to stand in one place and lift alternate knees in a controlled fashion or to exercise with a jumprope. From standing, the next progression would be to jogging in place and completing similar movements. Exercises should be limited in number at the beginning, gradually increasing over time. Skipping can also be useful if it is low and elastic. These exercises can be supplemented by leg flexion and extension movements on appropriate machines, squats, and stepping up and down on a bench while maintaining adequate body posture and breathing frequency.

Movements of the upper extremity should be executed with the remainder of the body stable in the standing, sitting, kneeling, and lying positions. Progressive isolation and control of major muscle groups from the shoulders should be the goal.

### 13.13.3.3  Exercises for the Pelvis

Conscious control of the position of the pelvis is critical for body posture and the position of the internal organs. Good postural control can be achieved by using a set of exercises in the standing, sitting, lying, and kneeling positions.

A more detailed description of exercises for various parts of the body is not the aim of this volume. Information can be gained from numerous textbooks on physical education. A textbook of physical education specifically for obese children is not currently available in the literature. Therefore, it is necessary to draw on all possible experiences and adapt or modify the information on different activities and exercises for normal-weight children to meet the needs of obese children, according to the above-mentioned guidelines and instructions.

## 13.14   How to Encourage Obese Children to Adhere to Regular Exercise

- Irrespective of the modest beginning and initial results it is always very important to demonstrate some positive improvement after a short period of time. There may not be any absolute change in body weight or BMI caused by simultaneous decrease of fat mass and increase of lean, fat-free body mass. Therefore, an evaluation of body composition measures including circumferences and skinfolds can be used to great effect. Reductions in centimeters at particular sites can be motivational and enable increased comfort in the clothes one wears. Lack of change in body weight may also be due to a simultaneous growth in height. All changes should be shared with the child and used as a major educational opportunity. Positive comments are of paramount importance to the child.

- It is necessary to persuade the obese child that only permanent adherence to increased physical activity and an exercise program will provide lasting reduction of overweight and excess fatness along with an increase in the level of physical performance and fitness. The opportunity for personal involvement of the obese child or adolescent in the weight management process through an appropriate psychological approach is the best way to successful treatment. It may also be useful to identify a group of charismatic individuals well known as local personalities to provide some 'star' quality.

- An enjoyable atmosphere in a nice environment needs to be fostered with a kind and friendly physical educator. With quality staff, the best results can be achieved. However, a degree of discipline is also necessary. Recognition of issues and concerns can help to increase interest in physical education classes and also enhance involvement in spontaneous exercise during leisure time.

- Positive evaluation and encouragement should be provided for each child on an individual basis. The presence of the other participants, or the family and friends is very important to most young people. This helps to encourage the child to continue to exercise and to maintain any increase in physical activity levels.

In summary, when no effect is obvious, one needs to determine whether to speak about the issue or not, or alternatively, to find something positive in the experience. Examples include better performance of an activity or physical task, or improvement of the silhouette or body posture. Some appreciation, praise, and encouragement are always very much valued.

## 13.15  Supportive Role of the Family

Parents and family members are usually the closest people to the child. Their emotional and psychological support is essential in all aspects of the weight management process and the education of the child.

Do not expect something different of the overweight or obese child; that is, anything expected of the overweight child should be expected of other family members. This applies to the consumption of food and all other activities. As mentioned in conjunction with nutrition, the best solution is for family members to actively participate, at least at the beginning of the new program. When all family members adopt and adhere to an active lifestyle, the more acceptable it is for the obese child. Exercising together with children is a good custom in some families, as is spending leisure time walking including all family members, and vacationing together. Often, simple options are the most enjoyable to encourage an increase in activity. For example, a more modest program in a park or recreational area close to the home can be sufficient since it is more ideally suited to participation in at least some activities. It is difficult or almost impossible to persuade a child to increase his/her physical activity output when looking at overweight parents who move only when they must.

Walking and suitable games can be shared on regular occasions as frequently as possible. Even small competitions based on gender and age can be fun and enable the involvement of all participants.

When caring parents have more than one obese child, their role may be made easier. More problems may be related to diet and exercise when one child is obese and another is not. However, when siblings are supportive, results can improve. A more active lifestyle can be useful for everybody. It is always better to adapt the program to the necessities of the obese child and increase the level of physical activity and exercise than the opposite way.

The obese member of the family should never be ridiculed or criticized. This applies particularly to siblings as well as peers at school. There is a risk that the obese child will be a target for joking and ridicule, some of which may be very unpleasant. This scenario rarely results in a defense reaction and an effort to improve status, with the aim to lose weight faster and achieve success in some other area. More commonly it results in the spontaneous isolation and self-pity with few positive outcomes with respect to the reduction of weight and fat.

Obese children usually cannot avoid negative reactions at school. They should at least be able to feel secure, at ease, and well appreciated at home. This applies particularly to the effort to adhere to the prescribed diet and exercise program. The encouragement of family members and kind assistance can significantly support a greater commitment to exercise.

## 13.16   Sample Activities That Provide the Basis of an Activity Program for Young Children

### 13.16.1   Games and Game Skills for Children

An introduction to games and game skills should be considered in an orderly sequence of stages. Progression through these stages is directly related to the individual child's stages of motor development.

### 13.16.1.1 Stage 1 Skills

Opportunity should be provided for free play with large, soft, light balls. Other useful ideas include running games, singing games, and other games that foster children's imagination.

### 13.16.1.2 Stage 2 Skills

Running and dodging

Hitting skills

- Hitting a ball off the top of a cone marker or off the ground.
- Continuous hitting of a balloon, trying to keep it in the air using either hand.

Catching

- Rolling a ball between partners who are stationary.
- Fielding a rolling ball.
- Catching a large ball (encouraging a basket catch on the chest).
- Catching a bean bag with two hands and the next time with only with one hand.

Throwing

- Underarm roll, trying to control direction and distance.
- One-handed roll concentrating on gripping the ball with fingers, combine with stopping and catching skills.

Bouncing

- Various tasks bouncing and catching a large ball.

### 13.16.1.3 Stage 3 Skills

Running and dodging

Hitting skills

- Bouncing a ball and hitting or striking with hand or bat.
- Hitting a ball against a fence or wall.
- Hitting a ball from a stationary position, for example, a T-ball stand.

Catching

- Catching bean bag with one hand, alternating sides.
- Two- and one-handed catches with various types of balls, for example, small to large.
- Add a partner or small group to test above-mentioned skills.
- Throwing and catching overhead.

Kicking
- Start with a large ball.
- Try to kick a large ball off the ground, alternate feet, progressively incorporating target and distance goals.
- Use alternate objects for balls, perhaps empty milk cartons and bean bags.

Bouncing
- Bouncing a large ball with both hands sitting, kneeling, or standing.
- Bouncing and catching on the move, start with walking then speed up.
- Pat bouncing while walking, then running.

### 13.16.1.4   Stage 4 Skills

Running and dodging

Hitting skills
- Involving progressive increases in difficulty: hitting a stationary ball, a ball pitched underarm, hitting a ball to a particular area of the field, experience hitting tasks using different bats and rackets.

### 13.16.2  Body Image or Body Awareness, Spatial Awareness, Eye–Hand and Eye–Foot Coordination

All children need to be provided with activities to develop body image (or body awareness), gross and fine muscle coordination, and rhythmic coordination. Some children will learn more slowly and some obese children will have difficulty in performing simple skills. Many children, of all shapes and sizes, and as a function of lack of opportunity or time spent in physical activity, may have difficulty in one or more of these areas.

Body image or body awareness: how the child views him or herself and the child's awareness of the relation of one body part to another.

Touch: child touches different parts of the body, while standing, sitting.

Body movement:
- Child moves various parts of the body as the teacher names each.
- Child crawls moving arm and leg of one side simultaneously.

Spatial awareness: the child's awareness of his/her body in space and in relation to directions such as up, down, forward, and backward. Once a child becomes thoroughly aware of his/her own body, he/she must begin to use body parts to explore space. He/she must feel what it is like to move through, in, out, over, around, and under various pathways and obstacles.

Eye–hand and eye–foot coordination: the child's ability to integrate muscles in tasks requiring the use of eyes and hands or hands and feet.

# 14

## Summary

## 14.1 Main Characteristics of Childhood Obesity

Obesity has now reached epidemic proportions and is evident much earlier in life. The numerous co-morbidities associated with obesity are also being recognized in childhood and adolescence as compared to the past when such problems were restricted to the adult years. This suggests that research, clinical support, and preventive measures must be developed to identify and work with individuals at risk while providing appropriate support for the wider community in a lifestyle approach to weight management.

The main reason for the limited success in the treatment and prevention of childhood obesity is that despite considerable research and clinical experience in the area, all of the causes have not yet been satisfactorily explained. Genetic make-up includes not only specific genes causing family clustering of obesity, but also predisposition to a certain food intake with respect to the amount of energy and the composition of the diet based on specific food preferences and aversions. The same may also apply to the level of spontaneous physical activity. Some evidence suggests that the genetic predisposition to obesity may be related to both the total volume as well as type of physical activity in which one participates.

The prevalence of obesity has increased, especially recently. This increase has occurred mainly in the industrially developed countries such as the U.S. and U.K., but children from higher socioeconomic groups in Third World countries are also at risk. The prevalence of childhood obesity in Asian, African, and Middle Eastern countries, and Oceania was initially lower, but has recently increased and may be quite similar in the larger urban agglomerations to some developed countries. With improving economic and social situations in these countries, the prevalence of childhood obesity is also increasing in other social strata. The same concerns exist for similar population groups of lower social status in the industrially developed countries.

Examples of childhood population groups from developing countries who emigrated and then became acculturated to their new country, as well as the increase in childhood obesity in the former East Germany, provide some important clarifications of the etiology of obesity. The speed with which obesity has worsened in such areas suggests that environmental causes are more likely to have been responsible for change rather than genetics. Therefore, particular attention must be paid to lifestyle changes.

Special attention has been paid to the nutrition and physical activity regimes of children in many countries. In some countries, obesity prevalence seems to have reached a plateau, for example, in the Czech Republic and in some countries of Eastern Europe. For a more accurate analysis of current trends, it would be necessary to repeat the assessment of the prevalence of childhood obesity using comparable criteria with the same methods and approaches in all countries, a process that has not yet been conducted.

A special type of obesity that occurs mainly, but not exclusively, in countries of the Third World, is that accompanying stunting of growth (that is, lower height for age) which follows early malnutrition. The mechanism of this type of obesity has not been fully elucidated but it seems that adaptation to restricted food intake early in life with a subsequent adequate or abundant food can cause increased metabolic efficiency accompanied by increased deposition of fat.

However, analyses of the present research data are compromised (much more than is the case in adults) because individual studies were conducted again with subjects of various ages, categorized into age groups at different stages of sexual maturity, which is also somewhat variable in different countries. Further, there has been a failure to report or inconsistent data on the duration and severity of obesity along with possible co-morbidities. The same shortcomings apply to studies on the results of treatment modalities. In addition, all children in spite of their many common features are unique. Comparisons of available methods are therefore potentially compromised if appropriate consideration has not been given to these issues including homogenous consented terminology. Nevertheless, a number of important pointers have been gained, each of which can be used to influence a more efficient treatment and also the prevention of childhood obesity.

Obesity is defined as an excessive accumulation and ratio of stored fat when compared to other tissues. Overweight refers to an increase of body weight above an arbitrary standard value usually defined in relation to height, and may not always be caused entirely by increased body fatness. Therefore, for the evaluation of obesity, the most important approach is measurement of the amount of body fat, both in absolute and relative terms.

A number of methods have been used in the assessment of body composition. The most important laboratory techniques used are hydrodensitometry (underwater weighing), dual energy X-ray absorptiometry (DXA), dilution methods using $D_2O$, total body conductivity measurements (TOBEC), $^{40}K$ measurements, magnetic resonance imaging (MRI), and creatinine excretion. Other techniques have also been used, for example, computer tomography (CT). However, the degree of irradiation has prevented more widespread use of this method during growth.

Field (bedside assessment techniques) body composition assessment has traditionally involved anthropometry. Most commonly, skinfold measurements are taken and summed or converted using regression equations based on the relationships of subcutaneous and total body fat to percent body fat values. Circumference measures, such as the arm and calculated fat and muscle areas, are also used extensively. Bioimpedance analysis (BIA) has more recently gained widespread acceptance.

The parameter most used in overweight and obesity assessment has been the body mass index (BMI). BMI growth charts have been developed in many countries based on the local growing population's measurements, e.g., in France, the U.S., U.K., Sweden, and the Czech Republic. BMI has also been validated using other measurements of body composition such as BIA, densitometry, and MRI. Correlations have always been significant, but the accuracy of the estimation of body fat using BMI alone is compromised, particularly in cases of more severe obesity.

When appropriately trained testers are available, the more direct measurement of body fatness by measuring skinfold thickness is still recommended. However, BMI or the skinfold measurement may be spurious as a technique in individuals who are obese. As a relatively simple index to employ, BMI provides for trend data to be used to track individual and group predisposition for the development of obesity with increasing age. One of the most important components in this respect is the adiposity rebound (AR), where BMI starts to increase again after a temporary decline during childhood. AR occurs earlier in obese children when compared to normal-weight peers and predicts the development of obesity in later years.

With respect to further morphological parameters, obese children usually show an accelerated growth in height along with increased weight. However, higher stature is only temporary and obese children do not always become taller adults. An increase in stored fat is often accompanied by increased development of lean, fat-free body mass, an increase in some bone dimensions (for example, bi-iliocristal breadth in boys), and bone age. These features have been revealed in some studies but not in others.

Fat deposited in the growing organism is not only indicative of increased relative (percentage) and absolute amounts (kg) of fat, but also of a different distribution pattern. These differences are reflected in various patterns of fat deposition on the trunk and extremities as evaluated by indices calculated from skinfold thickness measurements, e.g., the subscapular/triceps ratio. Similarly, the amount of intra-abdominal fat relative to subcutaneous fat is important and already increases the health risk during childhood. Intra-abdominal fat can be assessed by ultrasound, MRI, CT, and by simple anthropometric measurements such as the waist-to-hip ratio or the distance between the tip of the abdomen and L4 to L5 measured by pelvimeter.

Distribution of body fat varies significantly in normal-weight boys and girls but does not show any significant gender differences between obese boys and girls. Characteristic trends include an increased deposition of fat on the trunk as related to the extremities, or increased intra-abdominal fat as related to subcutaneous fat. This type of fat pattern is related significantly to a number of adverse biochemical and hormonal characteristics. These morphological features can also estimate possible variability in health risk in different types of obesity during growth.

Childhood obesity is associated not only with morphological change, but also changes in many other parameters. Among the most important of these are nutritional, functional, biochemical, hormonal, and psychological change. Many of these parameters vary markedly when comparisons are made with normal-weight peers, but may or may not be significant.

Both energy intake and energy expenditure have been studied. In the former, food habits and the composition of ingested foods have been considered. With respect to energy output, total energy expenditure (TEE), resting metabolic rate (RMR), and energy spent in physical activity levels (AEE) have been the areas of focus. However, such assessments have not necessarily been undertaken to elucidate their role in the development of obesity, or in the prevention, treatment, and management of the condition.

The main cause(s) of obesity is undisputed, an excess of energy intake is always present whatever the reason. An energy imbalance is of particular concern, especially in the case of genetically predisposed individuals. It must be remembered that obesity never occurs in conjunction with a markedly restricted food intake, as frequently occurs in poorer countries of the Third World and where malnutrition is rife. Similarly, obesity never occurs among young athletes involved in intensive aerobic sports training.

Many studies have shown neither increased food intake nor decreased resting or total energy output due to inactivity in assessments of children. However, some studies that have compared obese and normal-weight growing individuals have found some significant differences. The discrepancies between the results of individual studies may stem from differences in experiment design.

Various components of energy expenditure have also been studied in obese children of different ages and compared with those of normal-weight children. Resting metabolic rate (RMR, or resting energy expenditure, REE) is related mainly to body size and composition. Therefore, comparisons between direct measurements and indirect derivations of REE in obese and normal children have shown certain differences. Because all regression equations using body weight and/or height were derived from measurements of predominantly normal-weight children, direct measurements of RER are recommended for the evaluation of REE in obese children. Higher absolute values of REE have been found in obese children, but when values are adjusted to fat-free body mass, these values did not differ. The thermic effect of food (TEF) or thermic effect of meal (TEM) and REE were not related to different types of fat distribution. TEM as a percentage of RER (RMR) was lower in obese children.

Total energy expenditure (TEE) can be measured using a number of methods, i.e., direct and indirect calorimetry. More recently, doubly labelled water ($^2H_2$ $^{18}O$-DLW) has been used for the measurement of total energy expenditure over a number of days under free-living conditions. However, the cost of this method is prohibitive and non-specific in the sense that it cannot provide details of specific components of daily activity, only TEE (similar to heart monitors). Consequently, field measurements are usually used. More suitable options in this regard have included accelerometers, activity rating scales, and questionnaires.

Results gained in studies from this area are inconsistent. In relation to TEE, some studies have not shown any differences while others have found a higher TEE in the obese compared to normal-weight subjects, along with a higher volume of sedentary activities in obese subjects. This finding may be explained by the increased energy cost of all movements of an obese child. During the same physical workload, energy expenditure is higher in the obese. The same or higher TEE thus corresponds to lower physical activity in the obese compared to normal-weight subjects. When this was considered, it was concluded that the physical activity level was lower and the ratio of sedentary activities higher in the obese.

In some studies, a significant negative relationship between activity and fatness was shown. In subjects with a low activity level, the ratio of stored fat was higher, and the reverse situation appeared in active subjects who were leaner. These relationships were apparent from a very young age and became more pronounced as they got older. Overall, more studies have shown greater inactivity in obese individuals and this applied more frequently to those with one or two obese parents.

Similar conclusions were also gained by following Pima Indian children, who are genetically more predisposed to obesity. For example, the time spent viewing television predicted weight gain 8 years later. Another study showed that in spite of a comparable TEE, the levels of physical activity and energy expended were lower in obese children. Sport grades in school were lower and involvement in sports training was also lower in obese children. The effect of physical activity and exercise was most demonstrated markedly by longitudinal studies of the same subjects, where the differences in both activity and fatness were significant.

Physical fitness and performance are the functional characteristics that differentiate significantly obese and normal-weight individuals. Individual items of functional capacity are affected by excess fatness in different ways. Aerobic power measured on a treadmill test is the same in absolute values or higher in the obese compared to normal-weight subjects. However, maximum $O_2$ per kg of body weight is lower in the obese and is a true reflection of cardiorespiratory fitness of the obese. Values per kg FFM are the same or lower. Values for ventilatory threshold (VT, defined as the highest oxygen uptake at which the pulmonary ventilation stops increasing linearly) are lower in obese children.

Similarly, results in dynamic performance of an aerobic nature and endurance are also worse in the obese, that is, whenever relocation of total body weight is required, such as running and jumping. However, muscle strength, which is dependent on total and particularly lean body mass, is often the same or even higher in the obese. Performance in static tasks is most often not compromised by excess fatness. The same may also apply to some motor skills involving smaller muscle groups (such as in plate tapping) or the use of individual limbs (such as in throwing, which also involves an element of strength).

Lung function measurements such as forced expiratory flow, maximal voluntary ventilation, minute ventilation, vital capacity, expiratory reserve volume, residual volume, diffusing capacity, and other parameters have shown altered pulmonary function, indicating that bronchospasm of smaller airways occurs more frequently in obese children. Decreased distensibility of the chest wall was also considered.

Polysomnography also showed a positive relationship between the apnea index with fatness and a negative correlation between the degree of obesity and the degree of sleepiness on multiple sleep latency tests. Many obese adolescents also snore. Blood pressure correlated significantly with percent ideal weight, skinfold thickness, and BMI, particularly after an extended period with obesity. Obesity is associated with increased posterior wall thickness and left ventricular internal dimensions of the heart (assessed by echocardiographic parameters). These characteristics were found by the age of 6 years.

Plasma hemostatic measures such as D-dimer, fibrinogen, and plasminogen activator inhibitor-1 were associated with body fatness. These relationships show that general adiposity and visceral adipose tissue might play a role in regulating plasma hemostatic factors in obese children. BMI and fatness indicators correlated with the number of white blood cells, lymphocytes, and neutrophils.

Measurement of food intake has shown that children were able to select an adequate diet without adult supervision when given a choice of nutrients. Some studies have revealed that satisfactory mechanisms to preserve an adequate energy balance exist from an early age; however, this applies when satiety mechanisms with respect to the energy balance of an organism are involved. Various factors affecting food intake and choice early in life can change this situation. Studies in infants have shown that a vigorous infant feeding style was associated with greater adiposity. Infant food intake and nutritive sucking behavior at 3 months of age contributed to the measures of body size at 12 and 24 months. Mothers who preferred a chubby child more often had an obese offspring.

The composition of food also has a significant effect. The ratio of protein at the age of 2 to 3 years had a significant positive relationship with the age of adiposity rebound (AR), and then with BMI and body fatness at the age of 8 years and older. No other relationships with respect to food intake were revealed in a longitudinal study of French individuals. This reinforces the idea that the earlier the onset of AR, increased BMI, and fatness, the more probable obesity is later in life.

There is little evidence that obese children overeat. However, measurements of food intake have been conducted in a similar fashion to measurements of physical activity and EE; that is, only when obesity was fully developed and the observations concerned short periods of time, commonly not with simultaneous measurements of EE. Many studies have shown the same food intake in obese and normal-weight children. In some studies, food intake correlated with body weight and height only in obese children, not in normal-weight children, or mixed groups. Other studies have shown that when energy intake was expressed in relation to fat-free mass, it was lower in the obese. Further studies have shown that the composition of the diet may be more important for the development of obesity than total intake of energy; this especially concerned the intake of fat at any age. A positive association of fat intake and adiposity development was found in a greater number of studies. Children of heavier parents preferred more fat and mothers have a greater influence on their children's food intake.

The child's eating style is important. The eating index (reflecting the child's ability to precisely adjust food intake in response to changes in energy density of the diet) was correlated with body stores of fat. Children with greater adiposity were less able to regulate energy intake accurately. The thermic effect of food (meal, TEF or TEM) was lower in the obese children when compared to normal-weight peers.

Food consumption patterns during the day are also important. Fewer meals per day, skipping breakfast, and ingesting relatively more food in the second half of the day, especially at dinner, is more common in obese children. Severely or morbidly obese children eat more restaurant meals, pizzas, snacks, and soft drinks. Such children also eat faster and do not slow down their eating rate toward the end of the meal. Gastric electrical activity measured by electrogastrography was not different in obese children.

The utilization of macrocomponents and the oxidation of fat are associated with body fatness. Exogenous fat oxidation expressed as a proportion of total fat oxidation correlated significantly with the degree of adiposity. This can be considered as a protective mechanism to prevent further increase in body fat mass in the organism. Exogenous carbohydrate utilization was significantly greater and endogenous carbohydrate oxidation significantly lower in obese subjects when compared to normal-weight peers. Obesity in preadolescent children is associated with an absolute increase in whole-body protein turnover which is related to an increased lean, fat-free body mass (FFM). Both factors help explain higher REE in the obese compared to normal-weight children.

Body fatness was significantly associated with a number of biochemical parameters, as is the case in adults, particularly with serum lipid levels. A positive correlation between TC and TG, and the percentage of stored fat was found as early as preschool age. HDL-C was significantly higher in active preschool children with a trend for lower adiposity. More favorable serum lipid and lipoprotein levels were associated with lower levels of fatness and higher levels of physical fitness in children aged 4 to 5 years and older. Obesity was associated with unfavorable lipid profiles in adolescents in many countries (Italy, Poland, Czech Republic, France, the U.S., U.K., and many others). In obese Roman children, higher levels of ApoB, TG, TC, and LDL-C along with lower HDL-C levels were found. A higher TC/HDL-C ratio was found in obese children in Austria and in another group of Italian children in the lower quartile of polyunsaturated fatty acid intake. TC and TG had a significant positive correlation with BMI in boys; in girls, only TG correlated with BMI. *In vivo* lipolysis reflecting the mobilization of lipid stores from subcutaneous adipose tissue of obese children showed decreased sensitivity to epinephrine. Decreased mobilization of TG may contribute to excess fat accumulation during growth.

Hyperuricemia has been observed in obese children and some parameters concerning mineral metabolism were altered. These include alkaline-phosphatase, osteocalcin, parathyroid hormone, calcitonin, hydroxyproline, and cyclic AMP. All were under basal conditions significantly higher in obese children with lower urinary excretion of calcium and phosphorus. During an oral glucose tolerance test (OGTT), the changes in calcium, phosphate, serum parathyroid hormone, and calcitonin were different in obese children. In some studies, bone mineral content (BMC) was lower in the obese. Total antioxidant capacity and plasma levels of soluble antioxidant vitamins were reduced in obese subjects.

Other studies have characterized the levels of several hormones in the obese. Insulin resistance and hyperinsulinemia coexist in obese children. Both increased insulin secretion and decreased insulin clearance contribute to hyperinsulinemia in obese adolescents. Significant correlations between fasting insulin, body weight, and blood pressure were found. Further studies have confirmed that the most important metabolic complications of obesity are impaired glucose tolerance, hyperinsulinemia, insulin resistance, decreased insulin sensitivity, and eventually noninsulin dependent diabetes (NIDDM). A defect in oxidative and nonoxidative glucose metabolism was revealed in obese preadolescents at the higher infusion rate using an euglycemic hyperinsulinemic clamp. Assessment of circadian rhythms has shown that insulin rhythm was disturbed, but the secretion of insulin is as pulsatile as in adults. Higher levels of insulin were found in the saliva of obese children.

Insulin-like growth factor-1 (IGF-1) was significantly greater in obese children and this correlated with BMI. IGF-1 values increased significantly during puberty and were higher in the obese in the earlier stages of sexual maturation. Levels of insulin-like growth factor binding protein-3 (IGFBP-3) were not different in some studies. Similarly, the IGF-1/IGFBP-3 ratio was not different when comparing obese and normal-weight subjects.

IGFBP-1 level is strongly associated with insulin sensitivity and fatness in early prepubertal children. Insulin sensitivity, IGF-1, and obesity are important predictors of IGFBP-1 levels in pubertal children. IGFBP-1 is suppressed by insulin and may increase free IGF-1 levels and thus contribute to somatic growth, which is temporarily accelerated in obese children. The IGFBP-1 level may be a useful predictor for the early identification of the development of insulin resistance. The free form of IGF-1 in circulation in obese children is normal.

Significant positive relationships were found between BMI and somatomedine-C-insulin-like growth factor-1 (SM-C/IGF-1) and between immunoreactive insulin (IRI) and SM-C/IGF-1. Other studies revealed a significant correlation between BMI and IRI. These data seem to indicate that SM-IGF-1 in obese children is regulated by IRI, which is related to BMI. This regulating effect of insulin may be important in obese children since human growth hormone (HGH) production for stimulating factors is reduced. Increased IGF-1 may also contribute, due to negative feedback, to reduced growth hormone (GH) synthesis and secretion in obese children. Simple obesity is associated not only with a decrease in GH synthesis, but also increased GH clearance, along with increased insulin and IGF-1 levels. GH response to provocative stimuli is blunted and nocturnal GH concentrations are reduced. Obese children also have significantly lower urinary GH levels than age-matched normal-weight children. Obese children have increased growth hormone-binding protein (GHBP) activity. It may be speculated that this phenomenon can contribute to the compensation from the reduced GH secretion and accelerated GH clearance.

In prepubertal children with exogenous obesity, the GH-IGF-1 axis is significantly altered, even when most changes in the peripheral IGF system appear to be independent of modifications of GH secretion. GHBP correlated significantly with percent body fat, waist and hip circumferences, waist-to-hip ratio, body weight, serum leptin concentration, uric acid, insulin, TC, LDL-C, LDL-C/TC ratio, TG, and height standard deviation score (SDS). Multiple regression analysis containing age, gender, anthropometric variables, percent fat, and waist circumference as independent variables still revealed a significant association between GHBP and leptin, TG, TC and LDL-C, and LDL-C/HDL-C ratio. Body composition and visceral adiposity appear to be dominant negative determinants of GH production since the relationships between GH secretion and age and testosterone are attenuated or abolished by increased fatness.

A higher secretion of steroids was reported in obese children when compared to normal-weight children, but the differences were greatly reduced when the excretion rate was related to total body weight. Body weight was correlated with certain steroid groups and compounds representing the androgens, androsteron, then ethiocholanolon and dehydroepiandrosteron. Differences in steroid secretion may indicate certain alterations in the adrenal function of obese children, but there was no reason to expect any significant disturbances in their steroid metabolism. Another study showed that obese children had increased excretion of cortisol metabolites, along with increased secretion of androgen metabolites and pregnenediol, a metabolite of pregnanolon. In some obese children hypersecretion of some components of the steroid spectrum was more frequent in boys. Another study showed that the integrated concentration of cortisol is reduced in obese children. Hyperphagia and obesity are the common characteristics of hypercortisolism.

Menarche has been related to a certain level of fat deposition during puberty and usually occurs several months earlier in girls who are obese.

Changes in circulating leptin can serve as a hormonal sign which influences gonadotrophin secretion. LH and FSH responses to GnRH were negatively correlated with BMI and circulating leptin in perimenarcheal girls and young adult women, that is, decreased LH and FSH responses to GnRH were associated with increased adiposity. These findings were in agreement with a negative neuroendocrine effect of excess leptin on the central reproductive system in obese girls. Precocious puberty in obese children is assumed to be related to excess weight. Along with accelerated growth, bone age may also be advanced in obese children.

Obese children have significantly higher average concentrations of beta-endorphin along with increased insulin. Beta-endorphin increases more with greater fatness than insulin and is significantly associated with energy and macronutrient intake. Only in obese subjects was a correlation between these two hormones evident. The level of beta-endorphin may be used as an indicator of appetite in overweight and obese children. The reaction of somatostatin following a liquid meal is the same in obese and normal-weight subjects, in spite of a higher response of integrated insulin in the obese under the same conditions.

Leptin has become the focus of attention in the study of obese children. Body fat correlates significantly with serum leptin concentration in newborns, children of preschool and school age, and in adolescents is similar to that in adults. Obese children have significantly higher levels of leptin. This is more pronounced in girls who have a higher percentage of stored fat, a trend that appears *in utero*. The lack of a significant association between leptin and dietary parameters or serum lipids in normal preschool children seems to indicate that the serum leptin concentration expresses the amount of body fat rather than playing a role as a predictive factor of childhood obesity. Serum leptin levels also significantly correlate with BMI. Low birth weight (self-reported values) has been related to higher leptin values in adulthood, after controlling for age and adult weight. Retrospective analyses of birth weight values suggest that leptin resistance in adulthood might have a fetal origin. Comparisons of leptin levels at the ages of 12 and 18 months, and then at the age of 10.1 years, showed that the baseline leptin continued to predict greater values of BMI percentile change over time.

In obese 5-year-old Pima Indian children, serum leptin levels correlated significantly with TEE, both in absolute values and when adjusted for body size and physical activity level. A significant correlation was also found for serum leptin level and the percentage of fat. In adolescents aged 14.5 years, the average values of leptin were $21.1 \pm 12.1$ ng.ml$^{-1}$. At a given level of BMI, a one to fourfold range of leptin levels was revealed. Age, gender, or level of sexual maturation did not appear to explain these marked differences. In some studies, the values of leptin were four to five times higher in obese children and adolescents when compared to normal-weight children of the same age.

A significant correlation was also shown for leptin and subcutaneous fat deposits in children and a weaker correlation was surprisingly found for leptin and visceral fat mass. Higher values of leptin were found in girls, even after adjustment for fat mass. Testosterone had a potent negative effect on serum leptin levels in boys, but not in girls. Marked variations in serum leptin levels were significantly related to maturational stage. Leptin increases in girls and decreases in boys as puberty progresses. High androgen concentrations in obese boys are responsible for the low leptin level as compared to obese girls. A critical level of leptin is obviously needed to maintain menstruation.

Serum leptin is also significantly associated with percent fat intake, and a high fat and low carbohydrate intake was related to leptin levels. Circulating leptin has also been positively correlated with several cardiovascular risks. Correlations between leptin, BMI, and body fat percentage were also found in diabetic children. Some genetic studies revealed that it is unlikely that mutations in the coding region of the long isoform of the leptin receptor are a common cause of juvenile-onset obesity. Another study in extremely obese children did not show leptin deficiency mutation.

Psychological assessments have indicated that the onset of obesity can depend on psychological problems such as stress in the family, at school, and among the peer group. On the other hand, obesity that develops in the early years of life can also contribute to psychological problems during childhood and beyond. Younger children usually do not perceive they have a problem provided they are not ridiculed. Physical growth changes are slower and more gradual during childhood, but adolescence is the period when self-awareness of appearance and body shape is more important. In addition to biological changes due to puberty, psychological adjustments also complicate this period of life.

There are a number of psychological accompaniments of childhood obesity. A well-planned psychological approach can significantly contribute to the evaluation of the causes of obesity, as well as play a key role in the management of obesity in a particular child. Common features include a fear of participating with normal-weight peers in social activities, games, and recreational activities. Children often feel shy and self-conscious and avoid situations in which they may feel vulnerable or threatened, for example, in the gym or wearing swimwear. Their avoidance of physical activities and exercise further worsens their health and social status. Studies that have considered preferences for various forms of disability have consistently rated obesity poorly. Young children rate the obese lowest when compared with other forms of disability.

Obesity can contribute to an altered body image and related concerns. Body image, the picture that a person has of his/her appearance, may be disturbed, with fluctuating intensity over even short periods of time. Under positive conditions, the child may not be troubled by the disability although concern may never be far from his/her consciousness. When one has esteem-lowering experiences and is depressed, more emphasis may be focussed on his/her obesity, and the body becomes the explanation and symbol of unhappiness. Body perception disturbance is a form of disturbed perception of body image and is characterized by denial that the individual is the size that he/she is. The obese most commonly overestimate their body width compared with normal-weight individuals. Obese individuals are often evaluated as gluttonous and lacking self-control, undermining their body image and isolating them psychologically and socially. On the other hand, food may become the individual's hatred and result in anorexia.

Excess weight and fatness may result in various physiological handicaps and altered psychological characteristics; for example, studies using a hyperactivity subscale (Connor's Parents Questionnaire) on the effects of obesity on various behavioral characteristics showed that children can have abnormal scores. Results showed higher "sex problem" scores in obese girls. Further evaluations indicated subtle behavioral differences in obese children, and the proportion of obese children placed in special education and remedial class settings was twice that for children with normal body weight.

Increased BMI is associated with unfavorable changes in physical activity attitudes, activity preferences, perceived physical activity competence, self-concept, and body image. There also appears to be a concern with body weight and shape. In severely obese children in China, lower performance on IQ scores plus a higher Eysenck Personality Questionnaire (EPQ) score was found. Obese Chinese children also showed lower total IQ, speech IQ, operation IQ, and thyroid function along with increased baseline secretion of insulin and C-polypeptide. Gonad development and maturity occurred earlier in the obese. However, decreased thyroid function may indicate some hormonal abnormalities in these obese. Observations of this kind have not been reported in other populations of obese children.

Patients with early onset obesity demonstrated a greater frequency and higher levels of emotional distress and psychiatric symptomatology than individuals with later onset. Psychiatric problems in adulthood may be associated with early onset of obesity, serving as a predictor variable for possible psychological disturbances in obese populations later in life. On the other hand, it is false to assume that all obese individuals are psychologically and emotionally disturbed.

Many obese individuals do not perceive any problems and appear to cope more efficiently by pursuing other spheres of activity, e.g., greater diligence at school, stamp collecting, and/or playing a musical instrument. These activities do not require a level of activity and physical fitness that would be required for participation in sports.

Juvenile obesity is usually accompanied by a number of health problems. Childhood obesity contributes to approximately 30% of adult obesity. An obese child who becomes an obese adult may have more severe adult obesity than one whose obesity begins during the adult years. In such cases, morbidity and mortality from all causes are increased, and risk of cardiovascular diseases, cancer (mainly of the colon), diabetes, and arthritis is higher. Participants who died during a 40-year longitudinal study in Sweden and those who reported cardiovascular diseases were significantly heavier at puberty and in adulthood than those who remained healthier.

In a group of obese children, 28% had hyperlipidemia, 25% had elevated blood pressure, and 30% had asthma. Of these children, 63% had an obese mother, 31% had an obese father, and 50% had one or more obese siblings. Unfit children appear to be at an increased risk of high levels of serum lipids. This is primarily due to an increase in body fatness. In another study, it was shown that each 10 mm increase in the sum of 10 skinfolds was associated with a decrease of 1.4 mg.dL$^{-1}$ of HDL-C. Circulating leptin levels were significantly correlated not only with body weight, body fat, systolic blood pressure, and fasting blood sugar but also with TC, LDL-C, and TG. Increased blood pressure was apparent under resting conditions and abnormal blood pressure reactions appeared during workload. Heart rate during the same workload increased more in obese children compared to normal-weight peers, indicating a lower level of cardiorespiratory fitness. Associated health risks are greater the longer the individual has been obese and particularly when children approach adolescence.

The overweight and obese have an increased risk of insulin-dependent diabetes mellitus (IDDM). One study showed that the prevalence of IDDM was on average twofold greater from the age of 2 years onward when compared to normal-weight children of both genders. Insulin resistance with respect to glucose metabolism was evident in obese children and hyperinsulinemia was related to the development of hypertension.

The prevalence of multi-metabolic syndrome (MMS) is also seen in obese children and includes hypertension, hyperinsulinemia, hypercholesterolemia, low HDL-C, hypertriglyceridemia, and impaired glucose tolerance. These features were associated with resting tachycardia, low physical fitness, and reduced α-tocopherol and β-carotene plasma concentrations. In some obese children and adolescents, the development of a fatty liver has been observed, is related to hyperinsulinemia, and can be accompanied by further metabolic alterations.

There is an increased chance of obese children and adolescents developing some respiratory symptoms, correlating with body weight and triceps skinfold. This is also related to some alterations in respiratory function mentioned previously.

Impaired sexual development includes menstrual disorders (oligomenorrhea, amenorrhea, or irregular menses), and polycystic ovarian syndrome (PCOS) which may be manifested at perimenarcheal age. A significant positive relationship was found between waist-to-hip ratio and testosterone (T) levels, but not with insulin. A significant association was also found between BMI and T. These results seem to indicate that in girls with menstrual irregularities, overweight is associated with hyperinsulinemia along with an increase in androgen production, which may be a risk factor for PCOS.

It is common for parents to visit a medical doctor with their obese sons because they think their sexual development is retarded. Most commonly, the problem is related to an increased amount of fat deposited on the lower abdomen that makes evaluation of the degree of sexual maturation more difficult.

Obesity during the growing years is also accompanied by orthopedic problems. These include flat and hypermobile feet that minimize foot stability. Knee osteoarthritis also develops prematurely in severely obese individuals.

Blount's disease (tibia vara) is also the result of increased stress on young bone from excess weight. Genu varus and/or valgum often produces additional lower extremity exacerbations that include compensatory pronation, talar adduction, and a degree of toe-in.

Body posture can also be altered due to excess weight and weakness in postural muscles. Hyperlordosis and a protruding abdomen are the result of excess fat deposition, inadequate position of the vertebral column, and abdominal muscle tone. Shoulders are often uneven and a 'turtle neck' may also develop. Protruding scapulae and the eventual deviations of the vertebral column are less apparent than in normal children because of the extent of the subcutaneous fat layer. Muscle weakness accompanying a low level of physical fitness is the main cause.

## 14.2  Treatment and Management Principles

Treatment for obese children and adolescents must reflect the multidimensional nature of the condition. A clear explanation of the pathogenesis of obesity is a very difficult task, therefore a multidisciplinary approach is warranted. There are three key components of treatment during the growing years: diet, exercise, and psychological support.

Best results can be achieved through the cooperation of a team of professional health specialists including pediatricians, nutritionists, psychologists, and physical educators/exercise physiologists. To many people, such a team seems superfluous as the principles of treatment appear to be self-evident. However, if the treatment process was so simple, there would be a much lower prevalence of obesity and greater success in treating obesity at all ages.

When obesity has not advanced to a serious level, a logical recommendation is to monitor the individual's lifestyle, starting with nutrition, so that the child does not increase in weight and fatness. He or she would grow to optimal height and desirable value for BMI in relation to age and gender. However, this approach does not always provide desirable long-term results and is only temporary. Moreover, parallels exist between unsuccessful weight loss attempts and psychological problems that may include a predisposition to eating disorders. These problems are not only a personal difficulty for a child or adolescent, but can also seriously jeopardize the possibility of successful treatment.

As mentioned previously, each child has a unique personality, in spite of the many common traits of obesity. The first step in the treatment process is for the child to be properly examined for general health and morphological, nutritional, functional, biochemical, hormonal, and psychological status. This is critical in children who have a greater risk of familial obesity.

Behavior modification involves consideration of the amount and composition of the diet along with changes in physical activity that should be addressed using an individualized approach and support. This is always easier when started at a younger age and as close as possible to the commencement of obesity. For this reason, more detailed examinations of children who may be at risk should be undertaken, since to treat early and often may be the best. An individualized treatment strategy with the integration of basic scientific information with a clinical research outcome is the therapeutic approach recommended for obese children. According to the individual child, there may be significant differences in the reaction to various regimes of treatment. The same treatment will not have the equivalent effect on every obese individual. On the other hand, very similar results may be achieved with quite different approaches. Some studies have followed up on markers of possible success in treatment. Results showed that the best predictors of weight gain after 2 years were high protein oxidation, low activity EE, and high RQ during the TEF. This has led to the conclusion that EE, RMR, and components of substrate oxidation are predictors of an increase of body weight and fat in late childhood.

The supporting role of family during the treatment phase is essential. Children with obese parents are generally fatter than children with normal-weight parents. This indicates the important role of genetic factors as well as the family environment from the very beginning of life. Children of obese parents might lose more weight than the average, but they also regain weight more easily. Short-term results might be good, but such individuals are at a greater risk of not maintaining the positive results of the weight reduction treatment.

The treatment process must attempt to profit from cooperation of the family. A parent-directed weight reduction program can facilitate positive changes in their children with respect to weight and fat loss. The degree of compliance may also be expected to be much higher. It has been shown that the greater the number of sessions of group therapy attended by mothers, the greater the weight loss of the obese daughters being treated. Parents should therefore be direct participants in any intervention program. Children who were more successful initially in treatment had fewer siblings and were females. The situation can be different with older children as family size can interact with the treatment to determine the weight changes in other ways.

Other predictors of success include self-monitoring and the personal involvement of the child being treated. In this respect, appropriate parental assistance and psychological treatment to rectify poor lifestyle behaviors are essential. The major focus should be on a combined approach to reduce inactive behaviors while providing assistance to improve physical skills and maintain sound nutritional practices. The support of a group of similar obese individuals can help to improve adherence and thus improve treatment results. However, an individual approach may be more suitable for others. Decisions need to based on the personal characteristics of the child.

Arguably, the most important feature of weight management for the obese child is the diet. The establishment of recommended dietary allowances for obese children is a difficult task. Such determinations need to be made according to the individual characteristics of the child. This is one of the reasons for a comprehensive health appraisal that includes food intake information for each child. Dietary history must be assessed, at least to establish eating patterns during a typical week. This can best be achieved with the direct assessment technique of weighing food with the help of a dietitian, nurse, or comparably trained health professional. This is a very demanding and time-consuming approach and may be biased since individuals under direct control do not eat as they usually do, and/or are inaccurate in their record keeping. A combination of food diaries and/or food frequency records completed with the help of parents and teachers, and supplemented by interviews can accurately assess daily food intake and composition. Computer programs are used to assist with analyses as long as the program is representative of locally available foodstuffs.

The results of such individual analyses provide an indication of poor dietary habits and can therefore be of great assistance in the design of a special diet suitable for the obese child. The recommended allowance of energy should encompass the desired components for growth but be sufficiently conservative to allow for the mobilization and utilization of stored fat with regular participation in physical activity. The aim of the weight management process is to mobilize stored fat while maintaining normal growth in height and fat-free body mass and improve functional capacity.

In more serious cases of obesity, low energy diets may be used. This process should be reserved for a relatively small number of individuals and the energy intake defined as exactly as possible. The amount and ratio of the individual macro- and micronutrients must be adhered to the RDAs for a particular age and gender category. Special protein-sparing diets with an increased amount of protein (up to 2.5 g.kg$^{-1}$ ideal weight of the child) have been used with young people to promote significant weight loss and maintain fat-free body mass. However, some studies have shown that in spite of an increased intake of protein, total body potassium and nitrogen decreased, along with considerable weight loss. As lean body mass is generally greater in obese children, such a temporary loss may be tolerated if one considers other positive improvements in health status found at the same time. Nevertheless, the use of such diets, as is the case for the classical hypocaloric diet, should be conducted under medical supervision. The best scenario may be under inpatient conditions where physical activity can also be fostered. Very low energy diets (VLED) have also been used in children but this approach is not recommended for growing individuals.

The composition of any diet used in weight management may need to be modified, particularly with respect to the content of saturated fat. Diets with a low fat content have resulted in a decreased energy intake and increased weight loss. Some studies have shown that it is not necessary to supplement such a diet with polyunsaturated fatty acids (PUFA). Logical low-fat alternatives are skim milk and low-fat cuts of meat. However, the possibility for slight deficits in vitamin E needs to be considered.

Low-energy diets can result in significant changes in body composition and a decrease in BMI and REE. In some studies, no reduction of potassium and nitrogen was observed but such changes obviously depend on the degree of food reduction and changes in food composition. Nitrogen balance can fluctuate, but after a certain period will stabilize. Nitrogen losses show great variability in individual subjects, even under comparable conditions. This is further evidence of the individual nature of all components of lifestyle, including nutrition. In some studies, blood glucose, serum protein, and urea are reduced after such diets, but serum albumin does not change.

The thermic effect of food has been reported as being lower in obese children but can significantly increase after a reduction diet. This indicates a slight thermogenic defect in some obese children, representing a consequential rather than an etiological factor in such children. Total antioxidant capacity (TAC) and plasma levels of lipid-soluble antioxidant vitamins, which are also lower in obese individuals, have increased after reduction treatment using a hypocaloric diet. Some reducing diets have been supplemented by special ingredients, mostly fiber, wheat bran, or glucomannan. Weight loss with such supplementation has not differed from an unsupplemented diet but serum lipid features do change with a reduction of α-lipoprotein, and an increase in β-lipoprotein and TG.

Therefore, hypocaloric diets can be a risk, especially because of potential deficiencies in some essential items. However, some studies did not show any change in serum content of, for example, Fe, ferritin, and transferrin after such diets. A hypocaloric diet followed for 14 weeks did not have any significant effect on heart parameters, intraventricular septal thickness, left ventricular wall thickness, and left ventricular volume. After weight reduction, reduced heart rate and QT interval were found in obese children. Systolic and diastolic blood pressure also decreased. The effect of sodium intake in the regulation of blood pressure was followed and the results supported the hypothesis that blood pressure of obese adolescents is sensitive to sodium intake. This sensitivity may be due to the combined effects of hyperinsulinemia, hyperaldosteronism, and increased activity of the sympathetic nervous system, all characteristic of obesity.

A reduction in weight following a restricted diet also results in changes to some respiratory parameters such as peak expiratory flow and forced expiratory volume. With a diet-only approach, no changes may occur; however, hypopnea, obstructive sleep apnea, and respiratory disturbance index may improve significantly. As is the case in adults, serum lipid profiles improve significantly after weight loss due to caloric restriction. TC, LDL-C, TG, and apolipoprotein B decreased, and apolipoprotein A, HDL-C, and HDL-C/TC increased. After weight reduction, IGFII and BP2 increased, and IGF-1, BP1, BP3, and IGF-1/IGF3 decreased. The ratio of BP1/BP2 was ameliorated. The decrease in the IGF-1/BP3 ratio after weight loss indicated a decrease in biologically active IGF-1, which may contribute to the explanation of impaired growth velocity in obese children after a restricted diet. Similar changes were observed in another study; the ratio of IGFBP-2 to IGFBP-1 was inversely related to TC and LDL-C. IGFBP-2 was inversely correlated with waist-to-hip ratio. In other studies, a simultaneous reduction of TG, insulin, FFA, and apolipoprotein A1 and B was found. A significant decline in serum triiodothyronine (T3) concentration along with a decrease of RMR after weight loss due to a 6-week low-calorie diet was also observed. T3-concentration reduction combined with FFM loss could be responsible for an RMR decline.

Serum insulin usually decreases after weight loss along with reduction of insulin resistance and increased insulin sensitivity. Leptin also decreases; for example, a significant reduction from 16.5 to 10.0 ng.ml$^{-1}$ after a reduction of BMI was observed. Plasma apolipoprotein A and HDL-C were independent predictors of leptin concentrations during weight reduction. Similar favorable changes following weight reduction were also observed in children with NIDDM.

The use of physical activity and exercise without dietary change usually has a slower effect on childhood obesity. Exercise contributes to the maintenance and further development of fat-free body mass; therefore, it is highly recommended for the treatment of obesity during childhood, when a heavily restricted dietary intake can result in a slowing of growth in height and a reduction of muscle mass. The aim should be to increase habitual physical activity then progressively add more intense exercise. This is possible in a range of settings such as physical education classes and summer activity camps that are in widespread use in Europe, North America, and other parts of the world.

There is strong evidence of the positive effect of exercise on body composition, provided activity is dynamic, weight bearing, and aerobic. Eight to fourteen years of longitudinal observations of boys involved in various physical activities and exercise have shown significantly reduced deposition of stored fat and increased development of lean, fat-free mass along with changes in BMI and increased aerobic power in subjects who participated in a satisfactory level of sport training.

Observations in experimental situations with laboratory animals have enabled *in vitro* and *in vivo* measurement of selected characteristics of lipid metabolism modified by the adaptation to increased and/or decreased physical activity (usually running on a treadmill). Trained animals have shown an increased ability to mobilize and utilize fat metabolites, characteristics that were also evident under resting conditions. Consequent changes included decreased deposition of fat in spite of higher food intake. Limited observations of biopsies of adipose and/or muscle tissue in adult humans have supported these findings. In children, such studies have not been undertaken for obvious ethical reasons.

The effect of exercise is apparent when the intensity fluctuates or when activity is temporarily interrupted. Body weight and BMI usually do not change significantly, but subcutaneous and total body fat increase significantly following a reduction in TEE. The reverse is found when TEE is increased by exercise.

The effect of well-organized physical activity and exercise has been demonstrated in numerous longitudinal observations in obese children. Various strategies have been employed. A meaningful comparison of results is difficult as the subjects and mode of exercise treatment are invariably quite different. However, in many studies significant effects of exercise have been shown in relation to a decrease in body weight, BMI, and fatness (decrease in subcutaneous and visceral fat), along with an increase in aerobic power and physical performance. These changes fluctuated when the intensity of exercise therapy changed. There is a direct relationship between dose and response in terms of body composition and fitness parameters.

Boys exposed to various exercises showed decreases in serum lipids and an increase in HDL-C compared to boys treated only by a restricted diet. Even mild exercise, which may not result in weight loss, can improve glucose homeostasis, insulin dynamics, and risk factors for coronary heart disease. Exercise also favorably alters cardiac autonomic function by reducing the ratio of sympathetic to parasympathetic activity. Exercise is important for all obese individuals but particularly suitable for milder degrees of obesity and also for the prevention of the excess deposition of fat because exercise impairment in such individuals would commonly be minimal. A 4-year longitudinal study in obese boys who were measured each year before and after an exercise summer camp showed better results at the ages of 11 and 12 years (greater decrease of body weight and BMI, smaller decrease of lean, fat-free body mass and greater functional improvement) than at the ages of 13 and 14 years.

Many studies have not shown the same levels of improvement, and have therefore suggested or inferred that the role of exercise is superficial. It is important to qualify and question such findings. Some of the contradictions may be due to an insufficient intensity of exercise, or a treatment program that was too short. In many studies, dietary intake was not checked. Rather than the exercise being problematic, energy intake may have increased.

In summary, the best way to treat childhood obesity is to combine controlled diet and aerobic exercise treatment, and provide psychological support. Reduction of excess fat can be more pronounced with a monitored approach, with improvements in body composition, serum lipids, hormone profile, and cardiovascular fitness. Functional parameters and physical fitness level will also be maximized using such an approach.

Other approaches have also been used in the treatment of childhood obesity. Drug therapy has been reported without adverse health complications; however, this approach is not recommended for children. Gastric and plastic surgery have also been used in children and adolescents. Intragastric balloon therapy did not give satisfactory results in addition to being unsuitable for use during growth. Alternative approaches such as electroacupuncture have been used and positive results reported.

Suitably arranged school programs seem to be one of the best approaches for the optimal intervention using diet, exercise, and overall lifestyle modification. Outpatient and inpatient opportunities are quite rare and very costly.

Summer camps are used to good effect in many countries and have a strong tradition with good results. However, the number of such camps is also very limited given the large numbers of obese children. Such camps may also be considered unsatisfactory as the positive results gained during camp are often lost during the following school year; however, a reduced ratio of stored fat and lower BMI may persist.

Dietary strategies are an indispensable component of weight management for obese children and adolescents, but need to be well organized following appropriate appraisals of current status. Energy should be derived individually, according to the recommendations of WHO and similar sources of RDAs prepared for specific populations. The composition of the diet should follow the desired ratio of protein as 12 to 13%, fats up to 30% (with one third saturated, one third monounsaturated, and the remainder polyunsaturated fatty acids), and 57 to 60% carbohydrates.

According to the WHO, simple sugars should not exceed 10% of energy intake. However, this should be even lower in the case of obese children and the intake of sweets replaced by more appropriate food choices such as fruit. Vitamins and minerals must also correspond to the RDA for a particular age and gender group. When hypocaloric diets are prescribed, some vitamins and minerals may need to be supplemented. There must also be a sufficient intake of beverages, excluding sodas and sweetened soft drinks. Good quality drinking water is most desirable, although this can be a problem in some urban areas. Water or a small quantity of unsweetened, diluted fruit juice can be used as an alternative. Mineral waters must be used cautiously. Snack foods, sweets, and other highly processed products should be excluded.

Along with adequacy of food and drink, the frequency of meals is also important. The most desirable number of meals per day is questionable (at least 5) and is very much an individual issue. Nevertheless, an adequate breakfast and lunch should be the aim. Fresh fruit, low-fat yogurts, tomatoes, and other vegetables should be encouraged as snack items. Dinner should be served early, and wherever possible, a number of hours before going to bed. Ideally it should be at least 2 to 3 hours before (depending on when the child normally goes to sleep), and should not represent the largest meal of the day. A unified approach or recipe for success is not possible for all children. The above-mentioned guidelines should serve as an appropriate starting point for all children.

Physical activity must also be considered according to the individual needs of the child. The medical check-up should consider the functional capabilities of the child and be part of the determination of whether the child can and should participate in the normal physical education program at school. Differences of opinion exist regarding the merits of obese children participating in physical education. Some would argue that avoidance of physical education is recommended in the case of more severe or morbid obesity, particularly when the individual has more serious accompanying co-morbidities and orthopedic defects. Such children are likely to avoid physical education anyway if they perceive the setting to be threatening. A separate opportunity to move and experience physical activity with peers of a similar size and shape may be an excellent interim step to the longer-term aim of future mainstreaming of such children into normal activity settings, including at school.

Physical activity and exercise should commence in a controlled fashion. In the more serious cases of obesity, it is often best to start activity in an aquatic environment. The buoyancy provided by body fat helps to compensate for one's weight and enables concentration on specific body movements. Progressively, it is recommended that various exercises be completed in a lying position on the back or abdomen and then move to sitting and kneeling positions. Individual exercises should be thoroughly explained and supervised with technique checked and corrected where necessary. All activities should be completed slowly and safely in a non-threatening environment. When some success is made in the activity setting or perhaps a combination of weight loss and motor improvement, it is important to progress to the usual form of physical education and related activities as soon as possible. As mentioned above, the best procedure in the short term is for obese children to exercise together so they do not feel inferior to normal-weight peers, who can behave quite cruelly with a lack of understanding and empathy for their bigger classmates.

Initially, the aim of exercise should be to develop the cardiorespiratory system and increase the aerobic power of the child. A higher level of aerobic functioning facilitates the mobilization and utilization of fat metabolites, and such activity is highly suitable for reduction treatment. After an initial period of preparatory exercises when the child has adapted to a higher work output, has increased habitual physical activity, and has lost some weight, it is recommended that children run. This may initially occur in an intermittent fashion and be interspersed within games. Swimming is most suitable at the beginning of treatment or for maintenance following weight loss, as it is a useful all-around exercise. However, it does not contribute greatly to weight loss.

The continuous development of skills is a necessary precursor to an optimal involvement of the child in other exercises, games, and sport activities. Dance is also a very desirable supplement to an exercise regime as it can be made attractive for all children. Present styles of dancing guarantee a considerable increase in energy expenditure with the necessary intensity. Stretching activities should always be included in such as program.

In time, other disciplines such as track and field can be introduced and participation in various games such as football and basketball can be encouraged. Cycling is not highly recommended due to the increased risk of injury. However, using a stationary bicycle for supplementary exercises at the beginning of the treatment process can be useful.

The enhancement of motor skills should be a goal for all children. In reality, obese children fare poorly in most activity tasks but this is mainly attributed to lack of opportunity. A major challenge for all obese or overweight people is to manage their own weight in the available space during weight-bearing activities. Improvements in motor skill can be slow and in the obese may be achieved only following the loss of a considerable amount of weight.

Muscle strength is usually greater in the obese children, but specific strength of certain muscle groups can contribute to an improvement in body posture and the reinforcement of the supporting musculature of the vertebral column to prevent back pain. However, this also concerns children and youth of normal weight.

Children should be knowledgeable about everything they do, including the purpose of exercise. They should be encouraged even when no great results are apparent and stimulated to personally become involved in their physical activity regime. Self-monitoring of physical activity and exercise along with a proper diet and food patterning is the best way not only to achieve the weight loss, but also to permanently maintain desirable body composition improvements. Common everyday physical activities such as walking, climbing steps, working in the yard, etc., can contribute to an increase in energy expenditure.

The prescribed exercise should include the involvement of all muscle groups. A conditioning program should include a warm-up period, exercises for the development of the cardiorespiratory system, stretching, and skill activities. The environment, gym, or playground should be pleasant and attractive in order to provide an enjoyable atmosphere. The choice of an appropriate time to exercise during the day is also important, especially after a period of adaptation. However, this depends on the child's program at school, in the family, etc.

Breathing exercises and special exercises aimed toward improving the support of the vertebral column and posture should be included. The particular choice and mix of activities depend on the individual child, his/her personality, degree of obesity, health status, and level of physical fitness. The program should be modified according to all these characteristics in an attempt to achieve the best long-lasting results.

Finally, the role of the family must again be stressed. The best way is to adapt activity, similar to the focus with nutrition, to the needs of the child and to undertake at least part of the exercises and physical activities together. It is absolutely critical to avoid any ridiculing of the child for his or her effort. On the contrary, encouragement, praise, and appreciation are necessary ingredients for everyone. Obese children have enough negative experiences in the school and other environments, at least with the family they should feel at ease all of the time. It is highly desirable that the personality and behavior of the teacher who oversees the physical education of obese children be an outstanding individual.

The main aim of all work in the treatment and management of obesity is to achieve not only a reduction in weight, BMI, and excess fat, but also to improve the overall health status of the child. The development of optimal somatic characteristics, increased functional capacity, improved physical fitness, and an increase in self-esteem are further goals for obesity management during growth. They should be aimed toward the future physical, social, and psychological well-being of each child.

# 15

## General Conclusions and Perspectives

To conclude with some final comments, it is necessary to remind the reader that there continue to be numerous unanswered questions and unsolved problems, due to the multifactorial origin of obesity. First, the role of both endo- and exogenous environmental factors in the onset and development of obesity during growth has not yet been satisfactorily elucidated. The problem of childhood obesity cannot be solved by a single-factor analysis. In addition, relationships between the influences of various factors over time play very important roles. In spite of much already being achieved, it is necessary to consider what is left to be explained and solved.

When childhood obesity is generally defined, it can be concluded that an excess deposition of fat in childhood is a phenomenon that does not agree with the natural trends of growth. Under normal physiological conditions, this period of development is characterized, as compared with adult and advanced age, by a lower ratio of stored fat and higher ratio of lean, fat-free body mass. This applies to those with normal weight and BMI in the individual age categories. Two periods, the one just prior to the adiposity rebound (AR) occurring at the preschool age, and then during prepuberty, are characterized by quite a low deposition of fat. These periods are also defined as sensitive and critical periods of development. With increasing age, fat is deposited in greater quantities, even when body mass index remains the same. Therefore, childhood obesity does not correspond to expected trends during growth. The phrase "fattening is aging" is justified and is already evident during childhood and adolescence.

Excessive adiposity is associated with some other functional, biochemical, and hormonal changes that are in line with the conclusions on the above-mentioned body composition changes. A young growing organism is characterized by a higher level of aerobic power, expressed as the uptake of oxygen during a maximal workload, related to body weight (max $O_2.min^{-1}.kg^{-1}$). This parameter is considered one of the most essential physiological characteristics of cardiorespiratory fitness and functional capacity of the organism (which concerns not only athletes, but all human beings). Aerobic power increases during growth, but deteriorates under normal conditions only with increasing age. This characteristic is also considered a marker of "positive health" and is important for the well-being of any individual.

Values of aerobic power achieve their highest peaks during pre-puberty and puberty, and gradually decrease throughout adulthood and old age. The level of aerobic power is lower in the obese compared to normal-weight children. When this functional parameter is related to lean, fat-free body mass, it is usually the same, but under conditions of more severe obesity, it may be lower. However, aerobic power related to total body weight is a more meaningful parameter as an obese child cannot physically perform without his/her load of excess fat. This situation is noticeably reflected by significantly deteriorated performances in dynamic, weight-bearing activities in obese children, who, for example, run and jump with a lesser degree of ability than their lean peers. For practical purposes, it is therefore more important to express the level of physical fitness as aerobic power related to total body weight, including the undesirable amount of stored fat. With respect to physical performance, only muscle strength and some skills concerning smaller muscle groups of the extremities are not impacted negatively by obesity in children and youth. More detailed research concerning functional capacity in individuals during different periods of growth and obesity development can provide a key to its prevention and treatment.

A high level of spontaneous physical activity is one of the important characteristics of a growing organism, with it decreasing later in life. This is apparent in youngsters of all species who are playful and much more active than those of an older age. This is also associated with a relatively higher energy intake (as related to total and/or lean, fat-free body mass) and indicates a higher level of energy turnover in the growing organism. However, in obese children, the level of physical activity is usually lower compared to normal-weight children, in spite of the same or even higher total energy expenditure. This is not caused by higher motor activity, but by the higher cost of any movement during usual daily activities. Also, energy intake was found to be the same, or even lower than in lean peers.

Excess fatness corresponds to increased levels of total cholesterol, LDL-C and triglycerides, and lower HDL-C. This is another characteristic of older organisms compared to those during the growth period. Insulin level is higher and insulin sensitivity is lower in obese individuals, with the level of growth hormone being lower and its clearance higher resulting in reduced levels. Leptin levels are higher and correlate with total body fat. IGF is also higher in the obese. The interaction of hormonal activities during the process of excess fat deposition, as well as during its reduction will be another interesting problem to be elucidated.

Hormonal and biochemical changes are significantly associated with more frequent health problems in obese children and youth. This mainly concerns the increased risk for cardiovascular diseases: the early onset of atherosclerosis (which was defined as a pediatric problem), hypertension, and the like. Diabetes mellitus is also more frequent in obese children than in their normal-weight peers. All these problems appear in the obese much earlier than in lean individuals. Childhood obesity is significantly related to adult obesity and the morbidity and mortality of the above-mentioned diseases are more frequent in those who were obese in adolescence. More long-term epidemiological and clinical data on this topic are desirable. Naturally, leanness does not always guarantee optimal health. Nevertheless, excessive adiposity is always an unwanted risk factor.

Psychological problems manifest more often in obese children and youth, with later psychiatric complications appearing more frequently in individuals with an early onset of obesity. With respect to the human psyche, excess fatness brings certain types of deterioration that are usual in older individuals. The same applies to orthopedic problems, arthritis, and the deterioration of body posture and the vertebral column. Also, such problems usually concern individuals only during adulthood and advanced age. The role of excess adiposity during childhood in facilitating the development of all these health risks should be further explained, especially from the viewpoint of their prevention.

Changes caused by obesity during growth are, in certain aspects, very similar to those caused by aging. Excess adiposity speeds up the aging process, including health status. As life expectancy is usually shorter in the obese, it is possible to consider the status of an obese individual during growth as somebody who is, from certain points of view, much older than his/her chronological age. In conjunction with the mentioned deterioration of an obese child's status, the causes and mechanisms should be intensely studied with an intervention occurring as early as possible. When intervention is not guaranteed, the situation usually worsens with increasing age. Spontaneous rectification of the problem occurs only too rarely.

The role of genetics in the development of obesity is undeniable and significant, and has been already studied from many points of view. An obese child has, for example, more adipocytes in his/her adipose tissue from a young age, with this difference progressively increasing until young adulthood. Genetic factors can condition not only the predisposition for certain morphological features concerning obesity, but also food preferences and aversions, reaction to overfeeding, patterns of oxidized substrates, level of spontaneous physical activity and reaction to workload, and overall functional capacity including aerobic power and skeletal muscle oxidative potential. Some of the above-mentioned aspects were recently studied in greater detail, but with respect to available research data, a complex study covering more of the mentioned aspects in their mutual relationships with obesity has not been conducted over sufficiently long periods of growth. Such studies would be demanding but indispensable for the elucidation of the role of the individual factors and their interplay during obesity development.

However, as realized from a number of recent scientific studies on the rapidly increasing prevalence of obesity, the causes of this undesirable phenomenon cannot be only the result of changes to the genetic make-up. Environmental causes are considered mainly responsible for increasing obesity that begins during the growth period. Lifestyle has changed significantly over the last few decades and runs parallel with the greater prevalence of obesity.

Very little data exist on overeating in obese children. Also, studies most often revealed the same or even increased energy expenditure in the obese compared to normal-weight individuals. However, data exist on the decreased physical activity and reduced participation in sports activities and exercise in the obese compared to normal-weight peers. This seems to be a contradiction and can be explained by the fact that even the most common daily activities are executed in the obese at a higher energy cost due to the excess load caused an increased ratio of stored fat. This makes motor activity more challenging and usually results in a spontaneous reduction of movement and interest in exercise and sports. In addition, some studies give inaccurate results, especially when using questionnaires describing these activities; the same type and duration of physical activity noted by the obese and lean children are considerably different, especially with respect to the intensity of such an exercise. This can play a most important role in the differences between these groups. This also remains to be studied in greater detail and conducted not only during stabilized periods of obesity, but during its onset and initial phases of development.

As shown by some studies, the effect of physical activity on body fatness, aerobic power, serum lipids, health status, and the like can be guaranteed only when a certain level of exercise intensity over a specified period of time is achieved. Also, a certain type of exercise can result in desirable changes. Only dynamic, weight-bearing activities of an aerobic nature of sufficient intensity can stimulate the cardiorespiratory system to increase the utilization of energy from food, especially that from fats, as well as facilitate the mobilization and utilization of lipid metabolites from body fat deposits.

Most of the studies on energy expenditure describe the total amount spent during a certain period of time (most often, average values per 24 hr), but do not give information regarding the level of exercise intensity achieved. This can be determined by the increase in heart rate. However, when registering the number of heart beats during a certain period of time, which is also used as a measure of energy expenditure, the total sum for a single day (mostly during waking hours) is also given. Introducing more exact methods, enabling the assessment of heart rate and/or energy expenditure peaks over shorter intervals during the whole measured period could answer this essential question on exercise intensity and its efficiency. Obese children do not always show a lack of motor activity, but most commonly perform slower and less intensively compared to lean individuals due to strain and higher energy cost.

Similar problems appear in studies of dietary intake. Research data mostly concern the period of stabilized obesity and not the period of its onset. Fewer studies give data on the composition of the ingested food, from the point of view of macrocomponents. Food patterning, frequency of intake, and distribution of the meals with respect to their energy content during the day have rarely been followed up although these diet characteristics appear to play a very important role in the development of obesity during growth.

The onset of obesity can occur very early in life. The effect of some factors that cause obesity can influence a very young child, but most commonly do not manifest immediately, only later during development or even later during adulthood. It has been shown paradoxically that not only early hypernutrition, but also malnutrition can facilitate the development of obesity later in life. This also concerns the fetal period, due to a different dietary intake and nutritional status of the pregnant mother. This is partly reflected in the values of weight increment during pregnancy and varies considerably in individual countries; in some, they are relatively low, but in the others, they are much higher on average. Moreover, they can vary within an individual country and depend on a number of factors, such as the mother's level of education, social status, economic situation, etc. The custom of 'eating for two' does not consider that the two in question are not comparable with respect to body size and therefore energy needs. Also, the number of adipocytes was found to depend on early nutrition, both during the fetal and early postnatal period.

There are also marked interindividual differences in the composition of mother's milk (for example, in fat content and character, according to the nutrition of the mother during and prior to pregnancy). This can play an important role in food intake at the very beginning of life. There have not been any longitudinal studies following this aspect of the possible influence of the child's dietary intake and nutritional status, and contribution to possible predisposition to increased adiposity.

With regard to early nutrition, breast- and/or bottle-feeding has an essential role. Many studies have shown that breastfed children are less often obese in later age than bottle-fed children. This has been explained, inter alia, by the differences in the composition of mother's and cow's milk. Cow's milk contains, from the point of view of the energy ratio covered by various macrocomponents, greater amounts of proteins and lesser amounts of lipids and carbohydrates. It is also thought that a breast-fed baby stops accepting the mother's milk when satiated, meaning that the baby does not overeat. Under conditions of bottle-feeding, the mother often wants the bottle finished, sometimes resulting in the infant being fed more food than he/she really needs.

Pediatricians and researchers have also found very different feeding behaviors from the time a child first accepts mother's milk and/or bottle food. These findings could have been related to the development of adiposity only shortly after and not later, for example, during school age and/or adolescence. While studies continue, there is a question whether longitudinal follow-ups will be possible given the nature of the availability of the subjects, and/or their willingness to participate in such studies over many years. In addition, the interpretation of data collected is always very difficult, due to a great number of interfering factors during development, which affect individuals of various genetic backgrounds differently. A longitudinal study on the effects of various factors including food intake following pregnancy and early periods of life until adulthood could solve a number of questions, but this work would be too difficult to conduct for various reasons. However, without such knowledge, many of the questions and problems related to the onset and development of obesity at any age cannot be solved.

When considering WHO's RDAs for energy intake, it was shown that during the first year of life, children should ingest approximately 10% more energy when compared to their energy expenditure as assessed by doubly labelled water (DLW). With an energy intake lower than present RDAs, children still grew normally. Under conditions of bottle-feeding, a greater surplus of energy intake can be expected. It would be interesting to follow children fed in this way over much longer periods to verify the effect of early hypernutrition on the facilitation of obesity later in life.

From the point of view of food intake, it has been shown that recent trends in French children's eating patterns were not desirable. During the first 4 years of life, the ratio of energy from lipids most commonly increased while that of carbohydrates decreased, with the ratio of energy from proteins remaining about the same. A desirable trend for this period of development would be an increase in the ratio of carbohydrates and a decrease in lipids, along with adherence to or a decreased ratio of proteins in children's diet. The role of an increased ratio of dietary proteins as a cause of premature onset of adiposity rebound (AR), which can result in greater adiposity later in life, has already been demonstrated in longitudinal studies lasting 1 decade. Longitudinal studies of this type are still very rare and should be conducted in countries with different life conditions. Therefore, composition of the diet with respect to the relationships between individual macrocomponents seems to presently play a more important role in the onset and development of obesity than simple overeating and an excess intake of energy.

However, the contribution of additional factors over time seems to be obvious. It would be interesting to have longitudinal data on the energy expenditure and physical activity level in children with an earlier adiposity rebound compared to those with a later adiposity rebound. In this respect, not only the total amount of energy spent, but also how it is spent, that is, the intensity of exercise, is essential and needs to be studied in greater detail.

There is some evidence to suggest that humans are born with satisfactory mechanisms with respect to the amount and composition of the food ingested. This was shown by following the reactions of young children to a previous meal's varied energy intake and that of the next meal. The interference of adults, especially of the mother, is again essential. Adults can help to facilitate the development of both adequate and/or inadequate food habits from early childhood. However, this does not apply in all cases as it seems that some children are born with a different appetite and with different preferences and aversions, which are usually too difficult to modify. These issues also need to be studied in greater detail and for prolonged periods of time.

The role of the family environment, the type and amount of food offered, and the behaviors of other family members that leave more freedom for the child to eat according to his/her liking can significantly influence not only current food habits but those of later in life. George Bernard Shaw said that the two most important professions in the world that do not require any systematic education and professional preparation are politics and parenthood. Unfortunately, this is sometimes reflected in a very undesirable way.

The above-mentioned factors that are commonly mentioned in the literature can also have a different influence during the various periods of growth. Critical periods have been defined when the effect of any factor, either positive or negative, is far-reaching, not only in an immediate sense, but also in later life. The influence of such factors may not be immediately apparent, but after some period of latency they may be manifested as a delayed effect.

The period of the temporary decrease and then increase of BMI during childhood corresponds with the start of the adiposity rebound and significant changes in the proportionality of the growing organism. The timing of the adiposity rebound (AR) is a good predictor of later obesity. AR can start sooner or later depending on the individual child and preceding effects of further stimuli. The relationship to the actual level of spontaneous physical activity and energy output can also play an important role. The elucidation of all these mechanisms, which can change with respect to a different genetic basis, and the present and future characteristics of the growing organism including the predisposition for greater or lower adiposity, still remains to be answered. The solution in humans is particularly difficult due to the large variability of the characteristics and situations in which children grow up.

The last of the sensitive, critical periods are pre-puberty and puberty. During these periods, various stimuli can change more profoundly and with more lasting effects on the various characteristics of the adolescent.

There are more experimental data on the delayed effect of diet and physical activity over longer periods, as it is easier to follow-up individuals during more advanced periods of growth and continue this until at least young adulthood. For example, the correlations between the values of various parameters are always higher and more significant when measured over shorter periods of life, and are also due to the reduced possibility of interference from other conditions of life. Many unsolved problems remain on which research attention should be focused, despite more being known about the consequences during this period of development.

Questions also concern the prevalence, trends, and origins of obesity in individual countries. As mentioned in previous chapters, numerous data are available but the lack of consensus regarding criteria, procedures, terminology, and methods of measurements makes it difficult to conclusively define the possible differences and/or similarities in obesity prevalence in various parts of the world.

The increase of childhood obesity does not seem to be homogeneous. Existing evaluations seem to show that, for example, the prevalence of obesity increased most in the U.S. (+60%), less in the U.K. and Japan, and least in France (+28%). As mentioned previously, in France, but also in other countries, the prevalence of very severe obesity increased relatively more (nearly four times) than the prevalence of moderate obesity (more than once). Obviously, some individuals are more sensitive to environmental factors than others, which might be due to a combination of hereditary factors and inadequate energy balance and turnover. For example, children of obese parents preferred more fatty foods, had a higher energy intake, and, as a result, became more easily obese than children of lean parents with adequate and balanced food intakes.

Thus, the changes in trends in the prevalence of obesity seem to be diversified. As mentioned previously, it has been recently found that in certain countries, increasing prevalence in obesity is occuring more often in severe forms than the milder forms of obesity. At least in some countries, the average values and the range of normal BMI have not changed, but the prevalence of severe and/or morbid obesity increased in a more marked way. The average values of BMI in the child population in a particular country can be influenced by this phenomenon, but the differentiation has to be defined. This was considered as a special characteristic of the present situation, caused by a cluster of factors. They included familial and hereditary situations along with an impaired dietary intake (excess energy, particularly due to an increased fat intake, mainly saturated fat) and restricted physical activity. Mentioned changes in trends for different types and degrees of obesity during childhood deserve special attention. Despite morbidly obese children still representing a minority in the growing population, they are at the greatest health risk both at present and in the future, and therefore deserve more attention. A more detailed analysis of this phenomenon is also necessary.

When solving these problems, it is necessary to examine both decisive components of energy balance and turnover, that is, diet and physical activity level. As shown in the U.K., the prevalence of childhood obesity increased between 1950 and 1990, and energy and fat intake decreased after a peak in 1970. This may be explained, in part, by a decreased level of physical activity. However, very few studies have followed simultaneously, and for a longer period, both dietary intake and energy expenditure, especially when due to physical activity and exercise. The use of satisfactorily reliable and reproducible methods has not been always implemented.

In younger U.K. children (1.5 to 2.5 years of age), nutritional intake decreased by approximately 18%. However, the intake of protein increased by approximately 13%, fat decreased by approximately 5%, and the intake of carbohydrates changed only very slightly. These data show that food intake with respect to energy content and composition does not seem likely to contribute to weight gain. Other studies in Belgium, Denmark, Italy, France, and Spain mainly showed a composition of diet that could hardly explain an increased deposition of fat. This remains to be elucidated (especially the role of protein) and the contribution of reduced physical activity studied.

Another important problem in conjunction with all the above is that reported measurements were usually conducted during short periods of time (approximately 1 week), and during the period of stabilized obesity. In this respect, it would be necessary to measure these two items of energy balance simultaneously during the previously mentioned sensitive, critical periods, even when a temporary imbalance and decreased turnover of energy could cause more marked effects that may last until later periods of development.

Work with humans is particularly difficult due to the need to measure over prolonged periods of time, utilizing reliable methods. This may not be acceptable for those who may not presently require medical assistance. Ensuring the necessary cooperation of a homogeneous group of subjects willing to participate regularly in such a study is a very difficult task.

The dropout of subjects from such studies is always large, especially in subjects who are healthy and do not need, for example, medical or dietetic assistance. This can be partly compensated by recruiting a sufficiently large sample, but then there is always a risk of not having a similarly homogeneous group at the beginning and at the end of such a study. Including very high numbers of subjects in such a study poses organizational and financial challenges. Nevertheless, such studies are indispensable for the solution of both the prevention and treatment of obesity, especially obesity starting in early life.

There is some merit in analyses of data from various individual studies from different countries despite the heterogeneity of the groups involved.

Individual scientists and clinicians should not underestimate the need for further research on childhood obesity. While the level of attention focused on childhood obesity has increased recently, there is an urgent need for substantive surveys and analyses to avoid the previous ad hoc approach to study in this area. Generally scientific investigations have only involved smaller groups of subjects, especially when more sophisticated methodologies were implemented.

From the above, it is necessary to add the analyses on the effect of both diet and exercise as the main items of energy balance that can increase it to above basal levels. Very limited data exist on the effect of both diet and exercise as it was mainly obtained by studies using smaller samples with specific characteristics. Closer cooperation of nutrition and exercise scientists is desirable. There are also difficulties in comparing the results of the individual studies from different countries because of the heterogeneity of nutritional and physical activity assessments. More detailed clinical and laboratory measurements and epidemiological studies using simpler methods are necessary. Complex information on prevalence and distribution of childhood obesity in the individual continents, countries, social classes, and population groups, and studies examining the causes and mechanisms resulting in obesity during growth using more sophisticated laboratory approaches are indispensable. More efficient methods of prevention as well as treatment of excess fatness must be found.

Some examples from certain parts of the world have indicated some important aspects of the optimal growth patterns that can predispose better health, functional status, and longevity. Some experiences and analyses confirmed that the beginning of the factors identified above can occur at an early age. Growth and development characteristics in populations with a high ratio of long-living subjects (over 90 years, and in good health) excluded excess deposition of fat during development, increased food intake, excess animal proteins, and restriction of physical activity. On the other hand, longer periods of breast-feeding, slower growth rates, the eating of fresh food according to preference, and increased physical activity and workload since childhood until advanced age were the most important characteristics of those who could achieve a higher age with participation in full activity. Health parameters, serum lipids, psychological and social parameters, in such a population were on a more desirable level than in similar Abkhasian ethnic groups with comparable genetic traits living under city life conditions. In spite of the undeniably more fixed positive genetic make-up, way of life, and overall characteristic development deserve special attention as possible factors that contribute to the reduction of obesity and the achievement of a positive health prognosis until advanced adulthood.

Present conditions in western societies facilitate the prevention and treatment of many diseases and pathological situations, but seem to cause other problems that previously were much less frequent, when different conditions of life were customary. Present diet and physical activity regimes do not correspond to the needs of the human organism according to the phylogenetic trends. This particularly applies with respect to the conditions of life in large urban agglomerations and when considering children; recent trends in childhood obesity prevalence seem to bear witness to that.

Moreover, the lifestyle in the industrially developed countries and their large cities has been introduced, along with technological progress, to the countries of the Third World. There the situation, also with respect to obesity, has worsened significantly over the past 1 to 3 decades, and has started to be similar to the industrially developed countries. Obesity accompanying stunting is another example. This trend is highly undesirable and can be avoided.

Prevention is always better than cure. According to the recent knowledge on the effect of various factors influencing the growing organism in early periods of life, efficient interventions should be implemented at the very beginning of life. Lifestyle should be arranged in such a way that the development of obesity would be interfered with and prevented by efficient arrangements of dietary and physical activity regimes. There is evidence that this should start with the pregnant mother's way of life and continue from the beginning of postnatal life. Even if it does not always completely guarantee the prevention of increased adiposity, it can at least reduce the risk of obesity.

A concentrated effort and study involving a standardized program should be agreed to by representative institutions in as many countries as possible. There need to be vehicles by which research data can be summarized and organized so that a large number of people can benefit. There is now considerable interest in countries where previously no systematic follow-ups have been possible.

It is encouraging that some initiatives in this respect have recently been developed. Research projects concerning early nutritional and other determinants in relationship to the development of obesity risks were undertaken, with the aim of identifying the main causes and cluster situations resulting in childhood obesity. New reviews and monographs on obesity during growth appear, but more complex analysis will be necessary. It would be highly desirable to organize a representative study with a homogeneous program not only in Europe, but also in other parts of the world.

# Text References

1. Klish, W.J., Use of TOBEC instrument in the measurement of body composition in children, in *Recent Developments in Body Composition Analysis: Methods and Applications*, Kraal, J.G., and Vanitallie, T.B., Eds., Smith-Gordon/Nishimura, London, 1993, 111.

2. Hills, A.P., Physical activity and movement in children: it's consequences for growth and development, *Asia-Pacific J. Clin. Nutr.*, 4(1), 43, 1995.

3. WHO MONICA project, Geographical variation in the major risk factors of coronary heart diseases in men and women age 35–64 years, *World Health Statistics Q.*, 41, 115, 1988.

4. Mirtipati, A., Sothern, M., Suskind, R., Udakk, J., Blecker, U., and Tienboon, P., Body mass index of preschool youth with high socioeconomic status in Chiang Mai, Thailand, *Int. J. Obes. Relat. Metab. Disord.*, 22 (Suppl. 4), S4, 1998.

5. Brooke, O.G. and Abernathy, E., Obesity in children, *Human Nutr. Appl. Nutr.*, 39, 304, 1985.

6. Barlow, S.E. and Dietz, W.H., Obesity evaluation and treatment: Expert Committee Recommendations, The Maternal and Child Health Bureau, Health Resources and Services Administration and the Department of Health and Human Services, *Pediatrics*, 102, E39, 1998.

7. Yoshiike, N., Matsumura, Y., Zaman, M.M., and Yamaguchi, M., Descriptive epidemiology of body mass index in Japanese adults in a representative sample from the National Nutrition Survey 1990–1994, *Int. J. Obes. Relat. Metab. Dis.*, 22, 684, 1998.

8. Hernandez, B., Peterson, K., Sobol, A., Rivera, J., Sepulveda, J., and Lezana, M.A., Overweight in 12–49-year-old women and children under 5 years of age in Mexico, *Salud Publica Mex.*, 38, 178, 1996.

9. Hills, A.P., Byrne, N.M., Pařízková, J., Methodological considerations in the assessment of nutritional status and physical activity of children and youth, in *Physical Fitness & Nutrition in Children and Youth in Different Environments*, Pařízková, J. and Hills, A.P., Eds, Karger, Basel, 1998.

10. Hills, A.P. and Byrne, N.M., Exercise prescription for weight management, *Proc. Nutr. Soc.*, 57, 93, 1998.

11. Himes, J.H., Subcutaneous fat thickness as an indicator of nutritional status, in *Social and Biological Predictors of Nutritional Status, Physical Growth and Neurological Development*, Green, L.S. and Johnston, F.E., Eds., Academic Press, New York, 1980.

12. Hills, A.P. and Wahlqvist, M.L., What is overfatness? in *Exercise and Obesity*, Hills, A.P. and Wahlqvist, M.L., Eds., Smith-Gordon/London, 1994, 1.

13. Bray, G.A., The energetics of obesity, *Med. Sci. Sports Exerc.*, 15 (1), 30, 1983.

14. Kannel, W.B., Health and obesity: an overview, in *Health & Obesity*, Conn, H.L., Jr., De Felice, E.A., and Kuo, P., Eds., Raven Press, New York, 1983, 1.

15. Parry-Jones, W.L., Obesity in childhood and adolescents, in *Handbook of Eating Disorders, Part 2: Obesity*, Burrows, G.D., Beumont, P.J.V., and Casper, R.C., Eds., Elsevier, Amsterdam, 1988.

16. World Health Organization, Obesity: preventing and managing the global epidemic, Report of a WHO Consultation on Obesity, Geneva, 3–5 June, 1997, World Health Organization, Geneva 1998.

17. Gray, D.S. and Bray, G.A., Evaluation of the obese patient, in *Handbook of Eating Disorders, Part 2: Obesity*, Burrows, G.D., Beumont, P.J.V. and Casper, R.C., Eds., Elsevier, Amsterdam, 1988.

18. Pařízková, J., *Body Fat and Physical Fitness: Body Composition and Lipid Metabolism in Different Regimes of Physical Activity*, Martinus Nijhoff B.V. Medical Division, The Hague, 1977.

19. Allison, D.B., Faith, M.S., and Gorman, B.S., Publication bias in obesity treatment trials?, *Int. J., Obes. Metab. Disord.*, 20, 931, 1996.

20. Bouchard, C., Genetics of obesity and its prevention, in Nutrition and Fitness in Health and Disease, Simopoulos, A.P., Ed., *World Rev. Nutr. Dietetics*, Vol. 72, Karger, Basel 1993, 68.

21. Forbes, G.B., Diet and exercise in obese subjects: self-report versus controlled measurements, *Nutr. Rev.*, 51, 296, 1993.

22. Schoeller, D.A., Limitations in the assessment of dietary energy intake by self-report, *Metabolism*, 44, 18, 1995.

23. Klesges, R.C., Hanson, C.L., Eck, L.H., and Durff, A.C., Accuracy of self-reports of food intake in obese and normal-weight individuals: effects of parental obesity on reports of children's dietary intake, *Am. J. Clin. Nutr.*, 48, 1252, 1988.

24. Mayer, J., *Health*, Van Nostrand, New York, 1974.

25. Coleman, K.J., Saelens, B.E., Wiedrich-Smith, M.D., Finn, J.D., and Epstein, L.H., Relationships between TriTrac-R3D vectors, heart rate, and self-report in obese children, *Med. Sci. Sports Exerc.*, 29, 1535, 1997.

26. Widdowson, E.M., How much food does man require? An evaluation of human energy needs, *Experientia*, 44, 11, 1983.

27. Durnin, J.V.G.A., Energy balance in childhood and adolescence, *Proc. Nutr. Soc.*, 43, 271, 1984.

28. Posner, B.M., Franz, M.M., Quatromoni, P.A., Gagnon, D.R., Sytkowski, P.A., D'Agostino, R.B., and Cupples, L.A., Secular trends in diet and risk factors for cardiovascular disease: The Framingham Study, *J. Am. Diet. Assoc.*, 595, 171, 1995.

29. Widhalm, K., Obesity in childhood-diagnosis and therapy, *Pediatr. Padol.*, 20, 403, 1985 (in German).

30. Dietz, W.H., Jr., Prevention of childhood obesity, *Pediatr. Clin. North Am.*, 33, 823, 1986.

31. Dietz, W., Physical activity and childhood obesity, *Nutrition*, 7, 295, 1991.

32. Epstein, L.H., Methodological issues and ten-year outcomes for obese children, *Ann. N.Y. Acad. Sci.*, 699, 237, 1993.

33. Epstein, L.H., Myers, D.M., Raynor, H.A., and Saelens, B.E., Treatment of pediatric obesity, *Pediatrics*, 101, 554, 1998.

34. Korsten-Reck, U., Muller, H., Oberhauser, B., Rokitzki, L., and Keul, J., Sport and diet? An ambulatory program for obese children, *Offentl. Gesundheitswes.*, 52, 441, 1990 (in German).

35. Korsten-Reck, U., Muller, M., Pokan, R., Huonker, M., Berg, A., Oberhauser, B., Rokitzki, L., and Keul, J., Prevention and therapy of obesity with diet and sports, an ambulatory therapy program for overweight children, *Wien. Med. Wochenschr.*, 140, 232, 1994 (in German).

36. Guillaume, M., Lapidus, L., Bjorntorp, P., and Lambert, A., Physical activity, obesity, and cardiovascular risk factors in children. The Belgian Luxemburg Child Study II, *Obes. Res.*, 5, 549, 1997.

37. Williams, C.L., Bollella, M., and Carter, B.J., Treatment of childhood obesity in pediatric practice, *Ann. N.Y. Acad. Sci.*, 699, 207, 1993.

38. Suskind, R.M., Sothern, M.S., Farris, R.P., von Almen, T.K., Schumacher, H., Carlisle, L., Varg, A., Escobar, O., Loftin, M., Fuchs, G., et al., Recent advances in the treatment of childhood obesity, *Ann. N.Y. Acad. Sci.*, 699, 181, 1993.

39. Price, J.H., Desmond, S.M., Ruppert, E.S., and Stelzer, C.M., Pediatricians' perceptions and practice regarding childhood obesity, *Am. J. Prev. Med.*, 5, 95, 1989.

40. Kashani, I.A. and Nader, P.R., The role of pediatrician in the prevention of coronary heart disease in childhood, *Jap. Heart J.*, 27, 911, 1986.

41. Gutin, B. and Manos, T.M., Physical activity in the prevention of obesity, *Ann. N.Y. Acad. Sci.*, 699, 115, 1993.

42. ILSI Europe, Healthy lifestyles nutrition and physical activity, *ILSI Europe Concise Monogr. Ser.*, ILSI Europe, Brussels, 1998.

43. Cheung, L., Do media influence childhood obesity? *Ann. N.Y. Acad. Sci.*, 699, 104, 1993.

44. Dietz, W.H., Jr. and Gortmaker, S.L., Do we fatten our children at the television set? Obesity and television viewing in children and adolescents, *Pediatrics*, 75, 807, 1985.

45. Gortmaker, S.L., Dietz, W.H., Jr., Sobol, A.M., and Wehler, C.A., Increasing pediatric obesity in the United States, *Am. J. Dis. Child.*, 141, 535, 1987.

46. Gortmaker, S.L., Dietz, W.H., and Cheung, L.W., Inactivity, diet, and the fattening of America, *J. Am. Diet. Assoc.*, 90, 1247, 1990.

47. Bar-Or, O., Foreyt, J., Bouchard, C., Brownell, K.D., Dietz, W.H., Ravussin, E., Salbe, A.D., Schwenger, S., St. Jeor, S., and Torun, B., Physical activity, genetic, and nutritional considerations in childhood weight management, *Med. Sci. Sports Exerc.*, 30, 2, 1998.

48. Byrne, N.M. and Hills, A.P., Correlations of body composition and body-image assessments of adolescents, *Perceptual and Motor Skills*, 84, 1330, 1997.

49. Hills, A.P. and Byrne, N.M., Body composition, body satisfaction, eating and exercise behaviour of Australian adolescents, in *Physical Fitness and Nutrition during Growth*, Pařízková, J. and Hills, A.P., Eds., Karger, Basel, 1998, 44.

50. Dietz, W.H., You are what you eat? What you eat is what you are, *J. Adolesc. Health Care*, 11, 76, 1990.

51. Dietz, W.H., Therapeutic strategies in childhood obesity, *Horm. Res.* 39, 86, 1993.

52. Faozof, G., Saenz, S., and Gonzales, C., Television viewing and obesity in a sample of Argentinian children, *Int. J. Obes. Relat. Metab. Disord.*, 23 (Suppl. 5), S45, 1999.

53. Pařízková, J., Obesity and its treatment by diet and exercise, in *Nutrition and Fitness in Health and Disease*, Simopoulos, A.P., Ed., Karger, Basel, 1993, 78.

54. Hill, A.J. and Silver, E.K., Fat, friendless and unhealthy–9-year-old children's perception of body shape stereotype, *Int. J. Obes. Relat. Metab. Disord.*, 19, 423, 1995.

55. Pařízková, J., The impact of age, diet and exercise on man's body composition, _Ann. N.Y. Acad. Sci._, 110, 661, 1963.

56. Pařízková, J., Physical activity and body composition, in _Human Body Composition, Approaches and Applications_, Symposia of the Society for the Study of Human Biology, Vol. VII, Brozek, J., Ed., Pergamon Press, Oxford, 1963, 161.

57. Vamberová, M., Pařízková, J., and Vaněčková, M., Vegetative reaction to optimal work load as related to body weight and composition in adolescent boys and girls, _Physiol. Bohemoslov._, 20, 415, 1971.

58. Covington, C., Childhood obesity: too much, too little, too late, _Issues Compr. Pediatr. Nurs._, 19, iii, 1996.

59. Schonfeld-Warden, N. and Warden, C.H., Pediatric obesity. An overview of etiology and treatment, _Pediatr. Clin. North Am._, 44, 339, 1997.

60. Taubes, G., As obesity rates rise, experts struggle to explain why, _Science_, 280, 1367, 1998.

61. Pařízková, J., _Nutrition, Physical Activity, and Health in Early Life_, CRC Press, Boca Raton, 1996.

62. Power, C., Lake, J.K., and Cole, T.J., Measurement and long-term health risks of child and adolescent fatness, _Int. J. Obes. Relat. Metab. Disord._, 21, 507, 1997.

63. Dietz, W.H., Risk factors for childhood obesity, _Int. J. Obes. Relat. Metab. Disord._, 22 (Suppl. 4), S2, 1998.

64. Sugimori, H., Yoshida, K., Miykawa, M., Izuma, T., Takahashi, E., and Nauri, S., Temporal course of the development of obesity in Japanese obese children: A cohort study based on the Keio Study, _J. Pediat._, 134, 749, 1999.

65. Rolland-Cachera, M.F., Bellisle, F., and Sempé, M., The prediction in boys and girls of the weight/height$^2$ index and various skinfold measurements in adults: a two-decade follow-up study, _Int. J. Obes._, 13, 305, 1989.

66. Epstein, L.H., Valoski, A.M., Vara, L.S., McCurley, J., Wisniewski, L., Kalarchian, M.A., Klein, K.R., and Shrager, L.R., Effects of decreasing sedentary behavior and increasing activity on weight change in obese children, _Health Psychol._, 14, 109, 1995.

67. Garrow, J.S., Is it possible to prevent obesity? _Infusions Therapie_, 17, 28, 1990.

68. Pařízková, J., Interaction between physical activity and nutrition early in life and their impact on later development, _Nutr. Res. Rev._, 11, 71, 1998.

69. Leung, A.K. and Robson, W.L., Childhood obesity, _Postgrad. Med._, 87, 123, 1990.

70. Bouchard, C. and Blair, S.N., Introductory comments for the consensus on physical activity and obesity, _Med. Sci. Sports Exerc._, 31, 11, S498, 1999.

71. Gurney, M. and Gorstein, J., The global prevalence of obesity. An initial overview of available data, _World Health Statistics_, 41, 251, 1988.

72. Van Mil, E.G.A.H., Goris, A.H.C., and Westerterp, K.R., Physical activity and the prevention of childhood obesity — Europe versus the United States, _Int. J. Obes. Relat. Metab. Disord._, 23 (Suppl. 3), S41, 1999.

73. Delpeuch, F. and Maire, B., Obesity and developing countries of the south, _Med. Trp._, (Mars.), 57, 380, 1997.

74. Durnin, J.V.G.A., Lonergan, M.E., Good, J., and Ewan, A., A cross-sectional nutritional and anthropometric study with an interval of 7 years on 611 young adolescent children, _Br. J. Nutr._, 32, 169, 1974.

75. Sunnegardh, J., Bratteby, L.E., Hagman, U., Samuelson, G., and Sjolin, S., Physical activity in relation to energy intake and body fat in 8- and 13-year-old children in Sweden, _Acta Paediatr. Scand._, 75, 955, 1986.

76. Kimm, S.Y., Obesity prevention and macronutrient intakes in children in the United States, *Ann. N.Y. Acad. Sci.*, 699, 70, 1993.
77. Gibney, M.J., Epidemiology of obesity in relation to nutrient intake, *Int. J. Obes. Relat. Disord.*, 19 (Suppl. 5), S1, 1995.
78. Shear, C.L., Freedman, D.S., Burke, G.L., Harsha, D.W., Webber, L.S., and Berenson, G.S., Secular trends of obesity in early life: the Bogalusa Heart Study, *Am. J. Public Health*, 78, 75, 1988.
79. Troiano, R.P., Flegal, K.M., Kuczmarski, R.J., Campbell, S.M., and Johnson, C.L., Overweight prevalence and trend for children and adolescents, *Arch. Pediatr. Adolesc. Med.*, 149, 1085, 1995.
80. Klish, W.J., Childhood obesity: pathophysiology and treatment, *Acta Pediatr. Jpn.*, 37, 1, 1995.
81. Kuntzleman, C.T. and Reiff, G.G., The decline in American children's fitness level, *Res. Q. Exerc. Sport*, 63, 107, 1992.
82. Ogden, C.L., Troiano, R.P., Briefel, R.R., Kuczmarski, R., J., Flegal, K.M., and Johnson, C.L., Prevalence of overweight among preschool children in the United States, 1971 through 1994, *Pediatrics*, 99, 1098, 1997.
83. Mei, Z., Scanlon, K.S., Grummer-Strawn, L.M., Freedman, D.M., Yip, R., and Trowbridge, F.L., Increasing prevalence of overweight among US low-income preschool children: the Centers for Disease Control and Prevention of pediatric nutrition surveillance, 1983 to 1995, *Pediatrics*, 101, E12, 1998.
84. Campaigne, B.N., Morrison, J.A., Schumann, B.C., Falkner, F., Lakatos, E., and Sprecher, D., Indexes of obesity and comparisons with previous national survey data in 9- and 10-year-old black and white girls: the National Heart, Lung, and Blood Institute Growth and Health Study, *J. Pediatr.*, 124, 675, 1994.
85. McGill, H.C., Childhood nutrition and adult cardiovascular disease, *Nutr. Rev.*, 55, S2, 1997.
86. Noonan, S.S., Children and obesity: flunking the fat test, *N. J. Med.*, 94, 49, 1997.
87. Falkner, F., Obesity and cardiovascular disease risk factors in prepubescent and pubescent black and white females, *Crit. Rev. Food. Sci. Nutr.*, 33, 397, 1993.
88. Broussard, B.A., Johnson, A., Himes, J.H., Story, M., Fichtner, R., Hauck, F., Bachman-Carter, K., Prevalence of obesity in American Indian and Alaska Natives, Hayes, J., Frohlich, K., Gray, N. et al., *Am. J. Clin. Nutr.*, 53, (Suppl. 6) 1535, 1991.
89. Gilbert, T.J., Percy, C.A., Sugarman, J.R., Benson, L., and Percy, C., Obesity among Navajo adolescents. Relationship to dietary intake and blood pressure, *Am. J. Dis. Child.*, 146, 289, 1992.
90. Davis, K., Gomez, Y., Lambert, L., and Skipper, B., Primary prevention of obesity in American Indian children, *Ann. N.Y. Acad. Sci.*, 699, 167, 1993.
91. Foreyt, J.P. and Cousins, J.H., Primary prevention of obesity in Mexican American children, *Ann. J. Acad. Sci.*, 699, 137, 1993.
92. Alexander, M.A., Sherman, J.B., and Clark, L., Obesity in Mexican-American preschool children — a population group at risk, *Public Health Nurs.*, 8, 53, 1991.
93. Stevens, J., Alexandrov, A.A., Smirnova, S.G., Deev, A.D., Gershunskaya, Yu. B., Davis, C.E., and Thomas, R., Comparison of attitudes and behaviors related to nutrition, body size, dieting, and hunger in Russia, black-American, and white-American adolescents, *Obes. Res.*, 5, 227, 1997.

94. McNutt, S.W., Hu, Y., Schreiber, G.B., Crawford, P.B., Obarzanek, E., and Mellin, L., A longitudinal study of the dietary practices of black and white girls 9 and 10 years old at enrollment: the NHLBI Growth and Health Study, *J. Adolesc. Health*, 20, 27, 1997.

95. Johnson-Down, L.O., Loughlin, J., Koski, K.G., and Gray-Donald, K., High prevalence of obesity in low income and multi-ethnic schoolchildren: diet and physical activity assessment, *J. Nutr.*, 127, 2310, 1997.

96. Agrelo, F., Lobo, B., Bazan, M., Mas, L.B., Lozada, C., Jazan, G., and Orellana, L., Prevalence of thinness and excessive fatness in a group of school children in the city of Cordoba, Argentina, *Arch. Latinoam. Nutr.*, 38, 69, 1988 (in Spanish).

97. Esquivel, M., Romero, J.M., Berdasco, A., Gutierrez, J.A., Jumenez, J.M., Posada, E., and Ruben, M., Nutritional status of preschool children in Ciudad de la Habana from 1972 to 1993, *Rev. Panam. Salud Publica*, 1, 349, 1997 (in Spanish).

98. Kain, J., Uauy, R., and Diaz, M., Increasing prevalence of obesity among school children in Chile, *Int. J. Obes. Relat. Metab. Disord.*, 22 (Suppl. 4), S4, 1998.

99. Barros, A.A., Barros, M.B., Maude, G.H., Ross, D.A., Davies, P.S., and Preece, M.A., Evaluation of the nutritional status of 1st year school children in Campinas, Brazil, *Ann. Trop. Paediatr.*, 10, 75, 1990.

100. Mondini, L. and Monteiro, C.A., The stage of nutrition transition in different Brazilian region, *Arch. Latinoam. Nutr.*, 47, 17, 1997.

101. Guillaume, M., Lapidus, L., Beckers, F., Drouget, B., Lambert, A.E., and Björntorp, P., Prevalence of obesity in children in Belgian Luxembourg, *Int. J. Obes. Relat. Metab. Disord.*, 17 (Suppl. 2), S36, 1993.

102. Guillaume, M., Lapidus, L., Beckers, F., Lambert, A., and Bjorntorp, P., Familial trends of obesity through three generations: the Belgian-Luxembourg child study, *Int. J. Obes. Relat. Metab. Disord.*, 19 (Suppl. 3), S5, 1995.

103. Guillaume, M., Lapidus, L., and Lambert, A., Obesity and nutrition in children. The Belgian Luxembourg Child Study IV, *Eur. J. Clin. Nutr.*, 52, 323, 1998.

104. Woringer, W. and Schutz, Y., What is the evolution of the body mass index (BMI) in Swiss children from five to sixteen years, measured one decade apart? *Int. J. Obes. Relat. Metab. Disord.*, 22 (Suppl. 3), S209, 1998.

105. Petersen, C., Childhood overweight: an epidemiological study from Hamburg, Germany (N = 32610), *Int. J. Obes. Relat. Metab. Disord.*, 22 (Suppl. 3), S202, 1998.

106. Kromeyer-Hauschild, K. and Jaeger, U., Growth studies in Jena, Germany: Changes in body size and subcutaneous fat distribution between 1975 and 1995, *Am. J. Human Biol.*, 10, 579, 1998.

107. Prentice, A. and Jebb, S., Obesity in Britain: gluttony or sloth? *Brit. Med. J.*, 311, 437, 1995.

108. Chinn, S. and Rona, R.J., Trends in weight-for-height and triceps skinfold thickness for English and Scottish children, 1972–1982 and 1982–1990, *Pediatr. Perinat. Epidemiol.*, 8, 90, 1994.

109. Fomon, S.J., Haschke, F., Ziegler, E.E., and Nelson, S.E., Body composition of reference children from birth to age 10 years, *Am. J. Clin. Nutr.*, 35, 1169, 1982.

110. Ruxton, C.H.S., Reilly, J.J., Savage, S.A.H., and Kirk, T.R., Changes in height, weight and body fat in pre-pubescent Scottish children, *Int. J. Obes. Relat. Metab. Disord.*, 22 (Suppl. 4), S5, 1998.

111. Vol, S., Tichet, J., and Rolland-Cachera, M.F., Trends in the prevalence of obesity between 1980 and 1996 among French adults and children, *Int. J. Obes. Relat. Metab. Disord.*, 22 (Suppl. 3), S210, 1998.

112. Rolland-Cachera, M.F., Spyckerelle, Y., and Deschamps, P.J., Evolution of pediatric obesity in France, *Int. J. Obes. Relat. Metab. Disord.*, 16 (Suppl. 1), S5, 1992.

113. Rolland-Cachera, M.F. and Bellisle, F., No correlation between adiposity and food intake: why are working class children fatter? *Am. J. Clin. Nutr.*, 44, 779, 1986.

114. Rolland-Cachera, M.F., Deheeger, M., Akrout, M., and Bellisle, F., Influence of macronutrients on adiposity development: a follow-up study of nutrition and growth from 10 months to 8 years of age, *Int. J. Obes. Relat. Metab. Disord.*, 19, 573, 1995.

115. Astrup, A., Lunsgaard, C., and Stock, M.J., Is obesity contagious? *Int. J. Obes. Relat. Metab. Disord.*, 22, 375, 1999.

116. Charzewska, J. and Figurska, K., Incidence of obesity in 7- to 8-year-old boys in Warsaw, *Pediatr. Pol.*, 58, 127, 1983.

117. Koehler, B., Drzewicka, B., Wackerman-Ramos, A., Dobrowolska-Wiciak, B., Muchacka, M., Malecka-Tendera, E., Ladarew-Lach, I., Girczys, W., and Lacheta, M., Obesity in children from nurseries in the city of Katowice. Analysis of socioeconomic conditions and the nutrition of obese children, *Pediatr. Pol.*, 63, 159, 1988.

118. Stanimirova, N., Petrova, Ch., and Stanimirov, S., Frequency and characteristics of obesity during the different periods of childhood, *Int. J., Obes. Relat. Metab. Disord.*, 17 (Suppl. 2), S39, 1993.

119. Vígnerová, J., Bláha, P., Kobzová, J., Krejovsky, L., and Riedlová, J., Selected characteristics of school children with overweight, *Ès. Pediat.*, 1999 (in Czech).

120. Bláha, P., Vígnerová, J., and Lisá, L., Czech population under new socio-economic conditions, in *9th European Congress on Obesity*, Milano, Italy, 3-6 June 1999.

121. Elmadfa, I., Godina-Zarfl, B., Dichtl, M., and Konig, J., The Austrian study on nutritional status of 6- to 18-year-old pupils, *Bibl. Nutr. Dieta*, 51, 62, 1994.

122. Widhalm, K., Sinz, S., and Egger, E., Prevalence of obesity in Viennese school children: a longitudinal study of 900 11–18 yr. old children and adolescents, *Int. J. Obes. Relat. Metab. Disord.*, 22 (Suppl. 4), S5, 1998.

123. Pantano, L.C., Felice, M.A., Bevilacqua, L., Morandini, S.R., Raponi, A., and Morandini, L., Nutritional studies in a commune del Lazio. Anthropometric data and food consumption in childhood, *Minerva Pediatr.*, 44, 293, 1992 (in Italian).

124. Menghetti, E.P., Ambruzzi, A.M., Marulli, P., Cilona, A., and Mucedola, G., The nutritional aspects and incidence of obesity and hypertension in groups of Roman adolescents, *Minerva Pediatr.*, 45, 177, 1993 (in Italian).

125. Esposito-Del Puente, A., Contaldo, F., De Filippo, E., Scalfi, L., Di Maio, S., Franzese, A., Valerio, G., and Rubino, A., High prevalence of overweight in a children population living in Naples (Italy), *Int. J. Obes. Relat. Metab. Disord.*, 20, 283, 1996.

126. Visali, N., Olivieri, L., Mangia, M., Perna, E., Adorisio, E., and Sebastiani, L., Obesity in childhood. Update in one district of Rome, *Int. J. Obes. Relat. Metab. Disord.*, 22 (Suppl. 4), S5, 1998.

127. Mumbiela Pons, V., Sanmartin Zaragoza, S., and Gonzales Alvarez, C., Obesity in childhood and food habits, *Rev. Enferm.*, 20, 11, 1997.

128. Sanchez-Carracedo, D., Saldana, C., and Domenech, J.M., Obesity, diet and restrained eating in a Mediterranean population, *Int. J., Obes. Relat. Metab. Disord.*, 20, 943, 1996.

129. Plecas, D., Ristic, G., Jorga, J., and Popovic, D., Prevalence of obesity among children under five in Federal Republic of Yugoslavia, *Int. J. Obes. Relat. Metab. Disord.*, 22 (Suppl. 4), S6, 1998.

130. Pavlovic, M., Kadvan, A., Rapic, D., Kljakic, B., and Bjeloglav, D., The prevalence of overweight and obesity in children and adolescents from North Backa Region in Yugoslavia, *Scand. J. Nutr.*, 43 (Suppl. 34), S44, 1999.

131. Pavlovic, M., Dokic, D., Leketic, B., Jakovljevic, D., Gajic, I., Bolits, M., Rapic, D., Kljakic, B., and Bjeloglav, D., Nutrition and nutritional status in schoolchildren aged 10–18 from North Backa region in Yugoslavia, *Scand. J. Nutr.*, 43 (Suppl. 34, S78, 1999.

132. Tasevska, N., Dimitrovska, Z., Djorjev, D., and Kolevska, L., Prevalence of overweight and obesity in school-aged children, *Scand. J. Nutr.*, 43 (Suppl. 34), S46, 1999.

133. Rummukainen, I. and Rasanen, L., Overweight and pubertal maturation in adolescent girls living in the Arctic region of Finland, *Scand. J. Nutr.*, 43 (Suppl. 34), S41, 1999.

134. Thomsen, B.I., Ekstrom, C.T., and Sorensen, T.I.A., Development of the obesity epidemic in Denmark: cohort, time and age effects among boys born 1930–1975, *Int. I. Obes. Relat. Metab. Disord.* , 23, 693, 1999.

135. Hara, M., Trends in obesity, *Nippon Rinsho*, 46, 2361, 1988.

136. Takamura, M. et al., Change in infantile obesity among the population of Beijing in 1997 — comparison with the data of major Chinese cities in 1985, 1986, *Int. J. Obes. Relat. Metab. Disord.*, 22 (Suppl. 3), S204, 1998.

137. Popkin, B.M., Paeratakul, S., Zhai, F., and Ge, K., Dietary and environmental correlates of obesity in a population study in China, *Obes. Res.*, 3 (Suppl. 2), S135, 1995.

138. Popkin, B.M., Richards, M.K., and Adair, L.S., Stunting is associated with childhood obesity:dynamic relationships, in *Human Growth in Context*, Johnston, F.E., Zemel, B., and Eveleth, P.B., Eds., Smith-Gordon/Nishimura, London, 1999, 321.

139. Hongo, T., Suzuki, T., Ohba, T., Karita, K., Dejima, Y., Yoshinaga, J., Togo, M., Inshida, H., Suzuki, H., and Kisatsune, E., Nutritional assessment of a group of Japanese elementary school children in Tokyo: with special emphasis on growth, anaemia, and obesity, *J. Nutr. Sci. Vitaminol.*, 38, 177, 1992.

140. Yoshino, Y., Takamura, M., Iwata, F., Hara, M., Okada, T., Harada, K., and Ryo, S., Comparison of body compositions between Korean and Japanese schoolchildren? How different lifestyles may relate to these body compositions, *Int. J. Obes. Relat. Metab. Disord.*, 22 (Suppl. 4), S13, 1998.

141. Leung, S.S., Lau, J.T., Tse, L.Y., and Oppenheimer, S.J., Weight-for-age and weight-for-height references for Hong Kong children from birth to 18 years, I. *Pediatr. Child Health*, 32, 103, 1996.

142. Ho, S.C., Risk factor of obesity among Hong Kong youths, *Public Health*, 104, 249, 1990.

143. Chen, W., Childhood obesity in Taiwan, *Chung Hua Min Kuo Hsiao Erh Ko I Hsueh Husi Tsa Chin.*, 38, 438, 1997.

144. Ray, R., Lim, L.H., and Ling, S.L., Obesity in preschool children: an intervention programme in primary health care in Singapore, *Ann. Acad. Med. Singapore*, 23, 335, 1994.

145. Mo-suwan, L., Junjana, C., and Puetpaiboon, A., Increasing obesity in school children in a transitional society and the effect of the weight control program, *Southeast Asian J. Trop. Med. Public Health*, 24, 590, 1993.

146. Dhurandhar, N.V. and Kulkarni, P.R., Prevalence of obesity in Bombay, *Int. J. Obes. Relat. Metab. Disord.*,16, 367, 1992.

147. Neumark-Sztainer, D., Palti, H., and Butler, R., Weight concerns and dieting behaviors among high school girls in Israel, *J. Adolesc. Health*, 16, 53, 1995.

148. Pharaon, I., El Metn, J., and Frelut, M.L., Prevalence of obesity among Lebanese adolescent girls, *Int. J. Obes. Relat. Metab. Disord.*, 22 (Suppl. 4), S7, 1998.

149. Musaiger, A.O., Matter, A.M., Alekri, S.A., and Mahdi, A.R., Obesity among secondary school students in Bahrain, *Nutr. Health*, 9, 25, 1993.

150. Darwish, O.K., Khalil, M.H., Sarhan, A.A., and Ali, H.E., Aetiological factors of obesity in children, *Hum. Nutr. Clin. Nutr.*, 39, 131, 1985.

151. Oppert, J.M. and Rolland-Cachera, M.F., Prevalence, evolution dans le temps et consequence économique de l'obesité, *Med. Sci.*, 11, 939, 1998.

152. Bourne, L.T., Langenhoven, M.L., Steyn, K., Jooste, P.L., Laubscher, J.A., and Bourne, D.E., Nutritional status of 3–6-year-old African children in the Cape Peninsula, *East Afr. Med. J.*, 71, 695, 1994.

153. Hodge, A.M., Dowse, G.K., Toelupe, P., Collins, V.R., Imo, T., and Zimmet, P.Z., Dramatic increase in the prevalence of obesity in Western Samoa over 13 year period 1978–1991, *Int. J. Obes. Relat. Metab. Disord.*, 18, 419, 1994.

154. Hodge, A.M., Dowse, G.K., Koki, G., Mavo, B., Alpers, M.P., and Zimmet, P.Z., Modernity and obesity in coastal and Highland Papua New Guinea, *Int. J. Obes. Relat. Metab. Disord.*, 19, 154, 1995.

155. Lazarus, R., Baur, L., Webb, K., Blyth, F., and Glicksman, M., Recommended body mass index cutoff values for overweight screening programmes in Australian children and adolescents: comparisons with North American values, *J. Pediatr. Child Health*, 31, 143, 1995.

156. Lazarus, R., Baur, L., Webb, K., and Blyth, F., Body mass index in screening for adiposity in children and adolescents: systematic evaluation using receiver operating characteristic curves, *Am. J. Clin. Nutr.*, 63, 500, 1996.

157. Booth, M.L., Macaskill, P., and Baur, L.A., Sociodemographic distribution of measures of body fatness among children and adolescents in New South Wales, Australia, *Int. J. Obes. Relat. Metab. Disord.*, 23, 456, 1999.

158. Pařízková, J. and Hainer, V., Exercise therapy in growing and adult obese, in *Current Therapy in Sports Medicine*, Walsh, R.P., and Shephard, R.J., Eds., Decker, Toronto, 1989, 22.

159. Popkin, B.M., Richards, M.K., and Montiero, C.A., Stunting is associated with overweight in children of four nations that are undergoing the nutrition transition, *J. Nutr.*, 126, 3009, 1996.

160. Cameron, N., Changing prevalence of childhood obesity in developing countries, *Int. J. Obes. Relat. Metab. Disord.*, 22 (Suppl. 4), S1, 1998.

161. Pasquet, P., Meleman, F., Koppert, G., Temgoua, L., Manguelle-Dicoum, A., and Ricong, H., *Growth, Maturation and Nutrition Transition: with special reference to urban populations in Central Africa*, Abstr., 14th International Anthropological Congress of Ales Hrdlička "World Anthropology at the Turn of Centuries," Aug. 31st–Sept. 4th, 1999, Prague-Humpolec, 115.

162. Widdowson, E.M., Changes in pigs due to undernutrition before birth, and for one, two, and three years afterwards, and the effects of rehabilitation, in *Nutrition and Malnutrition, Identification and Measurement*, Roche, A.F. and Falkner, F., Eds., *Advances in Experimental Medicine and Biology, Vol. 49*, Plenum Press, New York and London, 1974, 165.

163. Hirsch, J. and Knittle, J.L., Cellularity of obese and nonobese human adipose tissue, *Fed. Proc.*, 29, 1516, 1970.

164. Knittle, J.L., Childhood obesity, *Bull N.Y. Acad. Sci. Med.*, 47, 579, 1971.

165. Brook, C.G.D., Lloyd, J.K., and Wolf, O.H., Relation between age of onset of obesity and size and number of adipose cells, *Brit. Med. J.*, ii, 25, 1972.

166. Brook, C.G.D., Evidence for a sensitive period in adipose-cell replication in man, *Lancet*, ii, 624, 1972.

167. Keys, A. and Brozek, J., Body fat in adult man, *Physiol. Rev.*, 33, 245, 1953.

168. Sawaya, A.L., Grillo, L.P., Verreschi, I., da Silva, A.C., and Roberts, S.B., Mild stunting is associated with higher susceptibility to the effects of high fat diets: studies in a shantytown population in São Paulo, Brazil, *J. Nutr.*, 128, S415, 1998.

169. Wiecha, J.L. and Casey, V.A., High prevalence of overweight and short stature among Head Start children in Massachusetts, *Public Health Rep.*, 109, 767, 1994.

170. Popkin, B.M. and Udry, J.R., Adolescent obesity increases significantly in second and third generation of US immigrants: The National Longitudinal Study of Adolescent Health, *J. Nutr.*, 128, 701, 1998.

171. Hauck, F.R., Gallaher, M.M., Yang-Oshida, M., and Serdula, M.K., Trends in anthropometric measurements among Mescalero Apache Indian preschool children 1968 through 1988, *Am. J. Dis. Child.*, 146, 1194, 1992.

172. Shephard, R.J., *Body Composition in Biological Anthropology, Cambridge Studies in Biological Anthropology 6*, Cambridge University Press, Cambridge, 1991.

173. McElroy, A. and Townsend, P.K., *Medical Anthropology in Ecological Perspective*, Westview Press, Harper Collins, Boulder, CO, 12, 1996.

174. Hjern, A., Kocturk-Runefors, T., Jeppson, O., Tegelman, R., Hojer, B., and Adlerkreutz, H., Health and nutrition in newly resettled refugee children from Chile and the Middle East, *Acta Paediatr. Scand.*, 80, 859, 1991.

175. Rovillé-Sausse, F., Increase of the body mass of children born to Maghrebi immigrant parents, *Int. J. Obes. Relat. Metab. Disord.*, 22 (Suppl. 4), S7, 1998.

176. Widhalm, K. and Schonegger, K., BMI: Does it really reflect body fat mass? *J. Pediatr.*, 134, 522, 1999.

177. Cole, T.J., Changing prevalence of childhood obesity in the Western world, *Int. J. Obes. Relat. Metab. Disord.*, 22 (Suppl. 4), S1, 1998.

178. Ceratti, F., Garavaglia, M., Piatti, L., Brambilla, P., Rondanini, G.F., and Bolla, P., Screening for obesity in a schoolchildren population of the 20th zone of Milan and an nutritional education intervention, *Epidemiol. Prev.*, 12, 1120, 1990 (in Italian).

179. Fanconi, G., Has malnutrition only bad consequences? What is the definition of health? in *Protein and Energy Malnutrition*, Von Muralt, A., Ed., Nestlé Foundation, Springer-Verlag, Berlin, 160, 1969, 57.

180. Cashdan, E., A sensitive period for learning about food, *Human Nature*, 5, 279, 1994.

181. Dietz, W.H., Critical periods in childhood for the development of obesity, *Am. J. Clin. Nutr.*, 59, 955, 1994.

182. Dietz, W.H., Childhood origins of adult obesity, *Int. J. Obes. Relat. Metab. Disord.*, 22 (Suppl. 3), S89, 1998.

183. Dietz, W.H., Childhood weight affects adult morbidity and mortality, *J. Nutr.*, 128, 411S, 1998.
184. Wisemandle, W., Siervogel, R.M., and Guo, S.S., Childhood levels of weight, stature, and body mass index for individuals with early and late onset of overweight, *Int. J. Obes. Relat. Metab. Disord.*, 22 (Suppl. 4), S3, 1998.
185. Barker, D.J.P., *Mothers, Babies, and Diseases in Later Life*, BMJ Publishing Group, London, 1994.
186. Barker, D.J.P., Fetal undernutrition and obesity in later life, *Int. J. Obes. Relat. Metab. Disord.*, 22 (Suppl. 3), S89, 1998.
187. Strauss, R.S., Effects of intrauterine environment on childhood growth, *Br. Med. Bull.*, 53, 81, 1997.
188. Zwiauer, K.F. and Widhalm, K.M., The development of obesity in childhood, *Klin. Pediatr.*, 196, 327, 1984 (in German).
189. Pařízková, J., Treatment and prevention of obesity by exercise in Czech children, in Physical Fitness and Nutrition during Growth, Pařízková, J. and Hills, A.P., Eds., *Med. Sport Sci.*, Vol. 43, Karger, Basel 1998, 145.
190. Allison, D.B., Paultre, F., Heymsfield, S.B., and Pi-Sunyer, F.X., Is the intrauterine period really a critical period for the development of obesity? *Int. J. Obes. Relat. Metab. Disord.*, 19, 397, 1995.
191. Maramatsu, S., Sato, Y., Miyao, M., Maramatsu, T., and Ito, A., A longitudinal study of obesity in Japan: relationship of body habitus between birth and age 17, *Int. J. Obes.*, 14, 39, 1990.
192. Lukas, A., Does early diet program future outcome? *Acta Paediatr. Scand.* (Suppl. 365), S58, 1990.
193. Hainer, V., Černá, M., Kunešová, M., Pařízková, J., and Kytnarová, I., Early postnatal nutrition in preterm infants and their anthropometric characteristics in later life, *Int. J. Obes. Relat. Metab. Disord.*, 23 (Suppl. 5), S45, 1999.
194. Jung, E. and Czajka-Narins, D.M., Birth weight doubling and tripling times: an updated look at the effects of birth weight, sex, race and type of feeding, *Am. J. Clin. Nutr.*, 42, 182, 1985.
195. Baughcum, A.E., Burklow, K.A., Deeks, C.M., Powers, S.W., and Whitaker, R.C., Maternal feeding practices and childhood obesity: a focus group study of low-income mothers, *Arch. Pediatr. Adolesc. Med.*, 152, 1010, 1998.
196. Engstrom, E.M. and Anjos, L.A., Relationship between maternal nutritional status and obesity in Brazilian children, *Rev. Saude Publica*, 30, 233, 1996 (in Portuguese).
197. Poskitt, E., Obesity in the young child: whither and whence? *Acta Paediatr. Scand.* (Suppl. 323), 24, 1986.
198. Baranowski, T., Bryan, G.T., Rassin, D.K., Harrison, J.A., and Henske, J.C., Ethnicity, infant-feeding practices, and childhood adiposity, *J. Dev. Behav. Pediatr.*, 11, 234, 1990.
199. Rolland-Cachera, M.F. and Deheeger, M., Fatness development in children born in 1955 or 1985: two longitudinal studies, *Int. J. Obes. Relat. Metab. Disord.*, 21 (Suppl. 2), S140, 1997.
200. Rolland-Cachera, M.F., Deheeger, M., Bellisle, F., Sempé, M., Guilloud-Bataille, M., and Patois, E., Adiposity rebound in children: a simple indicator for predicting obesity, *Am. J. Clin. Nutr.*, 39, 129, 1984.

201. Rolland-Cachera, M.F., Prediction of adult body composition from infant and child measurements, in *Body Composition Techniques in Health and Disease*, Davies, P.S.W. and Cole, T.J., Eds., Cambridge University Press, Cambridge, 1995, 100.

202. Widhalm, K., Fat nutrition during infancy and childhood, in *Nutrition in Pregnancy and Growth*, Porrini, M. and Walter, P., Eds, *Bibl. Nutr. Dieta*, Karger, Basel, 53, 116, 1996.

203. Rolland-Cachera, M.F., Deheeger, M., and Bellisle, F., Nutrient balance and body composition, *Reprod. Nutr. Dev.*, 37, 727, 1997.

204. Wit, J.M., Vaandrage, W., van den Hurk, T.A., Veen-Roelofs, J., and Messer, A.P., Obese children and their treatment, *Tijdschr. Kindergeneeskd.*, 55, 191, 1987.

205. Girardet, J.P., Tounian, P., le Bars, M.A., and Boreux, A., Obesity in children: value of clinical evaluation criteria, *Ann. Pediatr.* (Paris), 40, 297, 1993 (in French).

206. Birch, L.L., Johnson, S.L., Andersen, G., Peters, K.C., and Schulte, M.C., The variability of young children's energy intake, *N. Engl. J. Med.*, 24, 324, 1991.

207. Strauss, R.S. and Knight, J., Influence of the home environment on the development of obesity in children, *Pediatrics*, 103, E851, 1999.

208. Patterson, R.E., Typpo, J.T., Typpo, M.H., and Krause, G.F., Factors related to obesity in preschool children, *J. Am. Diet. Assoc.*, 86, 1376, 1986.

209. Stephen, A.M. and Sieber, G.M., Trends in individual fat consumption in the UK 1900–1985, *Br. J. Nutr.*, 71, 775, 1994.

210. Maillard, G., Charles, M.A., Thibault, N., Thomas, F., Lafay, L., Vray, M., Borys, J.M., and Eschwege, E., Diet and adiposity indices in prepubertal children, *Int. J. Obes. Relat. Metab. Disord.*, 22 (Suppl. 3), S204, 1998.

211. Schlicker, S.A., Borra, S.T., and Regan, C., The weight and fitness of United States children, *Nutr. Rev.*, 52, 11, 1994.

212. Maffeis, C., Role of energy metabolism in the pathophysiology of childhood obesity, *Int. J. Obes. Relat. Metab. Disord.*, 22 (Suppl. 3), S89, 1998.

213. Maffeis, C., Schutz, Y., Zaffanello, M., Piccoli, R., and Pinelli, L., Caloric intake, diet composition and habitual physical activity in obese children, *Int. J. Obes. Relat. Metab. Disord.*, 17 (Suppl. 2), 37, 1993.

214. Maffeis, C., Schutz, Y., Zaffanello, M., Piccoli, R., and Pinelli, L., Energy intake and energy expenditure in free-living condition prepubertal obese and control subjects, *Int. J. Obes. Relat. Metab. Disord.*, 17 (Suppl. 2), 37, 1993.

215. Maffeis, C., Zaffanello, M., and Schutz, Y., Relationship between physical inactivity and adiposity in prepubertal boys, *J. Pediatr.* 131, 288, 1997.

216. Rose, H.E. and Mayer, J., Activity, caloric intake, fat storage, and the energy balance of infants, *Pediatrics*, 41, 18, 1968.

217. Dietz, W.H. and Gortmaker, S.L., TV or not TV: fat is the question, *Pediatrics*, 91, 499, 1993.

218. Rössner, S., Television viewing, life style and obesity, *J. Intern. Med.*, 229, 301, 1991.

219. Kortzinger, I. and Mast, M., School-oriented intervention for the prevention of obesity as part of KOPS (Kiel Obesity Prevention Study), *Omt. J. Obes. Relat. Metab. Disord.*, 21, S2, 30, 1997.

220. Bernard, L., Lavallee, C., Gray-Donald, K., and Delisle, H., Overweight in Cree schoolchildren and adolescents associated with diet, physical activity, and high television viewing, *J. Am. Diet. Assoc.*, 95, 800, 1995.

221. Robinson, T.N., Hammer, L.D., Killen, J.D., Kraemer, H.C., Wilson, D.M., Hayward, C., and Taylor, C.B., Does television viewing increase obesity and reduce physical activity? Cross-sectional and longitudinal analyses among adolescent girls, *Pediatrics*, 91, 273, 1993.

222. DuRant, R.H., Baranowski, T., Johnson, M., and Thompson, W.O., The relationship among television watching, physical activity, and body composition of young children, *Pediatrics*, 94, 449, 1994.

223. Klesges, R.C., Shelton, M.L., and Klesges, L.M., Effects of television on metabolic rate: potential implications for childhood obesity, *Pediatrics*, 91, 281, 1993.

224. Buchowski, M.S. and Sun, M., Energy expenditure, television viewing and obesity, *Int. J. Obes. Relat. Metab. Disord.*, 20, 236, 1996.

225. Salbe, A.D., Weyer, C., Fontvieille, A.M., and Ravusssin, E., Low levels of physical activity and time spent viewing television at 9 years of age predict weight gain 8 years later in Pima Indian children, *Int. J. Obes. Relat. Metab. Disord.*, 22 (Suppl. 4), S10, 1998.

226. Taras, H.L., Sallis, J.F., Patterson, T.L., Nader, P.R., and Nelson, J.A., Television's influence on children's diet and physical activity, *J. Dev. Behav. Pediatr.*, 10, 176, 1989.

227. Ward, D.S., Trost, S.G., Felton, G., Saunders, R., Parsons, M.A., Dowda, M., and Pate, R.P., Physical activity and physical fitness in African-American girls with and without obesity, *Obes. Res.*, 5, 572, 1997.

228. DeLany, J.P., Role of energy expenditure in the development of pediatric obesity, *Am. J. Clin. Nutr.*, 68, 950S, 1998.

229. Goran, M.I. and Sun, M., Total energy expenditure and physical activity in prepubertal children: recent advances based on the application of the doubly labelled water method, *Am. J. Clin. Nutr.*, 68, S944, 1998.

230. Muecke, L., Simons-Morton, B., Huang, I.W., and Parcel, G., Is childhood obesity associated with high-fat foods and low physical activity? *J. Sch. Health*, 62, 19, 1992.

231. Hainer, V., Kunešová, M., Pařízková, J., Štich, V., and Stunkard, A., The response to VLCD treatment in obese female identical twins, *Int. J. Obes. Relat. Metab. Disord.*, 19, S2, 40, 1995.

232. Sorensen, T.I.A., Role of genes in the global epidemic of obesity, *Scand. J. Nutr.*, 43 (Suppl. 34), 15S, 1999.

233. Faith, M.S., Johnson, S.L., and Allison, D.B., Putting the behavior into the behavior genetics of obesity, *Behav. Genet.*, 27, 423, 1997.

234. Ledovskaya, N.M., Experience in the assessment of physical activity in twins, in *Physical Activity in Man and Hypokinesia*, Slonim, A.D. and Smirnov, K.M., Eds., Academy of Sciences of USSR, Siberian Dept., Institute of Physiology, Novosibirsk, 1972, 30 (in Russian).

235. Sklad, M., Similarity of movements in twins, *Wychowanie Fyziczne i Sport*, 3, 119, 1972.

236. Sorensen, T.I.A. and Lund-Sorensen, I.L., Genetic-epidemiological studies of causes of obesity, *Nord. Med.*, 106, 182, 1991 (in Danish).

237. Brock, K., Bogart, N., Baur, L., Bermingham, M., and Steinbeck, K., Is parental physical activity a predictor of prepubertal children's activity levels, *Int. J. Obes. Relat. Metab. Disord.*, 23 (Suppl. 5), S118, 1999.

238. Mossberg, H.O., Overweight in children and youths — a 40-year follow-up study, *Nord. Med.*, 106, 184, 1991.

239. Locard, E., Mamelle, N., Bilette, A., Miginiac, M., Munoz, F., and Rey, S., Risk factors of obesity in a five-year-old population, Parental versus environmental factors, *Int. J. Obes. Relat. Metab. Disord.*, 16, 721, 1992.

240. Laessle, R., Wurmser, H., and Pirke, K.M., Energy expenditure in preadolescent girls at high risk of obesity, *Int. J. Obes. Relat. Metab. Disord.*, 22 (Suppl. 3), S37, 1998.

241. Maffeis, C., Talamini, G., and Tato, L., Influence of diet, physical activity and parent's obesity on children's adiposity: a four-year longitudinal study, *Int. J. Obes. Relat. Metab. Disord.*, 22, 758, 1998.

242. Mo-suwan, L. and Gaeter, A.F., Risk factors for childhood obesity in a transitional society in Thailand, *Int. J. Obes. Relat. Metab. Disord.*, 20, 698, 1996.

243. Faith, M.S., Pietrobelli, A., Nunez, C., Heo, M., Heymsfield, S.B., and Allison, D.B., Genetic-environmental architecture of percent body fat measured by bioimpedance analysis in a pediatric twin sample, *Int. J. Obes. Relat. Metab. Disord.*, 22 (Suppl. 4), S13, 1998.

244. Lecomte, E., Herbeth, B., Nicaud, V., Rakotovao, R., Artur, Y., and Tiret, L., Segregation analysis of fat mass and fat-free mass with age- and sex- dependent effects: the Stanislas Family Study, *Genet. Epidemiol.*, 14, 51, 1997.

245. Maffeis, C., Micciolo, R., Must, A., Zaffanello, M., and Pinelli, L., Parental and perinatal factors associated with childhood obesity in northeast Italy, *Int. J. Obes. Relat. Metab. Disord.*, 18, 301, 1994.

246. Griffiths, M., Payne, P.R., Stunkard, A.J., Rivers, J.P., and Cox, M., Metabolic rate and physical development in children at risk of obesity, *Lancet*, 336 (8707), 76, 1990.

247. Eck, L.H., Klesges, R.C., Hanson, C.L., and Slawson, D., Children at familial risk for obesity: an examination of dietary intake, physical activity and weight status, *Int. J. Obes. Relat. Metab. Disord.*, 16, 71, 1992.

248. Mossberg, H.O., 40-year follow-up of overweight children, *Lancet*, 2, (8661), 491, 1989.

249. Goran, M.I., Carpenter, W.H., McGloin, A., Johnson, R., Hardin, J.M., and Weinsier, R.L., Energy expenditure in children of lean and obese parents, *Am. J. Physiol.*, 268, E917, 1995.

250. Allison, D.B., Heschka, S., Neale, M.C., and Heymsfield, S.B., Race effects in the genetics of adolescents' body mass index, *Int. J. Obes. Relat. Metab. Disord.*, 18, 363, 1994.

251. Broussard, B.A., Sugarman, J.R., Bachman-Carter, K., Stephenson, L., Strauss, K., and Gohdes, D., Toward comprehensive obesity prevention programs in Native American communities, *Obes. Res.*, 3, 289, 1995.

252. Klesges, R.C., Klesges, L.M., Eck, L.H., and Shelton, M.L., A longitudinal analysis of accelerated weight gain in preschool children, *Pediatrics*, 92, 126, 1995.

253. Klesges, R.C., Eck, L.H., Hanson, C.L., Haddock, C.K., and Klesges, L.M., Effects of obesity, social interactions, and physical environment on physical activity in preschoolers, *Health Psychol.*, 9, 435, 1990.

254. Klesges, R.C., Haddock, C.K., and Eck, L.H., A multimethod approach to the measurement of childhood physical activity and its relationship to blood pressure and body weight, *J. Pediatr.*, 116, 888, 1990.

255. Rolland-Cachera, M.F., Obesity among adolescents: evidence for the importance of early nutrition, in *Human Growth in Context*, Johnston, F.E., Zemel, B., and Eveleth, P.B., Eds., Smith-Gordon/Nishimura, London, 1999, 245.

256. Rolland-Cachera, M.F., Onset of obesity assessed from the weight/stature² curve in children: the need for a clear definition, *Int. J. Obes. Relat. Metab. Disord.*, 17, 245, 1993.

257. Rolland-Cachera, M.F., Bellisle, F., Deheeger, M., Pequignot, F., and Sempé, M., Influence of body fat distribution during childhood on body fat distribution in adulthood: a two decade follow-up study, *Int. J. Obes. Relat. Metab. Disord.*, 14, 473, 1990.

258. Beunen, G. and Thomis, M., Genetic determinants of sports participation and daily physical activity, *Int. J. Obes. Relat. Metab. Disord.*, 23 (Suppl. 3), S55, 1999.

259. Power, C. and Moynihan, C., Social class and changes in weight for height between childhood and early adulthood, *Int. J. Obes. Relat. Metab. Disord.*, 12, 445, 1988.

260. Gerald, L.B., Anderson, A., Johnson, G.D., Hoff, C., and Trimm, R.F., Social class, social support and obesity risk in children, *Child Care Health Dev.*, 20, 145, 1994.

261. Wolfe, W.S., Campbell, C.C., Frongillo, E.A., Haas, J.D., and Melnik, T.A., Overweight schoolchildren in New York State: prevalence and characteristics, *Am. J. Publ. Health*, 84, 807, 1994.

262. Jaeger, U. and Kromeyer-Hauschild, K., Rapid increase in prevalence of obesity in former East German children after reunification, *Int. J. Obes. Relat. Metab. Disord.*, 23 (Suppl. 5), S7, 1999.

263. Zellner, K., Kromeyer, K., and Jaeger, U., Growth studies in Jena, Germany: Historical background and secular changes in stature and weight in children 7–14 years, *Am. J. Human Biol.*, 8, 371, 1996.

264. Gutin, B., Exercise, body composition, and health in children, in *Perspectives in Exercise Science and Sports Medicine, Vol. 11, Exercise, Nutrition and Weight Control*, Lamb, D. and Murray, R., Eds., Cooper, Carmel, 1998, 295.

265. Prentice, A.M., Lucas, A., Vasquez-Velasquez, L., Davies, P.S., and Whitehead, R.G., Are current dietary guidelines for young children a prescription for over-feeding? *Lancet*, 2 (8619), 1066, 1988.

266. Davies, P.S., Energy requirements for growth and development in infancy, *Am. J. Clin. Nutr.*, (Suppl. 68), S939, 1998.

267. Alexy, U., Kersting, M., Sichert-Hellert, W., Manz, F., and Schoch, G., Energy intake and growth of 3- to 36-month-old German infants and children, *Ann. Nutr. Metab.*, 42, 68, 1998.

268. Huang, P.C. and Chiang, A.N., Anthropometric survey of students and school children in Taipei and group treatment of selected obese students, *Taiwan I Hsueh Hui Tsa Chih*, 86, 65, 1987 (in Chinese).

269. Sundaram, K.R., Ahuja, R.K., and Ramachandran, K., Indices of physical build, nutrition and obesity in school children, *Indian J. Pediatr.*, 55, 889, 1988.

270. Vígnerová, J., Lhotská, L., Bláha, P., and Roth, Z., Growth of Czech child population 0–18 years compared to the World Health Organization Growth Reference, *Amer. J. Human Biol.*, 9, 459, 1997.

271. Wetzel, N.V., Growth, in *Medical Physics*, The Year Book Publishers, Chicago, 1942, 513.

272. Tanner, J.M., Whitehouse, R.H., and Takaishi, M., Standards from birth to maturity for height, weight, height velocity and weight velocity: British children, *Arch. Dis. Childh.* Part I, 41, 454, 1966; Part II, 41, 613, 1966.

273. Kapalun, V., Evaluation of child's growth, in *Repetitorium of Medical Doctor*, Avicenum, Prague, 1967, 109 (in Czech).

274. World Health Organization, *Energy and Protein Requirements, Report of a Joint FAO/WHO/UNU Expert Consultation*, Rome 1981, World Health Organization, Techn. Report series No. 724, WHO Geneva, 1985, 180.

275. Cole, T.J., Do growth chart centiles need a face lift? *Brit. Med. J.*, 308, 641, 1994.

276. Waterlow, J.C., with contributions of Thomas, A.M. and Grantham-McGregor, S.M., *Protein Energy Malnutrition*, Edward Arnold, London, 1992.

277. Falorni, A., Galmacci, G., Bini, V., Faraoni, F., Molinari, D., Cabiati, G., Samasi, M., Celi, F., Di Stefano, G., Berioli, M.G., Contessa, G., and Bacosi, M.L., Using obese-specific charts of height and height velocity for assessment of growth in obese children and adolescents during weight excess reduction, *Eur. J. Clin. Nutr.*, 53, 181, 1999.

278. Rolland-Cachera, M.F., Cole, T.J., Sempé, M., Tichet, J., Rossignol, C., and Charraud, A., Variations of the body mass index in the French population from 0 to 87 years, in *Obesity in Europe*, Ailhaud, G. et al., Eds., John Libbey Ltd., London, 1991, 113.

279. Rolland-Cachera, M.F., Sempé, M., Guilloud-Bataille, M., Patois, E., Péquignot-Guggenbuhl, F., and Fautrad, V., Adiposity indices in children, *Am. J. Clin. Nutr.*, 36, 178, 1982.

280. Must, A., Dallal, G.E., and Dietz, W.H., Reference data for obesity: 85th and 95th percentiles of body mass index (wt/ht$^2$) and triceps skinfold thickness, *Am. J. Clin. Nutr.*, 53, 839, 1991.

281. Hammer, L.D., Kraemer, H.C., Wilson, D.M., Ritter, P.L., and Dornbusch, S.M., Standardized percentile curves of body mass index for children and adolescents, *Am. J. Dis. Child.*, 145, 259, 1991.

282. Bláha, P., Lhotská, L., Vígnerová, J., and Bosková, R., The 5th nationwide anthropological study of children and adolescents held in 1991 (Czech republic) selected anthropometric characteristics, *Československá Pediatr.*, 48, 621, 1993 (in Czech).

283. Cole, T.J., Freeman, J.V., and Preece, M.A., Body mass index reference curves for the UK, 1990, *Arch. Dis. Child.*, 73, 25, 1995.

284. Lindgren, G., Strandell, A., Cole, T., Healey, M., and Tanner, J., Swedish population reference standards for height, weight and body mass index attained at 6 to 16 years (girls) or 19 years (boys), *Acta Paediatr.*, 84, 1019, 1995.

285. Luciano, A., Bressan, F., and Zoppi, G., Body mass index reference curves for children aged 3–19 years from Verona, Italy, *Eur. J. Clin. Nutr.*, 51, 6, 1997.

286. Rolland-Cachera, M.F., Deheeger, M., and Guilloud-Bataille, M., Tracking the development of adiposity from one month of age to adulthood, *Ann. Human Biol.*, 14, 219, 1987.

287. Hajniš, K., New growth norms for Czech and Slovak children and youth, *Anthrop. Anz.*, 51, 207, 1993 (in German).

288. Siervogel, R.M., Roche, A.F., Guo, S., Mukherjee, D., and Chumlea, W.C., Patterns of changes in weight/stature$^2$ from 2 to 18 years: findings from long-term serial data for children in the Fels longitudinal study, *Int. J. Obes. Relat. Metab. Disord.*, 15, 479, 1991.

289. Williams, S., Davie, G., and Lam, F., Predicting BMI in young adults from childhood data using two approaches to modelling adiposity rebound, *Int. J. Obes. Relat. Metab. Disord.*, 23, 348, 1999.

290. Prokopec, M. and Bellisle, F., Body mass index variations from birth to adulthood in Czech Youths, *Acta Med. Auxol.*, 24, 87, 1992.

291. Prokopec, M. and Bellisle, F., Adiposity in Czech children followed from 1 month of age to adulthood: analysis of individual BMI patterns, *Ann. Human. Biol.*, 699, 253, 1993.

292. Pařízková, J. and Rolland-Cachera, M.F., High proteins early in life as a predisposition for late obesity and further health risks, *Nutrition*, 13, 818, 1997.

293. Rolland-Cachera, M.F., Cole, T.J., Sempé, M., Tichet, J., Rossignol, C., and Charraud, A., Body mass index variations: centiles from birth to 87 years, *Eur. J. Clin. Nutr.*, 45, 13, 1990.

294. Cronk, C.E., Roche, A.F., Kent, R., Berkey, C., Reed, R.B., Valadian, I., Eichorn, D., and McCammon, R., Longitudinal trends and continuity in weight/stature$^2$ from 3 months to 18 years, *Hum. Biol.*, 54, 729, 1982.

295. Dahlström, S., Viikari, J., Akerblom, H.K., Solakivi-Jaakkola, T., Huari, M., Dahl, M., Lahde, P.L., Pesonen, E., Pietikainen, M., Suoninen, P., and Louhivuori, K., Atherosclerosis precursors in Finnish children and adolescents. II. Height, weight, Body Mass Index, and skinfolds and their correlation to metabolic variables, in Atherosclerosis precursors in children, *Acta Paediatr. Scand.* (Suppl. 7), 318, 65, 1985.

296. Massé, G. and Moreigne, F., *Croissance et developpement de l'enfant a Dakar*, Centre International de l'Enfance, Paris, 1969.

297. Lemaire, B. and De Maegd, M., Prevalence de la malnutrition proteine-calorique, de l'anemie et du goitre dans, Imbo, Burundi (Afrique Centrale), in Les malnutritions dans le Tiers-Monde, *Colloque INSERM*, 136, 149, 1986.

298. Subash, B.D. and Chuttani, C.S., Indices of nutritional status derived from body weight and height among school children. *Ind. J. Pediatr.*, 45, 289, 1978.

299. Rolland-Cachera, M.F., Bellisle, F., Deheeger, M., Guilloud-Bataille, M., Pequignot, F., and Sempé, M., Adiposity development and prediction during growth in humans: a two decade follow-up study, in *Obesity in Europe*, John Libbey, London, 1988, 73.

300. Forbes, G.B., *Human Body Composition: Growth, Aging, Nutrition and Activity*, Springer-Verlag, New York, 1987.

301. Yiannakou, P., Rovagna, M.C., Zampetti, E., Porziani, M., Giorgi, F., Leoni, M., and Ceccarelli, G., Evaluation with the multifrequencies bioimpedance method of body water in the male prepubertal obese child, *Int. J. Obes. Relat. Metab. Disord.*, 22 (Suppl. 4), S13, 1998.

302. Schonegger, K. and Widhalm, K., Relationship between body fat measured by TOBEC and BMI in obese children and adolescents, *Int. J. Obes. Relat. Metab. Disord.*, 22 (Suppl. 4), S12, 1998.

303. Pařízková, J., Age related changes in dietary intake related to work output, physical fitness and body composition, *Am. J. Clin. Nutr.*, 5, (Suppl. 49), 962, 1989.

304. Pietrobelli, A., Faith, M.S., Allison, D.B., Gallagher, D., Chiumello, G., and Heymsfield, S.B., Body mass index as a measure of adiposity among children and adolescents: a validation study, *J. Pediatr.*, 132, 204, 1998.

305. Scharfer, F., Georgi, M., Wuhl, E., and Scharfer, K., Body mass index and percentage fat mass in healthy German school children and adolescents, *Int. J. Obes. Relat Metab. Disord.*, 22, 461, 1998.

306. Guillaume, M., Defining obesity in childhood: current practice, *Am. J. Clin. Nutr.*, 70, 126S, 1999.

307. Guo, S.S., Roche, A.F., Chumlea, W.C., Gardner, J.D., and Siervogel, R.M., The prediction value of childhood body mass index values for overweight at age 35 y, *Am. J. Clin. Nutr.*, 59, 810, 1994.

308. Smith, J.C., Sorey, W.H., Quebedeau, D., and Skelton, L., Use of body mass index to monitor treatment of obese adolescents, *J. Adolesc. Health*, 20, 466, 1997.
309. Heymsfield, S.B., Waki, M., Kehayias, J., Lichtman, S., Dilmanian, A., Kamen, Y., Wang, J., and Pierson, R.N., Chemical and elemental analysis of humans *in vivo* using improved body composition models, *Am. J. Physiol.*, 261, E103, 1991.
310. Heymsfield, S., Waki, M., Lichtman, S., and Baumgartner, R., Multicompartment chemical models of human body composition: recent advance and potential implications, in *Body Composition Analysis: Methods and Applications*, Kral, J.G. and Van Hallie, T.B., Eds., Int. monographs on nutrition, metabolism and obesity: 2, Smith-Gordon/Nishimura, London, 1993, 75.
311. Wang, Z.M., Human Body Composition Models and Methodology: Theory and Experiment, Thesis Landbouw Universiteit Wageningen, Grafisch Service Centrum Van Gils B.V., Wageningen, 1997.
312. Lohman, T.G., *Advances in Body Composition Assessment*, Human Kinetics, Champaign, IL, 1993.
313. Lohman, T.G., Roche, A.F., and Martorell, R., Eds., *Anthropometric Standardization, Reference Manual*, Human Kinetics Books, Champaign, IL, 1988.
314. Ellis, K.J. and Eastman, J.D., Eds., *Human Body Composition, In Vivo Methods, Models, and Assessment*, Plenum Press, New York, 1993.
315. Jebb, S.A. and Elia, M., Techniques for the measurement of body composition: a practical guide, *Int. J. Obes. Relat. Metab. Disord.*, 17, 611, 1993.
316. Pařízková, J., Obesity and physical activity, in *Nutricia Symposium on Nutritional Aspects of Physical Performance*, De Wijn, J.F. and Binkhorst, R.A., Eds., Nutricia Ltd., Zoetermeer, The Netherlands, 1972, 146.
317. Deurenberg, P., The dependency of bioeletcrical impedance on intra- and extracellular water distribution, in *Recent Development in Body Composition Analysis: Methods and Applications*, Kral, J.G.and VanItallie, T.B., Eds., Smith-Gordon/Nishimura, London, UK, 1993, 43.
318. Taylor, R.W., Gold, E., Manning, P., and Goulding, A., Gender differences in body fat content are present well before puberty, *Int. J., Obes. Relat. Metab. Disord.*, 21, 1082, 1997.
319. Mast, M., Kortzinger, I., Konig, E., and Muller, M.J., Gender differences in fat mass of 5–7 year old children, *Int. J. Obes. Relat. Metab. Disord.*, 22, 878, 1998.
320. Guo, S.S., Chumlea, W.C., Roche, A.F., and Siervogel, R.M., Age and maturity related changes in body composition during adolescence into adulthood: the Fels Longitudinal Study, *Int. J. Obes. Relat. Metab. Disord.*, 21, 1167, 1997.
321. Burniat, W., Childhood obesity: which specificities? *Int. J. Obes. Relat. Metab. Disord.*, 21 (Suppl. 2), S136, 1997.
322. Wabitsch, M., Christoffersen, C.T., Blum, W.F., Hornqvist, H., and Teller, W., Role of insulin-like growth factor I (IGF I) in growth and metabolism of human adipose tissue, *Eur. J. Pediatr.*, 156, 170, 1997.
323. Swinburn, B. and Ravussin, E., Energy balance or fat balance? *Amer. J. Clin. Nutr.*, 57, S766, 1993.
324. Elia, M. and Ward, L.C., New techniques in nutritional assessment: body composition methods, *Proc. Nutr. Soc.*, 58, 33, 1999.
325. Behnke, A.R., Feen, B.G., and Welham, W.C., The specific gravity of healthy men, *J. Am. Med. Assoc.*, 118, 495, 1942.
326. Brožek, J., Grande, F., Anderson, T., and Keys, A., Densitometric analysis of body composition: revision of some assumptions, *Ann. N.Y. Acad. Sci.*, 110, 113, 1963.

327. Lohman, T.G., Measurement of body composition in children, *J. O.P.E.R.D.*, 53, 67, 1982.

328. Pařízková, J., Morphologie du tissu gras, in *Problemes Actuels d'Endocrinologie et de Nutrition, L'Obésité*, Klotz, H. and Trémolières, J., Eds., Série 7, Expansion Scientifique Française, Paris 1963, 271.

329. Durnin, J.V.G.A. and Rahaman, M.M., The assessment of the amount of fat in the human body from skinfold thickness, *Br. J. Nutr.*, 21, 681, 1967.

330. Pařízková, J., Age trend in fatness in normal and obese children, *J. Appl. Physiol.*, 16, 173, 1961.

331. Matiegka, J., *Somatology of School Children*, Czechoslovak Academy of Sciences and ARTS (ČAVU), Prague, 1929 (in Czech).

332. Bláha, P., Lisá, L., and Krásničanová, H., Czech obese children — the reduction treatment, *Int. J. Obes. Relat. Metab. Disord.*, 21 (Suppl. 2), S123, 1997.

333. Pařízková, J., Longitudinal study of body composition and body build development in boys of various physical activity from 11 to 15 years of age, *Human Biol.*, 40, 212, 1968.

334. Pařízková, J., Longitudinal study of the relationship between body composition and anthropometric characteristics in boys during growth and development, *Glasnik Antropoloskog Drusstvo Jugoslavii*, 7, 33, 1970.

335. Pařízková, J., Total body fat and skinfold thickness in children, *Metabolism*, 10, 794, 1961.

336. Brook, C.G.D., Determination of body composition of children from skinfold measurement, *Arch. Dis. Child.*, 46, 182, 1975.

337. Kapoor, G., Aneja, S., Mumari, S., and Mehta, S.C., Triceps skinfold thickness in adolescents, *Indian J. Med. Res.*, 94, 281, 1991.

338. Fleta Zaragozano, J., Moreno Aznar, L.S.A., Mur de Frenne, L., Bueno Lozano, M., Feja Solana, C., Sarria Chueca, A., and Bueno Sanchez, M., Assessment of the submandibular adipose skinfold for the determination of nutritional status in children and adolescents, *An. Esp. Pediatr.*, 47, 258, 1997.

339. Hills, A.P. and Parker, A.W., Obesity management via diet and exercise intervention, *Child: Care, Health Development*, 14, 409, 1988.

340. Hills, A.P. and Parker, A.W., Anthropometric and body composition assessment of obese children, *J. Sport Sci.*, 8, 175, 1990.

341. Hills, A.P., Effects of diet and exercise on body composition of pre-pubertal children, *J. Phys. Ed. Sports Sci.*, 3, 22, 1991.

342. Hills, A.P. and Parker, A.W., Physical fitness of obese children, in *Physical Activity for a Better Lifestyle*, Rychtecky, A., Svoboda, B., and Tilinger, P., Eds., Proc. 6th ICHPER Eur. Congr., Prague, Czech Republic, 1993, 179.

343. Carter, J.E.L. and Phillips, W.H., Structural changes in exercising middle aged males during a 2-year period, *J. Appl. Physiol.*, 27, 787, 1969.

344. Pařízková, J. and Carter, J.E.L., Influence of physical activity on stability of somatotypes in boys, *Am. J. Phys. Anthropol.*, 44, 327, 1976.

345. Roche, A.F., *Growth, Maturation and Body Composition: the Fels Longitudinal Study, 1929–1991*, Cambridge University Press, Cambridge, 1992.

346. Roche, A.F., Heymsfield, S.B., and Lohmans, T.G., Eds., *Human Body Composition, Methods and Findings*, Human Kinetics Publishers, Champaign, IL, 1996.

347. Ellis, K.J., Shypailo, R.J., Pratt, J.A., and Pond, W.G., Accuracy of dual-energy X-ray absorptiometry for body composition measurements in children, *Am. J. Clin. Nutr.*, 60, 660, 1994.

348. Fisberg, M., Carvalho, C.N.M., Cintra, C., and Vitolo, M.R., Body composition assessment by dual-energy X-ray absorptiometry in Brazilian school children with severe obesity, *Int. J. Obes. Relat. Metab. Disord.*, 22 (Suppl. 3), S198, 1998.

349. Ward, L.C., Byrne, N.M., Rutter, K., Hennoste, L., Hills, A.P., Cornish, B.H., and Thomas, B.J., Reliability of multiple frequency bioelectrical impedance analysis: an intermachine comparison, *Am. J. Hum. Biol.*, 9, 1, 63, 1997.

350. Hills, A.P. and Byrne, N.M., Bioelectrical impedance: use and abuse, In *Nutrition and Physical Activity*, Coetsee, M.F. and Van Heerden, H.J., Eds., Proc. Int. Council Physical Activity Fitness Res., Itala, South Africa, 1997, 23.

351. Lukaski, H.C., Johnson, P.E., Bolonchuk, W.W., and Lykken, G.E., Assessment of fat free mass using bioelectrical impedance measurements of the human body, *Am. J. Clin. Nutr.*, 41, 810, 1985.

352. Lukaski, H.C., Bolonchuk, W.W., Hall, C.B., and Siders, W.A., Validation of tetrapolar bioelectrical impedance method to assess human body composition, *J. Appl. Physiol.*, 60, 1327, 1986.

353. Segal, K.R., van Loan, M., Fitzgerald, P.I., Hodgdon, J.A., Van Hallie, T.B., Lean body mass estimated by bioelectrical impedance analysis: a four site cross validation study, *Am. J. Clin. Nutr.*, 47, 7, 1988.

354. Kushner, R.F. and Schoeller, D.A., Estimation of total body water by bioelectrical impedance analysis, *Am. J. Clin. Nutr.*, 44, 417, 1986.

355. Davies, P.S.W., Preece, M.A., Hicks, C.J., and Halliday, D., The prediction of total body water using bioelectrical impedance in children and adolescents, *Ann. Hum. Biol.*, 15, 237, 1988.

356. Goran, M.I., Kaskoun, M.C., Carpenter, W.H., Poehlman, E.T., Ravussin, E., and Fontvieille, A.M., Estimating body composition of young children by using bioelectrical resistance, *J. Appl. Physiol.*, 75, 1776, 1993.

357. Schaefer, F., Georgi, M., Zieger, A., and Scharfer, K., Usefulness of bioelectric impedance and skinfold measurements in predicting fat-free mass derived from total body potassium in children, *Pediatr. Res.*, 35, 617, 1994.

358. Kabir, I., Malek, M.A., Rahman, M.M., Khaled, M.A., and Mahalanabis, D., Changes in body composition of malnourished children after dietary supplementation as measured by bioelectrical impedance, *Am. J. Clin. Nutr.*, 59, 5, 1994.

359. Cordain, L., Johnson, J.E., Bainbridge, C.N., Wicker, R.E., and Stockler, J.M., Potassium content of the fat free body in children, *J. Sports Med. Phys. Fitness*, 29, 170, 1989.

360. Prentice, A.M., Stable isotopes in nutritional science and the study of energy metabolism, *Scand. J. Nutr.*, 43, 56, 1999.

361. Klish, W.J., Forbes, G.B., Gordon, A., and Cochran, W.J., New method for the estimation of lean body mass in infants (EEME Instrument): validation in nonhuman models, *J. Pediatr. Gastroenterol.*, 3, 199, 1984.

362. Fiorotto, M., Cochran, W.J., and Klish, W.J., Fat-free mass and total body water of infants estimated from total body electrical conductivity measurements, *Pediatr. Res.*, 22, 417, 1987.

363. Sohlström, A., Wahlund, L.O., and Forsum, E., Adipose tissue distribution as assessed by magnetic resonance imaging and total body fat by magnetic resonance imaging, underwater weighing and body-water dilution in healthy women, *Am. J. Clin. Nutr.*, 58, 830, 1993.

364. Leger, J., Carel, C., Legrand, I., Paulsen, A., Hassan, M., and Czernichow, P., Magnetic resonance imaging evaluation of adipose tissue and muscle tissue mass in children with growth hormone (GH) deficiency, Turner's syndrome, and intrauterine growth retardation during the first year of treatment with GH, *J. Clin. Endocrinol. Metab.*, 78, 904, 1994.

365. Goran, M.I., Kaskoun, M., and Shuman, W.P., Intra-abdominal adipose tissue in young children, *Int. J. Obes. Relat. Metab. Disord.*, 19, 279, 1995.

366. Kunešová, M., Hainer, V., Hergetová, H., Žák, A., Pařízková, J., and Hořejš, J., Simple anthropometric measurements: Relation to body fat mass, visceral adipose tissue and risk factors of atherogenesis, *Sborník Lék.*, 96, 349, 1995.

367. Ellis, K.J., Measuring body fatness in children and young adults: comparison of bioelectrical impedance analysis, total body electrical conductivity, and dual-energy X-ray absorptiometry, *Int. J. Obes. Relat. Metab. Disord.*, 20, 866, 1996.

368. Vague, J., Degree of masculine differentiation of obesities: a factor determining predisposition to diabetes, atherosclerosis, gout and uric calculus disease, *Am. J. Clin. Nutr.*, 4, 20, 1956.

369. Skamenová, B. and Pařízková, J., Assessment of disproportional (spiderlike) and diffuse type of obesity by measurement of the total and subcutaneous body fat, *Čas. Lek čes.*, CII, 6, 142, 1963 (in Czech).

370. Marelli, G., Andreotti, M., Liuzza, R., Dalzano, M., and La Placa, G., Relation of body fat distribution to blood lipid pattern in severe childhood obesity, *Int. J. Obes. Relat. Metab. Disord.*, 17 (Suppl. 2), 38, 1993.

371. Moreno, L.A., Fleta, J., Mur, L., Feja, C., Sarria, A., and Bueno, M., Indices of body fat distribution in Spanish children aged 4.0 to 14.9 years, *J. Pediatr. Gastroenterol. Nutr.*, 25, 175, 1997.

372. Asayama, K., Hayashibe, H., Dobashi, K., Uchida, N., Nakane, T., Kodera, K., and Nakazawa, S., A new age-adjusted index of body fat distribution in children based on waist and hip circumferences and stature, *Int. J. Obes. Relat. Metab. Disord.*, 22 (Suppl. 4), S11, 1998.

373. Asayama, K., Hayashi, K., Hayashibe, H., Uchida, N., Nakane, T., Kodera, K., and Nakazawa, S., Relationship between an index of body fat distribution (based on waist and hip circumferences) and stature, and biochemical complications in obese children, *Int. J. Obes. Relat. Metab. Disord.*, 22, 1209, 1999.

374. Ilies, I., Mahunka, I., and Sari, B., Relationship between immunoreactive insulin and plasma somatomedin-C/insulin-like growth factor 1 concentration in childhood obesity, *Orv. Hetil.*, 135, 1633, 1994 (in Hungarian).

375. De Ridder, C.M., de Boer, R.W., Seidell, J.C., Nieuwenhoff, C.M., Jeneson, C.M., Bakker, C.J.G., Zonderland, M.L., and Erich, W.B.M., Body fat distribution in pubertal girls quantified by magnetic resonance imaging, *Int. J. Obes.*, 16, 443, 1992.

376. Brambilla, P., Agostini, G., Burgio, G., Beccaria, L., Sironi, S., Del Maschio, A., and Chiumello, G., Waist circumference can predict visceral adiposity in obese adolescents, *Int. J. Obes. Relat. Metab. Disord.*, 21 (Suppl. 2), S140, 1997.

377. Rolland-Cachera, M.F. and Deheeger, M., Correlations between anthropometric indicators of abdominal fat and fatness indices in children, *Int. J. Obes. Relat. Metab. Disord.*, 22 (Suppl. 4), S11, 1998.

378. Freedman, D.S., Serdula, M.K., Srinivasan, S.R., and Berenson, G., Relation of circumferences and skinfold thicknesses to lipid and insulin concentrations in children: the Bogalusa Heart Study, *Am. J. Clin. Nutr.*, 69, 308, 1999.

379. De Moura, E.C., Albano, O., Piovesan, M.C., Haten, R., Leite, F., and Avancini, C., Childhood obesity: a new issue for public health in Brazil, *Int. J. Obes. Relat. Metab. Disord.*, 22 (Suppl. 4), S3, 1998.
380. Rolland-Cachera, M.F. and Bellisle, F., Timing weight-control measures in obese children, *Lancet*, 335, 918, 1990.
381. Hsu, H.S., Chen, W., Chen, S.C., and Ko, F.D., Colored striae in obese children and adolescents, *Chung Hua Min Kuo Hsiao Erh. Ko I Hsueh Hui Tsa Chih.*, 37, 349, 1996.
382. Riganti, G., Colombo, A., Meloni, A., Gambarini, G., De Berti, M.P., and Salvatori, A., Diet composition in obese children and obesity related diseases, *Int. J. Obes. Relat. Metab. Disord.*, 17 (Suppl. 2), S39, 1993.
383. Vignolo, M., Milani, S., Di Battista, E., Naselli, A., Garzia, P., Zucchi, C., and Aicardi, G., Variability of height and skeletal maturation in simple obesity, *Int. J. Obes. Relat. Metab. Disord.*, 22 (Suppl. 4), S14, 1998.
384. Alcazar, M.L., Alvear, J., and Muzzo, S., Influence of nutrition on the bone development of children, *Arch. Latinoam. Nutr.*, 34, 298, 1984 (in Spanish).
385. De Simone, M., Farello, G., Palumbo, M., Gentile, T., Ciuffreda, M., Olioso, P., Cinque, M., and De Matteis, F., Growth charts, growth velocity and bone development in childhood obesity, *Int. J. Obes. Relat. Metab. Disord.*, 19, 851, 1995.
386. De Schepper, J., Van den Broeck, M., and Jonckheer, M.H., Study of lumbar spine bone mineral density in obese children, *Acta Paediatr.*, 84, 313, 1995.
387. Sothern, M., Loftin, M., Suskind, R., Udall, J., Wilson, J., Heusel, L., Hargis, J., and Blecker, U., The impact of mild, moderate and severe obesity on upper and lower bone mineral content, lean and fat body mass, *Int. J. Obes. Relat. Metab. Disord.*, 22 (Suppl. 3), S198, 1998.
388. Wade, A.J., Marbut, M.M., and Round, J.M., Muscle fibre type and etiology of obesity, *Lancet*, 335, 805, 1990.
389. Åstrand, P.O. and Rodahl, K., *Textbook of Work Physiology*, 2nd ed., McGraw-Hill, New York, 1977.
390. Raben, A., Mygind, E., Saltin, B., and Astrup, A., Decreased activity of fat-oxidizing enzymes in muscle of obesity prone subjects, *Int. J. Obes. Relat. Metab. Disord.*, 21 (Suppl. 2), S43, 1997.
391. James, W.P.T. and Schofield, E.C., *Human Energy Requirements*, Oxford Medical Publications, Oxford University Press, Oxford, 1990.
392. Maffeis, C., Schutz, Y., and Pinelli, L., Effect of weight loss on resting energy expenditure in obese prepubertal children, *Int. J. Obes. Relat. Metab. Disord.*, 16, 41, 1992.
393. Kaplan, A.S., Zemel, B.S., Neiswender, K.M., and Stallings, V.A., Resting energy expenditure in clinical pediatrics measured values versus prediction equations, *J. Pediatr.*, 127, 200, 1995.
394. Molnár, D., Jeges, S., Erhardt, E., and Schutz, Y., Measured and predicted resting metabolic rate in obese and nonobese adolescents, *J. Pediatr.*, 127, 571, 1995.
395. Molnár, D. and Schutz, Y., The effect of obesity, age, puberty and gender on resting metabolic rate in children and adolescents, *Eur. J. Pediatr.*, 156, 376, 1997.
396. Maffeis, C., Schutz, Y., Zoccante, L., Micciolo, R., and Pinelli, L., Meal-induced thermogenesis in lean and obese prepubertal children, *Am. J. Clin. Nutr.*, 57, 481, 1993.
397. Zwiauer, K., Muller, T., Kommer, N., and Widhalm, K., Effect of body fat distribution on resting energy expenditure and diet induced thermogenesis in adolescents, *Int. J. Obes. Relat. Metab. Disord.*, 17 (Suppl. 2), S41, 1993.

398. Davies, P.S.W., Day, J.M., and Lucas, A., Energy expenditure in early infancy and later body fatness, *Int. J. Obes. Relat. Metab. Disord.*, 15, 727, 1991.
399. Westertorp, K.R., Obesity and physical activity, *Int. J. Obes. Relat. Metab. Disord.*, 23 (Suppl. 1), S59, 1999.
400. Heath, G.W., Pate, R.R., and Pratt, M., Measuring physical activity among adolescents, *Public Health Report*, 108 (Suppl 1), 42, 1993.
401. Sallis, J.F., Self-report measures of children's physical activity, *J. School Health*, 61, 215, 1991.
402. Pate, R.R., Physical activity assessment in children and adolescents, *Crit. Rev. Food Sci. Nutr.*, 33, 321, 1993.
403. Simons-Morton, B.G., O'Hara, N.M., Parcel, G.S., Huang, I.W., Baranowski, T., and Wilson, B., Children's frequency of participation in moderate to vigorous physical activities, *Res. Q. Exer. Sport*, 61, 307, 1990.
404. Montoye, H.J., Kemper, H.C.G., Saris, W.H.M., and Washburn, R.A., *Measuring Physical Activity and Energy Expenditure*, Human Kinetics, Champaign, IL, 1996.
405. Pařízková, J., Adaptation of functional capacity and exercise, in *Nutritional Adaptation in Man*, Blaxter, K. and Waterlow, J.C., Eds., John Libbey, London, Paris, 1985, 127, Chap. 11.
406. Hills, A.P., Byrne, N.M., and Ramage, A.J., Submaximal markers of exercise intensity, *J. Sports Sci.*, 16, S71, 1998.
407. Terrier, P., Aminian, K., and Schutz, Y., Can accelerometry accurately predict energetic cost of walking in uphill and downhill conditions? *Int. J. Obes. Relat. Metab. Disord.*, 23 (Suppl. 5), 1999.
408. Epstein, L.H., Paluch, R.A., Coleman, K.J., Vito, D., and Anderson, K., Determinants of physical activity in obese children assessed by accelerometer and self-report, *Med. Sci. Sports Exerc.*, 28, 1157, 1996.
409. Hills, A.P. and Byrne, N.M., Exercise, daily physical activity, eating and weight disorders in children, In *Paediatric Exercise and Medicine*, Armstrong, N. and van Mechelen, W., Eds., Oxford University Press, Oxford, 2000.
410. Puhl, J., Greaves, K., Hoyt, M., and Baranowski, T., Children's Activity Rating Scale (CARS): description and calibration, *Res. Q. Exerc. Sport*, 61, 26, 1990.
411. DuRant, R.H., Baranowski, T., Rhodes, T., Gutin, B., Thompson, W.O., Carroll, R., Puhl, J., and Greaves, K.A., Association among serum lipid and lipoprotein concentration and physical activity, physical fitness, and body composition in young children, *J. Pediatr.*, 123, 185, 1993.
412. Roberts, S.B., Savage, J., Coward, W.A., Chew, B., and Lucas, A., Energy expenditure and intake in infants born to lean and overweight mothers, *N. Engl. J. Med.*, 318, 727, 1988.
413. Griffiths, M., Rivers, J.P., and Payne, P.R., Energy intake in children at high and low risk of obesity, *Hum. Nutr. Clin. Nutr.*, 41, 425, 1987.
414. DeLany, J.P., Harsha, D.W., Kime, J.C., Kumler, J., Melancon, L., and Bray, G., Energy expenditure in lean and obese prepubertal children, *Obes. Res.*, 3 (Suppl. 1), 67, 1995.
415. Treuth, M.S., Hunter, G.R., Pichon, C., Figueroa-Colon, R., and Goran, M.I., Fitness and energy expenditure after strength training in obese prepubertal girls, *Med. Sci. Sports Exerc.*, 30, 1130, 1998.
416. Caspersen, C.J., Nixon, P.A., and DuRant, R.H., Physical activity epidemiology applied to children and adolescents, *Exerc. Sport Sci. Rev.*, 26, 341, 1998.
417. Astrup, A., The role of energy expenditure in the development of obesity, *Int. J. Obes. Relat. Metab. Disord.*, 22, S68, 1998.

418. Zurlo, F., Ferraro, R.T., and Fontvieille, A.M., Spontaneous physical activity and obesity: cross-sectional and longitudinal studies in Pima Indians, *Am. J. Physiol.*, 263, E296, 1992.
419. Berkowitz, R.I., Agras, W.S., Korner, A.F., Kraemer, H.C., and Zeanah, C.H., Physical activity and adiposity: A longitudinal study from birth to childhood, *J. Pediatr.*, 106, 734, 1985.
420. Maffeis, C., Schutz, Y., Zoccante, L., and Pinelli, L., Meal-induced thermogenesis in obese children with or without familial history of obesity, *Eur. J. Pediatr.*, 152, 128, 1993.
421. Epstein, L.H., Wing, R.P., Cluss, P., Fernstrom, M.H., Penner, B., Perkins, K.A., Nudelman, S., Marks, B., and Valoski, A., Resting metabolic rate in lean and obese children: relationship to child and parent weight and percent-overweight change, *Am. J. Clin. Nutr.*, 49, 331, 1989.
422. Elliot, D.L., Goldberg, L., Kuehl, K.S., and Hanna, C., Metabolic evaluation of obese and nonobese siblings, *J. Pediatr.*, 114, 957, 1989.
423. Roberts, S.B., Abnormalities of energy expenditure and the development of obesity, *Obes. Res.*, 3 (Suppl. 2), 155, 1995.
424. Davies, P.S.W., Connolly, C., and Day, J.M.E., Energy expenditure in infancy and later body composition, *Int. J. Obes. Relat. Metab. Disord.*, 17 (Suppl. 2), S35, 1993.
425. Vara, L. and Agras, S., Caloric intake and activity levels are related in young children, *Int. J. Obes.*, 13, 613, 1989.
426. Pařízková, J., Human growth, physical fitness and nutrition under various environmental conditions, in Human Growth, Physical Fitness and Nutrition, Shephard, TR.J., and Pařízková, J. Eds., *Medicine and Sport Science*, Vol. 31, Karger, Basel, 1991, 1.
427. Kelley, G.A., Gender differences in the physical activity levels of young African-American adults, *J. Natl. Med. Assoc.*, 87, 545, 1995.
428. Greene, L.C., Livingstone, M.B.E., McGloin, A.F., Webb, S.E., and Gibson, J.M.A., Comparison of total energy expenditure among children at low and high risk of obesity, *Int. J. Obes. Relat. Metab. Disord.*, 22 (Suppl. 4), 1998.
429. Obarzanek, E., Schreiber, G.B., Crawford, P.B., Goldman, S.R., Barrier, P.M., Frederick, M.M., and Lakatos, C., Energy intake and physical activity in relation to indices of body fat: The National Heart, Lung and Blood Institute Growth and Health Study, *Am. J. Clin. Nutr.*, 60, 15, 1996.
430. Calderon, L.L., Johnston, P.K., Lee, J.W., and Haddad, E.H., Risk factors for obesity in Mexican-American girls: dietary factors, anthropometric factors, and physical activity, *J. Am. Phys. Assoc.*, 96, 1177, 1996.
431. Ekelund, U.M., Yngve, A., and Sjostrom, M., The relationship between physical activity and body fat in adolescents, in *Physical Activity and Obesity*, Satellite Symposium of the 8th Int. Congress on Obesity, Maastricht, The Netherlands Aug. 26–9, 1998, (Abstr.) 28, 1998.
432. Bandini, L.G., Schoeller, D.A., and Dietz, W.H., Energy expenditure in obese and nonobese adolescents, *Pediatr. Res.*, 27, 198, 1990.
433. Salbe, A.D., Fonteinvielle, A.M., Harper, I.T., and Ravussin, E., Low levels of physical activity in 5-year-old children, *J. Pediatr.*, 131, 423, 1997.
434. Fontvieille, A.M., Kriska, A., and Ravussin, E., Decreased physical activity in Pima Indian compared with Caucasian children, *Int. J. Obes. Relat. Metab. Disord.*, 17, 445, 1993.

435. Freymond, D., Larson, K., Bogardus, C., and Ravussin, E., Energy expenditure during normo- and overfeeding in peripubertal children of lean and obese Pima Indians, *Am. J. Physiol.*, 257, E647, 1989.

436. Schutz, Y., The role of physical inactivity in the etiology of obesity, *Ther. Umsch.*, 46, 281, 1989.

437. Maffeis, C., Zaffanello, M., Pinelli, L., and Schutz, Y., Total energy expenditure and patterns of activity in 8–10-year-old obese and nonobese children, *J. Pediatr. Gastroenterol. Nutr.*, 23, 256, 1996.

438. Maffeis, C., Schutz, Y., Schena, F., Zaffanello, M., and Pinelli, L., Energy expenditure during walking and running in obese and nonobese prepubertal children, *J. Pediatr.*, 123, 193, 1993.

439. Maffeis, C., Schutz, Y., Zaffanello, P., Piccoli, R., and Pinelli, L., Elevated energy expenditure and reduced energy intake in obese prepubertal children: paradox of poor dietary reliability in obesity? *J. Pediatr.*, 124, 348, 1994.

440. Chen, W., Chen, P., Chen, S.C., Shih, W.T., and Hu, H.C., Lack of association between obesity and dental caries in three-year-old children, *Acta Pediatr. Sin.*, 39, 109, 1998.

441. Caldarone, G., Spada, R., Berlutti, G., Callari, L., Fiore, A., Giampietro, M., and Lista, R., Nutrition and exercise in children, *Ann. Inst. Super. Sanita*, 31, 445, 1995.

442. Borra, S.T., Schwartz, N.E., Spain, C.G., and Natchipolsky, M.M., Food, physical activity and fun: inspiring American kids to more healthy lifestyles, *J. Am. Diet. Assoc.*, 95, 816, 1995.

443. Wolf, A.M., Gortmaker, S.L., Cheung, L., Gray, H.M., Herzog, D.B., and Colditz, G.A., Activity, inactivity, and obesity: racial, ethnic, and age differences among schoolgirls, *Am. J. Public Health*, 83, 1625, 1993.

444. Chiloiro, M., Guerra, V., Riezzo, G., Caroli, M., and Martucci, T., Play in obese and nonobese children in Southern Italy, *Int. J. Obes. Relat. Metab. Disord.*, 22 (Suppl. 4), S10, 1998.

445. Huttunen, N.P., Knip, M., and Paavilainen, T., Physical activity and fitness in obese children, *Int. J. Obes.*, 10, 519, 1986.

446. Romanella, N.E., Wakat, D.K., Lloyd, B.H., and Kelly, L.E., Physical activity and attitudes in lean and obese children and their mothers, *Int. J. Obes.*, 15, 407, 1991.

447. Bandini, L.G., Schoeller, D.A., Edwards, J., Young, V.R., Oh, S.H., and Dietz, W.H., Energy expenditure during carbohydrate overfeeding in obese and nonobese adolescents, *Am. J. Physiol.*, 256, E357, 1989.

448. Vermorel, M., Vernet, J., Bitar, A., Fellmann, N., and Couderty, J., Variability of physical activity and energy expenditure in adolescents: which consequences on occurrence of obesity? *Int. J. Obes. Relat. Metab. Disord.*, 22 (Suppl. 4), S8, 1998.

449. DeLany, J.P., Harsha, D., and Bray, G.A., Parameters of energy metabolism predicting change in body fat over 2 years in boys, *Int. J. Obes. Relat. Metab. Disord.*, 22 (Suppl. 3), S36, 1998.

450. Kemper, H.C.G., Post, G.B., Twisk, J.W.R., and van Mechelen, W., Lifestyle and obesity in adolescence and young adulthood: results from the Amsterdam Growth and Health Longitudinal Study (AGAHLS), *Int. J. Obes. Relat. Metab. Disord.*, 23 (Suppl. 3), S34, 1999.

451. Sallis, J.F., Patterson, T.L., McKenzie, T.L., and Nader, P.R., Family variables and physical activity in preschool children, *J. Dev. Behav. Pediatr.*, 9, 57, 1988.

452. Kemper, H., Snel, J., Verschuur, R., and Storm van Essen, L., Tracking of health and risk indicators of cardiovascular diseases from teenager to adult: Amsterdam Growth and Health Study, *Prev. Med.*, 19, 642, 1990.

453. Du Rant, R.H., Dover, E.V., and Alpert, B.S., An evaluation of five indices of physical working capacity in children, *Med. Sci. Sp. Exerc.*, 15 (1), 83, 1983.

454. McArdle, W.D., Katch, F.I., and Katch, V.L., *Exercise Physiology. Energy, Nutrition and Human Performance*, 3rd ed., Lea & Febiger, Philadelphia, 1991.

455. Sallis, J.F., Epidemiology of physical activity and fitness in children and adolescents, *Crit. Rev. Food Sci. Nutr.*, 33, 403, 1993.

456. Maffeis, C., Schena, F., Zafanello, M., Zoccante, L., Schutz, Y., and Pinelli, L., Maximal aerobic power during running and cycling in obese and non-obese children, *Acta Pediatr.*, 83, 113, 1994.

457. Pařízková, J., Hainer, V., Štich, V., Kunešová, M., and Ksantini, M., Physiological capabilities of obese individuals and implications for exercise, in *Exercise and Obesity*, Wahlquist, M. and Hills, A.P., Eds., Smith-Gordon/Nishimura, London, 1995, 131.

458. DeMeersman, R.E., Stone, S., Schaefer, D.C., and Miller, W.W., Maximal work capacity in prepubescent obese and nonobese females, *Clin. Pediatr.*, 24, 199, 1985.

459. Zanconato, S., Baraldi, E., Santuz, P., Rigon, F., Vido, L., Da Dalt, L., and Zacchello, F., Gas exchange during exercise in obese children, *Eur. J. Pediatr.*, 148, 614, 1989.

460. Tamiya, N., Study of physical fitness in children, and its application to pediatric clinics and sports medicine, *Hokkaido Igaku Zasshi*, 66, 849, 1991 (in Japanese).

461. Malova, N.A., Simonova, L.A., and Fetisov, G.V., Hygienic rationale for diagnosis and correction of excessive body weight in schoolchildren with physical training, *Vestn. Ross. Akad. Med. Nauk.*, 51, 9, 1993 (in Russian).

462. Rowland, T.W., Effects of obesity on aerobic fitness in adolescent females, *Am. J. Dis. Child.*, 145, 764, 1991.

463. Fernandez, A.C., Cintra, I.P., Stella, S., Fisberg, M., and Carlos Silva, A., Correlation between percentage of fat and physical performance in obese children, *Int. J. Obes. Relat. Metab. Disord.*, 22 (Suppl. 4), S12, 1998.

464. Fernandez, A.C., Cintra, I.P., Stella, S., Fisberg, M., and Carlos Silva, A., The lean body mass as determinant of physical performance in children, *Int. J. Obes. Relat. Metab. Disord.*, 22 (Suppl. 3), S199, 1998.

465. Cooper, D.M., Poage, J., Barstow, T.J., and Springer, C., Are obese children truly unfit? Minimizing the confounding effect of body size on the exercise response, *J. Pediatr.*, 335, 805, 1990.

466. Pongprapai, S., Mo-suwan, L., and Leelasamran, W., Physical fitness of obese schoolchildren in Hat Yai, southern Thailand, *Southeast Asian J. Trop. Med. Public Health*, 25, 354, 1994.

467. Katch, V., Becque, M.D., Marks, C., Moorehead, C., and Rocchini, A., Oxygen uptake and energy output during walking of obese male and female adolescents, *Am. J. Clin. Nutr.*, 47, 26, 1988.

468. Taylor, W. and Baranowski, T., Physical activity, cardiovascular fitness, and adiposity in children, *Res. Q.Exerc. Sport*, 62, 157, 1991.

469. Reybrouck, T., Weymans, M., Vinckx, J., Stijns, H., and Vanderschueren-Lodeweyckx, M., Cardiorespiratory function during exercise in obese children, *Acta Paediatr. Scand.*, 76, 342, 1987.

470. Reybrouck, T., Vinckx, J., Van den Berghe, G., and Vanderschueren-Lodewyckx, M., Exercise therapy and hypocaloric diet in the treatment of obese children and adolescents, *Acta Paediatr. Scand.*, 79, 84, 1990.

471. Reybrouck, T., Mertens, L., Schepers, D., Vinckx, J., and Gewillig, M., Assessment of cardiorespiratory exercise function in obese children and adolescents by body mass-independent parameters, *Eur. J. Appl. Physiol.*, 75, 478, 1997.

472. Thoren, C., Seliger, V., Máček, M., Vávra, J., and Rutenfranz, J., The influence of training on physical fitness in healthy children with chronic diseases, in *Current Aspects of Perinatology & Physiology of Children*, Linnewaeh, C., Ed., Springer, Berlin, 1973.

473. Ward, D.S., and Bar-Or, O., Role of the physician and physical education teacher in the treatment of obesity at school, *Pediatrician*, 13, 44, 1986.

474. Ho, T.F., Tay, J.S., Yip, W.C., and Rajan, U., Evaluation of lung function in Singapore obese children, *J. Singapore Paediatr. Soc.*, 31, 46, 1989.

475. Inselma, L.S., Milanese, A., and Deurloo, A., Effect of obesity on pulmonary function in children, *Pediatr. Pulmonol.*, 16, 130, 1993.

476. Kaplan, T.A. and Montana, E., Exercise-induced bronchospasm in nonasthmatic obese children, *Clin. Pediat.*, 12, 220, 1993.

477. Bosisio, E., Sergi, M., di Natale, B., and Chiumello, G., Ventilatory volumes, flow rates, transfer factor and its components (membrane component, capillary volume) in obese adults and children, *Respiration*, 45, 321, 1984.

478. Barlett, H.L., Kenney, W.L., and Buskirk, E.R., Body composition and expiratory volume of pre-pubertal lean and obese boys and girls, *Int. J. Obes. Relat. Metab. Disord.*, 16, 653, 1992.

479. Fung, K.P., Lau, S.P., Chow, O.K., Lee, J., and Wong, T.W., Effects of overweight on lung function, *Arch. Dis. Child.*, 65, 512, 1990.

480. Marcus, C.L., Curtis, S., Koerner, C.B., Joffe, A., Serwint, J.R., and Loughlin, G.M., Evaluation of pulmonary function and polysomnography in obese children and adolescents, *Pediatr. Pulmonol.*, 21, 176, 1996.

481. Mallory, G.B., Jr., Fiser, D.H., and Jackson, R., Sleep-associated breathing disorders in morbidly obese children and adolescents, *J. Pediatr.*, 115, 892, 1989.

482. McMurray, R.G., Harrel, J.S., Levine, A.A., and Gansky, S.A., Childhood obesity elevates blood pressure and total cholesterol independently of physical activity, *Int. J. Obes. Relat. Metab. Disord.*, 19, 881, 1995.

483. Salvatoni, A., Deiana, M., Riganti, G., and Nespoli, L., Is blood pressure more related to insulin sensitivity or to body weight? *Int. J. Obes. Relat. Metab. Disord.*, 21 (Suppl. 2), S140, 1997.

484. Andre, J.L., Deschamps, J.P., and Gueguen, R., Relationship between blood pressure and weight characteristics in childhood and adolescence. I. Blood pressure, weight and overweight, *Rev. Epidemiol. Santé Publique*, 30, 1, 1982.

485. Labarthe, D.R., Mueller, W.H., and Eissa, M., Blood pressure and obesity in childhood and adolescence: Epidemiological aspects, *Ann. Epidemiol.*, 1, 337, 1991.

486. Adeyanju, M., Cresswell, W.H., Stone, D.B., and Macrina, D.M., A three-year study of obesity and its relationship to high blood pressure in adolescents, *J. Sch. Health*, 57, 109, 1987.

487. Kohno, T., Tanaka, H., and Honda, S., Therapeutic assessment of childhood obesity with body composition measured by bioelectrical impedance analysis, *Fukuoka Igaku Zasshi*, 85, 267, 1994 (in Japanese).

488. Urbina, E.M., Gidding, S.S., Bao, W.H., Elkasabany, A., and Berenson, G.S., Association of fasting blood sugar level, insulin level, and obesity with left ventricular mass in healthy children and adolescents. The Bogalusa Heart Study, I, *Am. Heart J.*, 138, 122, 1999.

489. Ferguson, M.A., Gutin, B., Owens, S., Litaker, M., Tracy, R.P., and Allison, J., Fat distribution and hemostatic measures in obese children, *Am. J. Clin. Nutr.*, 67, 1136, 1998.

490. Perrone, L., D'Alfonso, C.D., Del Giudice, G., Marotta, A., Boccia, E., Ponticiello, E., and Di Toro, R., Relationships among white blood cell count and anthropometric indexes of adiposity in obese children and adolescents, *Int. J. Obes. Relat. Metab. Disord.*, 22 (Suppl. 4), S27, 1998.

491. Birrer, R.B. and Levine, R., Performance parameters in children and adolescent athletes, *Sp. Med.*, 4, 211, 1987.

492. Borms, J., The child and exercise: an overview, J. *Sports Sci.*, 4, 3, 1986.

493. Docherty, D. and Bell, R., The relationship between flexibility and linearity measures in boys and girls 6–15 years, *J. Human Movement Stud.*, 11, 279, 1985.

494. Krahenbuhl, G.S. and Martin, S.L., Adolescent body size and flexibility, *Res. Q.*, 48, 797, 1977.

495. Watson, A.W.S. and O'Donovan, D.J., Factors relating to the strength of female adolescents, *J. Appl. Physiol.*, 43, 5, 834, 1977.

496. McLeod, W.P., Hunter, S.C., and Etchison, B., Performance measurement and percent body fat in the high school athlete, *Am. J. Sp. Med.*, 11 (6), 390, 1983.

497. Laubach, L.L. and McConville, J.T., The relationship of strength to body size and topology, *Med. Sci. Sp.*, 1, 189, 1969.

498. Lamphiear, D.E. and Montoye, H.J., Muscular strength and body size, *Human Biol.*, 48, 147, 1976.

499. Kim, H.K., Matsuura, Y., and Inagaki, A., Physical fitness and motor ability in obese boys 12 through 14 years of age, *Ann. Physiol. Anthropol.*, 12, 17, 1993 (in Japanese).

500. Suzuki, M. and Tatsumi, M., Effect of therapeutic exercise on physical fitness in a school health program for obese children, *Nippon Koshu Eisei Zasshi*, 40, 17, 1993 (in Japanese).

501. Wear, C.L. and Miller, K., Relationship of physique and developmental level to physical performance, *Res. Q.*, 33 (4), 615, 1962.

502. Palgi, Y., Gutin, B., Young, J., and Alejandro, D., Physiologic and anthropometric factors underlying endurance performance in children, *Int. J. Sports Med.*, 5, 67, 1984.

503. Gutin, B., Trinidad, A., Norton, C., Giles, E., Stewart, K., and Giles, A., The dominance of body fat in explaining endurance performance of 11–12-year-old girls, *Res. Q.*, 49, 44, 1978.

504. Jaffe, M. and Kosakov, C., The motor development of fat babies, *Clin. Pediatr.*, 21, 619, 1982.

505. Sawada, Y., On the body composition of obese children and in particular, sexual, age, and regional differences of skinfold thickness, *J. Hum. Ergol.* 7, 103, 1978.

506. Malina, R.M., Beunen, G.P., Claessens, A.L., Lefevre, J., Vanden Eynde, B.V., Renson, R., Vanreusel, B., and Simons, J., Fatness and physical fitness of girls 7 to 17 years, *Obes. Res.*, 3, 221, 1995.

507. Hills, A.P. and Parker, A.W., Electromyography of walking in obese children, *Electromyogr. Clin. Neurophysiol.*, 33 (4), 225, 1993.

508. Petrolini, N., Iughetti, L., and Bernasconi, S., Difficulty in visual coordination as a possible cause of sedentary behaviour in obese children, *Int. J. Obes. Relat. Metab. Disord.*, 19, 928, 1995.

509. Hunt, S.M. and Groff, J.L., *Advanced Nutrition and Human Metabolism*, West Publ., Los Angeles, 1990.

510. Dwyer, J., Dietary assessments, in *Modern Nutrition in Health and Disease*, Shils, M.E., Olson, J.A., and Shike, M., Eds., Lea & Febiger, Philadelphia, 1994.

511. Hammer, L.D., The development of eating behavior in childhood, *Pediatr. Clin. North Am.*, 39, 379, 1992.

512. Alberton, A.M., Tobelmann, R.C., Engstrom, A., and Asp, E.H., Nutrient intakes of 2- to 10-year-old American children: 10-year study, *J. Am. Diet. Assoc.*, 92, 1492, 1992.

513. Kennedy, E. and Goldberg, J., What are American children eating? Implications for public policy, *Nutr. Rev.*, 53, 111, 1995.

514. Agras, W.S., Kraemer, H.C., Berkowitz, R.I., Korner, A.F., and Hammer, L.D., Does a vigorous feeding style influence early development of adiposity? *J. Pediatr.*, 110, 799, 1987.

515. Lahlou, N., Landais, P., De Boissieu, D., and Bougeners, P.F., Circulating leptin in normal children and during the dynamic phase of juvenile obesity: relation to body fatness, energy metabolism, caloric intake, and sexual dismorphism, *Diabetes*, 46, 989, 1997.

516. Kaskoun, M.C., Johnson, R.K., and Goran, M.I., Comparison of energy intake by semiquantitative food-frequency questionnaire with total energy expenditure by the doubly labelled water method in young children, *Am. Clin. Nutr.*, 60, 43, 1994.

517. Johnson, S.L. and Birch, L.L., Parent's and children's adiposity and eating style, *Pediatrics*, 94, 653, 1994.

518. Greco, M., Croci, M., Tufano, A., Sassano, G., Panigoni, G., Costa, M., Morricone, L., Longari, V., Mazzochi, M., and Caviezel, F., Caloric intake and distribution of the main nutrients in a population of obese children, *Minerva Endocrinol.*, 15, 257, 1990.

519. Forbes, G.B. and Brown, M.R., Energy need for weight maintenance in human beings: effect of body size and composition, *J. Am. Diet. Assoc.*, 89, 499, 1989.

520. Hardy, S.C. and Kleinman, R.E., Fat and cholesterol in the diet of infants and young children: implications for growth, development, and long-term health, *J. Pediatr.*, 125, S69, 1994.

521. Barker, D.J.P., The fetal and infant origin of adult diseases, *Br. Med. J.*, 301, 1111, 1990.

522. Pařízková, J., How much energy is consumed and spent for optimal growth and development? *Nutrition*, 12, 820, 1996.

523. Valoski, A. and Epstein, L.H., Nutrient intake of obese children in a family-based behavioral weight control program, *Int. J. Obes.*, 14, 667, 1990.

524. Ortega, R.M., Requejo, A.M., Andres, P., Lopez-Sobaler, A.M., Redondo, R., and Gonzales-Fernand, M., Relationships between diet composition and body mass index in a group of Spanish adolescents, *Br. J. Nutr.*, 74, 765, 1995.

525. Nguyen, N.V., Larson, D.E., Johnson, R.K., and Goran, M.I., Fat intake and adiposity in children of lean and obese parents, *Am. J. Clin. Nutr.*, 63, 507, 1996.

526. Park, H.S., Choi, M.K., Lee, M.S., Sung, M.K., and Sung, J.C., Association with leptin, cardiovascular risk factors, and nutrition in Korean girls, *Int. J. Obes. Relat. Metab. Disord.*, 22 (Suppl. 4), S27, 1998.

527. Tucker, L.A., Seljaas, G.T., and Hager, R.L., Body fat percentage of children varies according to their diet composition, *J. Am. Diet. Assoc.*, 97, 981, 1997.

528. Gazzaniga, J.M. and Burns, T.L., Relationship between diet composition and body fatness, with adjustment for resting energy expenditure and physical activity, in preadolescents children, *Am. J. Clin. Nutr.*, 58, 21, 1993.

529. Byrne, N.M. and Hills, A.P., Assessment of eating practices in adolescence, *Proc. Nutr. Soc.* (Australia), 19, 106, 1995.

530. Lifshitz, F. and Moses, N., Growth failure: A complication of dietary treatment of hypercholesterolemia, *Am. J. Dis. Child.*, 143, 537, 1989.

531. Ferrante, E., Vania, A., Mariani, P., Pitzalis, G., De Pascale, A., Monti, S., Falconieri, P., Bonamico, M., and Imperato, C., Nutritional epidemiology during school age, *Ann. Inst. Super. Sanita*, 31, 435, 1995.

532. Anderson, G.H., Sugars, sweetness, and food intake, *Am. J. Clin. Nutr.*, 62 (Suppl. 1), 195S, 1995.

533. MacKeown, J.M., Cleaton-Jones, P.E., Edwards, A.W., Turgeon, O., and Brien, H., Energy, macro- and micronutrient intake of 5-year-old urban black South African children in 1984 and 1995, *Pediatr. Perinatal Epidemiol.*, 12, 297, 1998.

534. Wandel, M., Nutrition-related diseases and dietary change among Third World immigrants in northern Europe, *Nutr. Health*, 9, 117, 1993.

535. Bianco, L., Barbera, S., Bianchini, M., Crea, M.R., and Spagnoli, T.D., Eating behavior in children and youth, *Int. J. Obes. Relat. Metab. Disord.*, 17 (Suppl. 2), 34, 1993.

536. Dennison, B.A., Fruit juice consumption by infants and children: a review, *J. Am. Coll. Nutr.*, 15, 4S, 1996.

537. Widhalm, K., Prevention of morbid obesity in adolescents: a new pediatric clinical syndrome? *Int. J. Obes. Relat. Metab. Disord.*, 23 (Suppl. 5), S7, 1999.

538. Maffeis, C., Schutz, Y., and Pinelli, L., Postprandial thermogenesis in obese children before and after weight reduction, *Eur. J. Clin. Nutr.*, 46, 577, 1992.

539. Salas-Salvado, J., Barenys-Manent, M., Recasens Gracia, M.A., Marti-Henneberg, C., Influence of adiposity on the thermic effect of food and exercise in lean and obese adolescents, *Int. J. Obes. Relat. Disord.*, 17, 717, 1993.

540. Katch, V.L., Moorehead, C.P., Becque, M.D., and Rocchini, A.P., Reduced short-term effects of a meal in obese adolescent girls, *Eur. J. Appl. Physiol.*, 65, 535, 1992.

541. Bellisle, F., Rolland-Cachera, M.F., Deheeger, M., and Guilloud-Bataille, M., Obesity and food intake in children: evidence for a role of metabolic and/or behavioral daily rhythm, *Appetite*, 11, 111, 1988.

542. Maffeis, C., Zantedeschi, P., Filippi, L., Bonscard, G., Grezzani, A., Pinelli, L., and Zaffanello, M., Patterns of food intake and obesity in Italian children, *Int. J. Obes. Relat. Metab. Disord.*, 23 (Suppl. 5), S44, 1999.

543. Ortega, R.M., Requejo, A.M., Lopez-Sobaler, A.M., Quintas, M.E., Andres, P., Redondo, M.R., Navia, B., Lopez-Bonilla, M.D., and Rivas, T., Differences in the breakfast habits of overweight/obese and normal weight schoolchildren, *Int. J. Vitam. Nutr. Res.*, 68, 125, 1998.

544. Araya, H.L., Alvina, M.W., Vera, G.A., Sola, J.C., Diaz, C., and Pak, N.D., Effect of protein and carbohydrate preloads on food and energy intakes in preschool children with different nutritional status, *Arch. Latinoam. Nutr.*, 45, 25, 1995 (in Spanish).

545. Agostoni, C., Rottoli, A., Trojan, S., and Riva, E., Dairy products and adolescent nutrition, *J. Int. Med. Res.*, 22, 67, 1994.
546. Murata, M., Nutrition for the young — its current problems, *Nutr. Health*, 8, 143, 1992.
547. Berkeling, B., Ekman, S., and Rössner, S., Eating behaviour in obese and normal weight 11-year-old children, *Int. J. Obes. Relat. Metab. Disord.*, 16, 355, 1992.
548. Widhalm, K., Zwiauer, K., and Eckharter, I., External stimulus dependence in food intake of obese adolescents: studies using a food dispenser, *Klin. Pediatr.*, 202, 168, 1990 (in German).
549. Riezzo, G., Chiloiro, M., and Guerra, V., Electrogastrography in healthy children: evaluation of normal value, influence of age, gender and obesity, *Dig. Dis. Sci.*, 43, 1646, 1998.
550. Bartkiw, T.P., Children's eating habits: a question of balance, *World Health Forum*, 14, 404, 1993.
551. Gustafson-Larson, A.M. and Terry, R.D., Weight-related behaviors and concerns of fourth-grade children, *J. Am. Diet. Assoc.*, 92, 818, 1992.
552. Maffeis, C., Pinelli, L., and Schutz, Y., Increased fat oxidation in prepubertal obese children: a metabolic defence against further weight gain? *J. Pediatr.*, 126, 15, 1995.
553. Maffeis, C., Armellini, F., Schena, S., Sidoti, G., Bissoli, L., Zantedeschi, P., Zafanello, M., and Schutz, Y., Fat oxidation and adiposity in children: Exogenous versus endogenous fat utilisation, *Int. J. Obes. Relat. Metab. Disord.*, 22 (Suppl. 3), S37, 1998.
554. Molnár, D. and Schutz, Y., Fat oxidation in nonobese and obese adolescents: Effect of body composition and pubertal development, *J. Pediatr.* 132, 98, 1998.
555. Rueda-Maza, C.M., Maffeis, C., Zaffanello, M., and Schutz, Y., Total and exogenous carbohydrate oxidation in obese prepubertal children, *Am. J. Clin. Nutr.*, 64, 844, 1996.
556. Tounian, P., Girardet, J.P., Frelut, M.L., Veinberg, F., and Fontaine, J.L., Resting energy expenditure and food-induced thermogenesis in obese children, *J. Pediatr. Gastroenterol. Nutr.*, 16, 451, 1993.
557. Berenson, G.S., Srinivasan, S.R., Wattigney, W.A., and Harsha, D.W., Obesity and cardiovascular risk in children, *Ann. N.Y. Acad. Sci.*, 699, 93, 1993.
558. Wattigney, W.A., Harsha, D.W., Srinivasan, S.R., Webber, L.S., and Berenson, G.S., Increasing obesity impact on serum lipids and lipoproteins in young adults, *Arch. Intern. Med.*, 151, 2017, 1991.
559. Yamamoto, A., Sawada, S., Uyama, M., Matsuzawa, Y., Yamamura, T., Yokoyama, S., Kameda, K., Kasagi, F., and Horibe, H., Serum lipid levels in elementary and junior high schoolchildren and their relationship to obesity, *Prog. Clin. Biol. Res.*, 255, 107, 1988.
560. Simon, J.A., Morrison, J.A., Similo, S.L., McMahon, R.P., and Schreiber, G.B., Correlates of high-density lipoprotein cholesterol in black and white girls: the NHLBI Growth and Health Study, *Am. J. Public Health*, 85, 1698, 1995.
561. Fripp, R.R., Hodgson, J.L., Kwiterovitch, P.O., Werner, J.C., Schuler, H.G., and Whitman, V., Aerobic capacity, obesity, and atherosclerotic risk factors in male adolescents, *Pediatrics*, 75, 813, 1985.
562. Petridou, E., Malamou, H., Doxiadis, S., Pantelakis, S., Kanellopoulou, G., Toupadaki, N., Trichopoulou, A., Flytzani, V., and Trichopoulos, D., Blood lipids in Greek adolescents and their relationship to diet, obesity, and socioeconomic factors, *Ann. Epidemiol.*, 5, 286, 1995.

563. Giovannini, M., Bellu, R., Ortisi, M.T., Incerti, P., and Riva, E., Cholesterol and lipoprotein levels in Milanese children: relation to nutritional and familial factors, *J. Am. Coll. Nutr.*, 11, Suppl. 28S, 1992.

564. Obuchowitz, A. and Szczepanski, Z., Evaluation of the biochemical indicators of risk of atherosclerosis in children with simple obesity, *Pediatr. Pol.*, 61, 409, 1986.

565. Malecka-Tendera, E., Piskorska, D., Wazowski, R., Muchacka-Bianga, M., and Klimek, K., Relationship between lipid profile and body mass index in non-obese pubertal children, *Int. J. Obes. Relat. Metab. Disord.*, 21 (Suppl. 2), S140, 1997.

566. Malecka-Tendera, E., Wrzesniewski, N., Kurkowska, M., and Kudla, M., Overweight in adolescent girls with menstrual irregularities is a risk factor for polycystic ovary syndrome (PCOS), *Int. J. Obes. Relat. Metab. Disord.*, 22 (Suppl. 4), S26, 1998.

567. Šonka, J., Kostiuk, P., Hilgertová, J., Límanová, Z., and Drozdová, V., Hormonal and metabolic adaptation to a reducing regimen in children, *Acta Univ. Carolinae*, 39, 33, 1993.

568. Lísková, S., Hošek, P., and Stožický, F., The metabolic syndrome and cardiovascular risk factors in obese children, *Int. J. Obes. Relat. Metab. Disord.*, 22 (Suppl. 4), S25, 1998.

569. Ferrer-Gonzales, J., Belda Galiana, I., Segarra Aznar, F.M., Fenollosa Entrena, B., and Dalmau Serra, J., The development of lipid and anthropometric parameters in the treatment of pre-pubertal obese patients, *An. Esp. Pediatr.*, 48, 267, 1998 (in Spanish).

570. Sveger, T., Flodmark, C.E., Fex, G., and Henningsen, N.C., Apolipoproteins A-I and B in obese children, *J. Pediatr. Gastroenterol. Nutr.*, 9, 497, 1989.

571. Lecerf, J.M., Labrunie, M., and Charles, M.A., Triglycerides increase and LpA1 decreases with weight in obese boys and with waist:hip ratio in obese girls, *Int. J. Obes. Relat. Metab. Disord.*, 22 (Suppl. 4), S24, 1998.

572. Menghetti, E., Di Feo, G., Mucedola, G., Montaleone, M., Marulli, P., Liberti, A., Cellitti, R., Spagnolo, A., and Pascone, R., Obesity and hypercholesterolemia in primary school in Rome, *Minerva Pediatr.*, 47, 303, 1995.

573. Guillaume, M., Differences in associations of fatness status, familial and nutritional factors with blood lipids between boys and girls, *Int. J. Obes. Relat. Metab. Disord.*, 22 (Suppl. 4), S24, 1998.

574. Asayama, K., Hayashiba, H., Dobashi, K., Uchida, N., Kawada, Y., and Nakazawa, S., Relationships between biochemical abnormalities and anthropometric indices of overweight, adiposity and body fat distribution in Japanese elementary school children, *Int. J. Obes. Relat. Metab. Disord.*, 19, 253, 1995.

575. Moreno, L.A., Quintela, I., Sarría, A., Fleta, J., and Bueno, M., Body fat distribution and postprandial lipidemia in obese adolescents, *Int. J. Obes. Relat. Metab. Disord.*, 22 (Suppl. 4), S24, 1998.

576. Bougnères, P., Le Stunff, C., Pecqueur, C., Pinglier, E., Adnot, D., and Ricquier, D., In vivo resistance of lipolysis to epinephrine. A new feature of childhood onset obesity, *J. Clin. Invest.*, 99, 2568, 1997.

577. Grugni, G., Guzzaloni, G., Mazzilli, G., Moro, D., and Morabito, F., Hyperuricemia and obesity in young female subjects, *Int. J. Obes. Relat. Metab. Disord.*, 22 (Suppl. 4), S27, 1998.

578. Schutz, Y., Rueda-Maza, C.M., Zaffanello, M., and Maffeis, C., Whole-body protein turnover and resting energy expenditure in obese, prepubertal children, *Am. J. Clin. Nutr.*, 69, 857, 1999.

579. Zamboni, G., Soffiati, M., Giavarina, D., and Tato, L., Mineral metabolism in obese children, *Acta Paediatr. Scand.*, 77, 741, 1988.

580. Molnár, D., Decsi, T., Burus, I., Torok, K., and Erhardt, E., Effect of weight reduction on plasma total antioxidative capacity in obese children, *Int. J. Obes. Relat. Metab. Disord.*, 22 (Suppl. 4), S23, 1998.

581. Decz, T., Molnár, D., and Koletzko, B., The effect of under- or overnutrition on essential fatty acid metabolism in childhood, *Eur. J. Clin. Nutr.*, 52, 541, 1998.

582. Strauss, R.S., Comparison of serum concentration of alpha-tocopherol and beta-carotene in a cross-sectional sample of obese and nonobese children (NHANES III), *J. Pediat.*, 124, 160, 1999.

583. Beckett, P.R., Wong, W.W., and Copeland, K.C., Developmental changes in the relationship between IGF-1 and body composition during puberty, *Growth Hormone IGF Res.*, 8, 283, 1998.

584. Bideci, A., Cinaz, P., Hasanoglu, A., and Elberg, S., Serum levels of insulin-like growth factor-I and insulin-like growth factor binding protein-3 in obese children, *J. Pediat. Endocrinol. Nutr. Metab.*, 10, 295, 1997.

585. Yasunaga, T., Furukawa, S., Katsumata, N., Horikawa, R., Tanaka, T, Tanae, A., and Hibi, I., Nutrition related hormonal changes in obese children, *Endocr. J.*, 45, 221, 1998.

586. Hasegawa, T., Hasegawa, Y., Takada, M., Ishii, T., Sato, S., and Matsuo, N., Free form of insulin-like growth factor-1 in circulation is normal in children with simple obesity, *Hormone Res.*, 49 (Suppl. 1), 51, 1998.

587. Park, M.J., Kim, H.S., Kong, J.H., Kim, D.H., and Chung, C.Y., Serum levels of insulin-like growth factor (IGF-I), free IGF-I, IGF binding protein (IGFBP-1), IGFBP-3 and insulin in obese children, *J. Pediat. Endocrinol. Metab.*, 12, 139, 1999.

588. Falorni, A., Bini, V., Molinari, D., Papi, F., Celi, F., Di Stefano, G., Berioli, M.G., Bacosi, M.L., and Contessa, G., Leptin serum levels in normal weight and obese children and adolescents: relationships with age, sex, pubertal development, body mass index and insulin, *Int. J. Obes. Relat. Metab. Disord.*, 21, 881, 1997.

589. Falorni, A., Bini, V., Cabiati, G., Papi, F., Arzano, S., Celi, F., and Sanasi, M., Serum levels of type I procollagen C-terminal propeptide, insulin-like growth factor-I (IGF-I), and IGF binding protein-3 in obese children and adolescents: relationship to gender, pubertal development, growth, insulin and nutritional status, *Metab. Clin. Endocrinol.*, 46, 862, 1997.

590. Travers, S.H., Labarta, J.I., Gargoski, S.E., Rosenfeld, R.G., Jeffers, B.W., and Eckel, R.H., Insulin-like growth factor binding protein-I levels are strongly associated with insulin sensitivity and obesity in early pubertal children, *J. Clin. Endocrinol. Metab.*, 83, 1935, 1998.

591. Saitoh, H., Kamoda, T., Nakahara, S., Hirano, T., and Nakamura, N., Serum concentrations of insulin, insulin-like growth factor (IGF-1), IGF binding protein (IGFBP)-1 and -3 and growth hormone binding protein in obese children: fasting IGFBP-1 is suppressed in normoinsulinemic obese children, *Clin. Endocrinol.*, 48, 487, 1998.

592. Attia, N., Tamborlane, W.V., Heptulla, R., Maggs, D., Grozman, A., Sherwin, R.S., and Caprio, S., The metabolic syndrome and insulin-like growth factor I regulation in adolescent obesity, *J. Clin. Endocrinol. Metab.*, 83, 1467, 1998.

593. Vanderschueren-Lodeweyck, M., The effect of simple obesity on growth and growth hormone, *Horm. Res.*, 40, 23, 1993.

594. Sartorio, A., Ferrero, S., Silvestri, G., Petri, A., Rapa, A., and Bona, G., Reference values for urinary growth hormone excretion in normally growing nonobese and obese children, *Int. J. Obes. Relat. Metab. Disord.*, 23 (Suppl. 5), S118, 1999.

595. Bona, G., Petri, A., Rapa, A., Conti, A., and Sartorio, A., The impact of gender, puberty and body mass on reference values for urinary growth hormone (GH) excretion in normal growing non-obese and obese children, *Clin. Endocrinol.*, 50, 775, 1999.

596. Argente, J., Caballo, N., Barrios, V., Pozo, J., Munoz, M.T., Chowen, J.A., and Hernandez, M., Multiple endocrine abnormalities of the growth hormone and insulin-like growth factor axis in prepubertal children with exogenous obesity: effect of short- and long-term weight reduction, *J. Clin. Endocrin. Metab.*, 82, 2076, 1997.

597. Kratzsch, J., Dehmel, B., Pulzer, F., Keller, E., Englaro, P., Blum, W.F., and Wabitsch, M., Increased serum GHBP levels in obese pubertal children and adolescents: relationship to body composition, leptin and indicators of metabolic disturbances, *Int. J. Obes. Relat. Metab.*, 21, 1130, 1997.

598. Volta, C., Bernasconi, S., Iughetti, L., Ghizzoni, L., Rossi, M., Costa, M., and Cozzini, A., Growth hormone response to growth hormone-releasing hormone (GHRH), insulin, clonidine and arginine after GHRH pretreatment in obese children: evidence of somatostatin increase, *Eur. J. Endocrinol.*, 132, 716, 1995.

599. Vedhuis, J.D. and Iranmanesh, A., Physiological regulation of the human growth hormone (GH), insulin-like-growth factor type I (IGF-I) axis: predominant impact of age, obesity, gonadal function and sleep, *Sleep*, 19 (Suppl. 10), S221, 1996.

600. Caprio, S., Bronson, M., Sherwin, R.S., Rife, F., and Tamborlane, W.V., Co-existence of severe insulin resistance and hyperinsulinaemia in preadolescent obese children, *Diabetologia*, 39, 1489, 1996.

601. Rocchini, A.P., Katch, V., Schork, A., and Kelch, R.P., Insulin and blood pressure during weight loss in obese adolescents, *Hypertension*, 10, 267, 1987.

602. Jiang, X., Srinivasan, S.R., and Berenson, G.S., Relation of obesity to insulin secretion and clearance in adolescents: the Bogalusa Heart Study, *Int. J. Obes. Relat. Metab. Disord.*, 20, 951, 1996.

603. Radetti, G., Bozzola, M., Pasquino, B., Paganini, C., Aglialoro, A., Livieri, C., and Barreca, A., Growth hormone bioactivity, insulin-like growth factors (IGFs) and IGF binding proteins in obese children, *Metab. Clin. Exper.*, 47, 1490, 1998.

604. Yasunaga, T., Furukawa, S., Katsumata, N., Horikawa, R., Tanaka, T., Tanae, A., and Hibi, I., Nutrition related hormonal changes in obese children, *Endocr. J.*, 45, 221, 1998.

605. Le Stunf, C. and Bougnères, P., Early changes in postprandial insulin secretion, not in insulin sensitivity, characterize juvenile obesity, *Diabetes*, 43, 696, 1994.

606. Hoffman, R.P. and Armstrong, P.T., Glucose effectiveness, peripheral and hepatic insulin sensitivity, in obese and lean prepubertal children, *Int. J. Obes. Relat. Metab. Disord.*, 20, 521, 1996.

607. Gonzales Moran, I., Sarria Chueca, A., Bueno Sanchez, M., and Abos Olivares, M.D., Circadian rhythms of cortisol and insulin in nutritional obesity in children, *An. Esp. Pediatr.*, 30, 79, 1989 (in Spanish).

608. Radetti, G., Ghizzoli, L., Paganini, C., Inghetti, L., Caselli, G., and Bernascoin, S., Insulin pulsatility in obese and normal prepubertal children, *Hormone Res.*, 50, 78, 1998.

609. Kamarýt, J., Stejskal, J., Mrskos, A., and Lavický, P., Insulin, glucose, proteins, and amylase in the saliva of obese children, *Česk. Pediatr.*, 44, 517, 1989.

610. Olefski, J., Kolterman, O.G., and Scarlett, J., Insulin action and resistance in obesity and non-insulin-dependent type II diabetes mellitus, *Am. J. Physiol. Endocrinol. Metab.*, 6, E15, 1982.

611. Juricskay, Z. and Molnár, D., Steroid metabolism in obese children. I. The relationship between body composition and adrenal function, *Acta Paediatr. Hung.*, 29, 383, 1988.

612. Juricskay, Z. and Molnár, D., Steroid metabolism in obese children. II. Steroid excretion of obese and normal weight children, *Acta Paediatr. Hung.*, 29, 395, 1988.

613. Chalew, S.A., Nagel, H., Burt, D., and Edwards, C.R.W., The integrated concentration of cortisol is reduced in obese children, *J. Pediat. Endocrinol. Metab.*, 10 (Suppl. 2), 287, 1997.

614. Kiess, W., Englaro, P., Hanitsch, S., Rascher, W., Attanasio, A., and Blum, W.F., High leptin concentrations in serum of very obese children are further stimulated by dexamethasone, *Horm. Metab. Res.*, 28, 708, 1996.

615. Klein, K.O., Larmore, K.A., de Lancey, E., Brown, J.M., Considine, R.V., and Hassink, S.G., Effect of obesity on estradiol level, and its relationship to leptin, bone maturation and bone mineral density in children, *J. Clin. Endocrinol. Metab.*, 83, 3469, 1998.

616. Bouvattier, C., Lahlou, N., Roger, M., and Bougnères, P., Hyperleptinaemia is associated with impaired gonadotrophin response to GnRH during late puberty in obese girls, not boys. *Eur. J. Endocrinol.*, 138, 653, 1998.

617. Jabbar, M., Pugliese, M., Fort, P., Recker, B., and Lifshitz, F., Excess weight and precocious pubarche in children: alteration of the adrenocortical hormones, *J. Am. Coll. Nutr.*, 10, 289, 1991.

618. Obuchowitz, A. and Obuchowitz, E., Plasma beta-endorphin and insulin concentrations in relation to body fat and nutritional parameters in overweight and obese prepubertal children, *Int. J. Obes. Relat. Metab. Disord.*, 21, 783, 1997.

619. Rosskamp, R., Becker, M., and Zallet, M., Circulating somatostatin concentrations in childhood. Studies in normal weight and obese children and patients with growth hormone deficiency, *Monatsschr. Kinderheilkd.*, 134, 849, 1986.

620. Apter, D., Leptin in puberty, *Clin. Endocrinol.*, 47, 175, 1997.

621. Frelut, M.L., Childhood obesity: from clinics to leptin, *Int. J. Obes. Relat. Metab. Disord.*, 21 (Suppl. 2), S137, 1997.

622. Zhang, Y.Y., Proenca, R., Maffei, M., Barone, M., Leopold, L., and Friedman, J.M., Positional cloning of the mouse obese gene and its human homolog, *Nature*, 372, 425, 1994.

623. Ma, Z., Gingerich, R.L., Santiago, J., V., Klein, S., Smith, C.H., and Landt, M., Radioimmunoassay of leptin in human plasma, *Clin. Chem.*, 42, 942, 1996.

624. Stehling, O., Doring, H., Ertl, J., Preibisch, G., and Schmidt, I., Leptin reduces juvenile fat stores by altering the circadian cycle of energy expenditure, *Am. J. Physiol.*, 271, R1170, 1997.

625. Van Gaal, L.F., Wauters, M.A., Mertens, H., Considine, R.V., and De Leuw, I.H., Clinical endocrinology of human leptin, *Int. J. Obes. Relat. Metab. Disord.*, 23 (Suppl. 1), 29, 1999.

626. Ambrosius, W.T., Compton, J.A., Bowsher, R.R., and Pratt, J., H., Relation of race, age, and sex hormone differences to serum leptin concentrations in children and adolescents, *Horm. Res.*, 49, 240, 1998.

627. Jacquet, D., Leger, J., Levy-Marchal, C., Oury, J.F., and Czernichow, P., Ontogeny of leptin in human fetuses and newborns: effects of intrauterine growth retardation on serum leptin concentrations, *J. Clin. Endocrinol. Metab.*, 83, 1243, 1998.

628. Hassink, S., G., de Lancey, E., Sheslow, D.V., Smith-Kirwin S., M., O'Connor, D.M., Considine, R., Opentanova, I., Dostal, K., Spear, M.L., Leef, K., Ash, M., Spoitzer, A.R., and Funanage, V.L., Placental leptin: an important new growth factor in intrauterine and neonatal development? *Pediatrics*, 100, E1, 1997.

629. Helland, I.B., Reseland, J.E., Saugstad, O.D., and Drevon, C.A., Leptin levels in pregnant women and newborn infants: gender differences and reduction during the neonatal period, *Pediatrics*, 101, E12, 1998.

630. Maffeis, C., Vettor, R., Moghetti, P., Matti, P., Vecchini, S., Zantedeschi, P., Zaffanello, M., and Tato, L., Leptin concentration in cord blood: relationship to gender and hormones, *Int. J. Obes. Relat. Metab. Disord.*, 22 (Suppl. 4), S28, 1998.

631. Shekhavat, P.S., Garland, J.S., Shivpuri, C., Mick, G.J., Sasidharan, P., Pelz, J.C., and McCormick, K.L., Neonatal cord blood leptin: its relationship to birth weight, body, mass index, maternal diabetes, and steroids, *Pediatr. Res.*, 43, 338, 1998.

632. Hakanen, M., Bergendahl, M., Tuominen, J., Koulu, M., Ronnemaa, T., and Simell, O., Serum leptin concentration and dietary aspects in lean, normal weight and obese children during the first five years of life, *Int. J. Obes. Relat. Metab. Disord.*, 22 (Suppl. 4), S27, 1998.

633. Lissner, I., Karlsson, C., Lindroos, A.K., Sjöstrom, L., Carlsson, B., Carlsson, L., and Begtsson, C., Relations between leptin and body weight history in Swedish female populations, using serum stored 29 years, *Int. J. Obes Relat. Metab. Disord.*, 22 (Suppl. 3), S37, 1998.

634. Steinbeck, K.S., Byrnes, S.E., Bermingham, M., Brock, K., and Baur, L.A., Leptin as a predictor of weight gain in prepubertal children, *Int. J. Obes. Relat. Metab. Disord.*, 22 (Suppl. 3), S200, 1998.

635. Salbe, A.D., Nicolson, M., and Ravussin, E., Total energy expenditure and the level of physical activity correlate with plasma leptin concentrations in five-year-old children, *J. Clin. Invest.*, 99, 592, 1997.

636. Considine, R.V., Weight regulation, leptin and growth hormone, *Horm. Res.*, 48 (Suppl. 5), 116, 1997.

637. Frelut, M.L., Bihain, B., Yen, F., Willig, T.N., and Navarro, J., Leptin plasma concentrations in morbidly obese children suggest heterogenous responsiveness. Impact of weight loss, *Int. J. Obes. Relat. Metab. Disord.*, 21 (Suppl. 2), S142, 1997.

638. Palmert, M.R., Radovick, S., and Beopple, P.A., The impact of reversible gonadal sex steroid suppression on serum leptin concentrations in children with central precocious puberty, *J. Clin. Endocrinol. Metab.*, 83, 1091, 1998.

639. Coutant, R., Lahlou, N., Bouvattier, C., Bougnères, P., and Title, P., Circulating leptin level and growth hormone response to stimulation tests in obese and normal children, *Eur. J. Endocrinol.*, 139, 591, 1998.

640. Matkovic, V., Ilich, J.Z., Badenhop, N.E., Skugor, M., Clairmont, A., Klisovic, D., and Landoll, J., Gain in body fat is inversely related to the nocturnal rise in serum leptin level in young females, *J. Clin. Endocrinol. Metab.*, 82, 1368, 1997.

641. Argente, J., Barrios, V., Chowen, J.A., Sinha, M.K., and Considine, R.V., Leptin plasma levels in healthy Spanish children and adolescents, children with obesity, and adolescents with anorexia nervosa and bulimia nervosa, *J. Pediatr.*, 131, 833, 1997.

642. Wabitsch, M., Blum, W.F., Muche, R., Braun, M., Hube, F., Rascher, W., Heinze, E., Teller, W., and Hauner, H., Contribution of androgens to the gender difference in leptin production in obese children and adolescents, *J. Clin.*, 100, 808, 1997.

643. Kopp, W., Blum, W.M., von Prittwitz, S., Ziegler, A., Lubbert, H., Emons, G., Herzog, W., Herpertz, S., Deter, H.C., Remschmidt, H., and Hebebrand, J., Low leptin levels predict amenorrhea in underweight and eating disordered females, *Mol. Psychiatry*, 2, 335, 1997.

644. Ellis, K.J. and Nicolson, M., Leptin levels and body fatness in children: effects of gender, ethnicity, and sexual development, *Pediatr. Res.*, 42, 484, 1997.

645. Verrotti, A., Basciani, F., Morgese, G., and Chiarelli, F., Leptin levels in nonobese and obese children and young adults with type I diabetes mellitus, *Eur. J. Endocrinol.*, 139, 49, 1998.

646. Caprio, S., Tamborlane, W.V., Silver, D., Robinson, C., Leibel, R., McCarthy, S., Grozman, A., Belous, A., Maggs, D., and Sherwin, R.S., Hyperleptinemia: an early sign of juvenile obesity. Relations to body fat depots and insulin concentrations, *Am. J. Physiol.*, 271, E626, 1996.

647. Montague, C.T., Farooqi, I.S., Whitehead, J.P., Soos, M.A., Rau, H., Wareham, N.J., Sewter, C.P., Digby, J.E., Mohammed, S.N., Hurst, J.A., Cheetham, C.H., Earley, A.R., Barnett, A.H., Prins, J.B., O'Rahilly, S., Congenital leptin deficiency is associated with severe early-onset obesity in humans, *Nature*, 387, 903, 1997.

648. Hinney, A., Bornscheuer, S., Depenbusch, M., Mierke, B., Tolle, A., Mayer, H., Siegfried, W., Remschmidt, H., and Hebebrand, J., Absence of leptin deficiency mutation in extremely obese German children and adolescents, *Int. J. Obes. Relat. Metab. Disord.*, 21, 1190, 1997.

649. Echwald, S.M., Sorensen, T.D., Sorensen, T.I., Tybjaerg-Hansen, A., Andersen, T., Chung, W.K., Leibel, R.L., and Pedersen, O., Amino acid variants in the human leptin receptor: lack of association to juvenile onset of obesity, *Biochem. Biophys. Res. Commun.*, 233, 248, 1997.

650. Garrow, J.S., Health risks of obesity, in *British Nutrition Foundation, Obesity*, Blackwell Sciences, Oxford, 1999.

651. Dietz, W.H., Childhood obesity, in *Obesity*, Björntorp, P. and Brodoff, B.M., Lippincott, Philadelphia, 1992, 606.

652. Hills, A.P. and Byrne, N.M., Body composition and body image: implications for weight-control practices in adolescents, *Int. J. Obes.*, 21 (Suppl. 2), S115, 1997.

653. Hills, A.P. and Byrne, N.M., Exercise prescription, body satisfaction and exercise motivation of girls and boys, *Med. Sci. Sports Exer.*, 30, S120, 1998.

654. Gortmaker, S.L., Must, A., Perrin, J.M., Sobol, A.M., and Dietz, W.H., Social and economic consequences of overweight in adolescence and young adulthood, *N. Engl. J. Med.*, 329, 1008, 1993.

655. Lissau, I. and Sorensen, T.I.A., Parental neglect during childhood and increased risk of obesity in young adulthood, *Lancet*, 343, 324, 1994.

656. Stunkard, A.J., Perspectives on human obesity, in *Perspectives in Behavioral Medicine: Eating, Sleeping and Sex*, Stunkard, A.J. and Baum, A., Eds., Hillsdale, NJ, 1989, 9.

657. Bruch, H., *Eating Disorders*, Basic Books, New York, 1973.

658. Wadden, T.A., Foster, G.D., Stunkard, A.J., and Linowitz, J.R., Dissatisfaction with weight and figure in obese girls; discontent but not depression, *Int. J. Obesity*, 13, 89, 1989.

659. Drummer, G., Rosen, L., Heusner, W., Roberts, P., and Counsilman, J., Pathogenic weight-control behaviours of young competitive swimmers, *Physician Sports Med.*, 15 (5), 75, 1987.

660. Smolak, L., Levine, M.P., and Gralen, S., The impact of puberty and dating on eating problems among middle school girls, *J. Youth Adolesc.*, 22 (4), 355, 1993.

661. Stein, D.M. and Riechert, P., Extreme dieting behaviors in early adolescence, *J. Early Adolesc.*, 10 (2), 108, 1990.

662. Wertheim, E.H., Paxton, S.J., Maude, D., Szmukler, G.I., Gibbons, K., and Hiller, L., Psychosocial predictors of weight loss behaviors and binge eating in adolescent girls and boys. *Int. J. Eating Disord.*, 12, 151, 1992.

663. Killen, J.D., Taylor, C.B., Hammer, L.D., Litt, I., Wilson, D.M., Rich, T., Haywood, C., Simmonds, B., Kraemer, H., and Varady, A., An attempt to modify unhealthful eating attitudes and weight regulation practices of young adolescent girls, *Int. J. Eating Disord.*, 13, 369, 1993.

664. Brodie, D.A. and Slade, P.D., The relationship between body image and body fat in adult women, *Psycholog. Med.*, 18, 623, 1988.

665. Bruce, B. and Agras, W.S., Binge eating in females: a population-based investigation, *Int. J. Eating Disord.*, 12, 365, 1992.

666. Cash, T.F. and Green, T.F., Body weight and body image among college women: perception, cognition, and affect, *J. Personal. Assess.*, 50, 290, 1986.

667. Litrell, M.A., Damhorst, M.L., and Littrell, J.M., Clothing interests, body satisfaction, and eating behavior of adolescent females: related or independent dimensions? *Adolescence*, 25 (97), 77, 1990.

668. Andersen, A.E. and DiDomenico, L., Diet vs. shape content of popular male and female magazines: a dose-response relationship to the incidence of eating disorders? *Int. J. Eating Disord.*, 11 (3), 283, 1992.

669. Schilder, P., *The Image and Appearance of the Human Body: Studies in the Constructive Energies of the Psyche*, International Universities Press, New York, 1950.

670. Kolb, L.C., Disturbances of the body-image, Reiser, M.F., Ed., *American Handbook of Psychiatry*, 2nd ed., Basic Books, New York, 1975, 810.

671. Schontz, F.C., *Perceptual and Cognitive Aspects of Body Experience*, Academic Press, New York, 1969.

672. Fisher, S. and Cleveland, S.E., *Body Image and Personality*, 2nd ed., Dover, New York, 1968.

673. Thompson, J.K., Penner, L.A., and Altabe, M., Procedures, problems, and progress in the assessment of body images, in *Body Images: Development, Deviance, and Changes*, Cash, T.F. and Pruzinsky, T., Eds., Gilford Press, New York, 1990, 21.

674. Koff, E., Rierdan, J., and Stubbs, M., Gender, body image, and self-concept in early adolescence, *J. Early Adolesc.*, 10 (1), 56, 1990.

675. Burns, R.B., *The Self Concept*, Longmans, London, 1979.

676. Altabe, M. and Thompson, J.K., Size estimations versus figural ratings of body image disturbance: relation to body dissatisfaction and eating dysfunction, *Int. J. Eating Disord.*, 11, 4, 397, 1992.

677. Altabe, M., and Thompson, J.K., Body image changes during early adulthood, *Int. J. Eating Disord.*, 13, 323, 1992.

678. Offman, H.J. and Bradley, S.J., Body image of children and adolescents and its measurement: an overview, *Canad. J. Psychiatry*, 37, 417, 1992.

679. Byrne, N.M. and Hills, A.P., Should body-image scales designed for adults be used with adolescents? *Percept. Motor Skills*, 82, 747, 1996.

680. Fisher, S., The evolution of psychological concepts about the body, in *Body Images: Development, Deviance, and Change*, Cash. T.F. and Pruzinsky, T., Eds., Gilford Press, New York, 1990, 3.

681. Garfinkel, P.E., Goldbloom, D., Davis, R., Olmsted, M.P., Garner, D.M., and Halmi, K.A., Body dissatisfaction in bulimia nervosa: relationship to weight and shape concerns and psychological functioning, *Int. J. Eating Disord.*, 11, 151, 1992.

682. Garner, D.M. and Garfinkel, P.E., Body image in anorexia nervosa: measurement, theory, and clinical implications, *Int. J. Psychiatry Med.*, 11, 263, 1981.

683. Brownell, K.D., Dieting and the search for the perfect body: where physiology and culture collide, *Behav. Ther.*, 22, 1, 1991.

684. Brownell, K.D., Rodin, J., and Wilmore, J.H., Eating, body weight, and performance in athletes: an introduction, in *Eating, Body Weight, and Performance in Athletes*, Brownell, K.D., Rodin, J., and Wilmore, J.H., Eds., Lea & Febiger, London, 1992, 7.

685. Danforth, E. and Sims, E.A.H., Obesity and efforts to lose weight, *N. Engl. J. Med.*, 327, 1497, 1992.

686. Williamson, D.A., *Assessment of Eating Disorders. Obesity, Anorexia, and Bulimia Nervosa*, Elmsford, Pergamon Press, New York, 1990.

687. Slade, P.D. and Russell, G.F.M., Awareness of body dimensions in anorexia nervosa: Cross-sectional and longitudinal studies, *Psycholog. Med.*, 3, 188, 1973.

688. Thompson, J.K., Larger than life, *Psychol. Today*, April 20 and 28, 1986.

689. Thompson, J.K. and Thompson, C.M., Body size distortion and self-esteem in asymptomatic, normal weight males and females, *Int. J. Eating Disord.*, 5, 1061, 1986.

690. Rosen, J.C., Body-image disturbance in eating disorders, in *Body Images: Development, Deviance, and Change*, Cash, T.F. and Pruzinsky, T., Eds., Guilford Press, New York, 1990, 190.

691. Gralen, S.J., Levine, M.P., Smolak, L., and Murnen, S.K., Dieting and disordered eating during early and middle adolescence: do the influences remain the same? *Int. J. Eating Disord.*, 9, 501, 1990.

692. Streigel-Moore, R.H., Silberstein, L.R., Frensch, P., and Rodin, J., A prospective study of disordered eating among college students, *Int. J. Eating Disord.*, 8, 499, 1989.

693. Byrne, N.M., and Hills, A.P., *An evaluation of body image assessment protocols with implications for age and gender differences*, Proc. Australasian Soc. Study Obesity, Melbourne, 1993.

694. McDonald, K. and Thompson, J.K., Eating disturbance, body image dissatisfaction, and reasons for exercising: gender differences and correlational findings, *Int. J. Eating Disord.*, 11, 289, 1992.

695. Williamson, D.A., Davis, C.J., Bennett, S.M., Goreczny, A.J., and Gleaves, D.H., Development of a simple procedure for assessing body image disturbances, *Behav. Assess.*, 11, 433, 1989.

696. Williamson, D.A., Kelley, M.L., Davis, C.J., Ruggiero, L., and Blouin, D.C., Psychopathology of eating disorders: a controlled comparison of bulimic, obese, and normal subjects, *J. Consult. Clin. Psychol.*, 53 (2), 161, 1985.

697. Attie, I. and Brooks-Gunn, J., The development of eating problems in adolescent girls: a longitudinal study, *Develop. Psychol.*, 25, 70, 1989.

698. Thornton, B. and Ryckman, R.M., Relationship between physical attractiveness, physical effectiveness, and self-esteem: a cross-sectional analysis among adolescents, *J. Adolesc.*, 14, 85, 1991.

699. Simmons, R.G., Blyth, D.A., and McKinney, K.L., The social and psychological effects of puberty on white females, in *Girls at Puberty: Biological and Psychosocial Perspectives*, Brooks-Gunn, J.and Petersen, A.C., Eds., Plenum, New York, 1983, 229.

700. Alsaker, F.D., Pubertal timing, overweight, and psychological adjustment, *J. Early Adolesc.*, 12, 396, 1992.

701. Richards, L.H., Regina, C.C., and Larson, R., Weight and eating concerns among pre- and young adolescent boys and girls, *J. Adolesc. Health Care*, 11, 203, 1990.

702. Schonfeld, W.A., Body image disturbance in adolescence, *Arch. Gen. Psychiatry*, 15, 6, 1966.

703. Bernstein, N.R., Objective bodily damage: disfigurement and dignity, in *Body Images: Development, Deviance, and Change*, Cash, T.F., and Pruzinsky, T., Gilford Press, New York, 1990, 131.

704. Zoppi, G., Luciano, A., Vinco, A., and Residori, P., Obesity in pediatrics: statistical analysis of school performance of obese children, *Pediatr. Med. Chir.*, 17, 559, 1995 (in Italian).

705. Tershakovec, A.M., Weller, S.C., and Gallagher, P.R., Obesity, school performance and behavior of black, urban elementary school children, *Int. J. Obes. Relat. Metab. Disord.*, 18, 323, 1994.

706. Kolody, B. and Sallis, J.F., A prospective study of ponderosity, body image, self-concept, and psychological variables in children, *J. Dev. Behav. Pediatr.*, 16, 1, 1995.

707. Li, X., A study of intelligence and personality in children with simple obesity, *Int. J. Obes. Relat. Metab. Disord.*, 19, 355, 1995.

708. Mills, J.K. and Adrianopoulos, G.D., The relationship between childhood onset obesity and psychopathology in adulthood, *J. Psychol.*, 127, 547, 1993.

709. Emmons, L., Dieting and purging behavior in black and white high school students, *J. A. Diet. Assoc.*, 92, 306, 1992.

710. Davies, E. and Furnham, A., The dieting and body shape concerns of adolescent females, *J. Child Psychol. Psychiatry*, 27, 417, 1986.

711. Fallon, A. and Rozin, P., Sex differences in perceptions of desirable body shape, *J. Abnorm. Psychol.*, 94, 102, 1985.

712. Cok, F., Body image satisfaction in Turkish adolescents, *Adolescence*, 25, 409, 1990.

713. Spring, B., Pingitore, R., Brucker, E., and Penava, S., Obesity: idealized or stigmatized? Sociocultural influences on the meaning and prevalence of obesity, Hills, A.P. and Wahlquist, M.L., Eds., *Exercise and Obesity*, Smith-Gordon/London, 1994, 49.

714. Pasquet, P., Brigant, L., Froment, A., Koppert, G.A., Bard, D., de Garine, I., and Apfelbaum, M., Massive overfeeding and energy balance in men: the Guru Walla model, *Am. J. Clin. Nutr.*, 56, 483, 1992.

715. Rodin, J. and Larson, L., Social factors and the ideal body shape, in *Eating, Body Weight, and Performance in Athletes*, Brownell, K.D., Rodin, J., and Wilmore, J.H., Eds., Lea & Febiger, London, 1992, 7.

716. Wiseman, C., Gray, J., Mosimann, J., and Ahrens, A., Cultural expectations of thinness in women: an update, *Int. J. Eating Disord.*, 11, 85, 1992.

717. Koff, E. and Rierdan, J., Perceptions of weight and attitudes toward eating in early adolescent girls, *J. Adolesc. Health*, 12, 307, 1991.

718. Rosen, J., Gross, J., and Vara, L., Psychological adjustment of adolescents attempting to lose or gain weight, *J. Consult. Clin. Psychol.*, 55, 742, 1987.

719. Butters, J.W. and Cash, T.F., Cognitive-behavioral treatment of women's body-image dissatisfaction, *J. Consult. Clin. Psychol*, 55, 889, 1987.

720. Olmstead, M.P., Cocina, D.V., Rockert, W., and Johnston, L., Psychoeducational principles in the treatment of bulimia and anorexia nervosa, Garner, D.M. and Garfinkel, P.E., Eds., *Handbook of Psychotherapy for Anorexia Nervosa and Bulimia*, Guilford Press, New York, 1985, 513.

721. Loosemore, D.J. and Moriarty, D., Body dissatisfaction and body image distortion in selected groups of males, *CACHPER J.*, Nov./Dec., 11, 1990.

722. Fisher, M., Schneider, M., Pegler, C., and Napolitano, B., Eating attitudes, health-risk behaviours, self-esteem, and anxiety among adolescent females in a suburban high school, *J. Adolesc. Health*, 12, 377, 1991.

723. Silberstein, L., Striegel-Moore, R., Timko, C., and Rodin, J., Behavioural and psychological implications of body dissatisfaction: Do men and women differ? *Sex Roles*, 19, 219, 1988.

724. Wilmore, J.H., Eating and weight disorders in the female athlete, *Int. J. Sport Nutr.*, 1, 104, 1991.

725. Sturney, P. and Slade, P.D., Body image and obesity, a critical psychological perspective, in *Handbook of Eating Disorders*, Part 2, Burrows, G.D., Beumont, P.J.V., Casper, R.C., Eds., Elsevier, Amsterdam, 1988.

726. Rössner, S., Childhood obesity and adulthood consequences, *Acta Pediatr.*, 87, 1, 1998.

727. Davis, K., Christoffel, K.K., Vespa, H., Pierleoni, M.P., and Papanastassiou, R., Early frequent treatment in prevention of childhood obesity. How we do it, *Ann. N.Y. Acad. Sci.*, 699, 260, 1993.

728. Davis, K., Christoffel, K.K., Vespa, H., Pierleoni, M.P., and Papanastassiou, R., Obesity in preschool and school-age children. Early frequent treatment is best, *Ann. N.Y. Acad. Sci.*, 699, 262, 1993.

729. Becque, M.D., Katch, V.L., Rocchini, A.P., Marks, C.R., and Moorehead, C., Coronary risk incidence of obese adolescents: reduction by exercise plus diet intervention, *Pediatrics*, 81, 605, 1988.

730. DiPietro, L., Mossberg, H.O., and Stunkard, A.J., A 40-year history of overweight children in Stockholm: life-time overweight, morbidity and mortality, *Int. J. Obes. Relat. Metab. Disord.*, 18, 585, 1994.

731. Unger, R., Kreeger, L., and Christoffel, K.K., Childhood obesity. Medical and familial correlates and age of onset, *Clin. Pediatr.*, 29, 368, 1990.

732. Must, A., Jacques, P.F., Dallal, G.E., Bajema, C.J., and Dietz, W.H., Long-term morbidity and mortality of overweight adolescents. A follow-up of the Harvard Growth Study of 1922 to 1935, *N. Engl. J. Med.*, 327, 1350, 1992.

733. Freeman, W., Weir, D.C., Whitehead, J.E., Rogers, D.I., Sapiano, S.B., Floyd, C.A., Kirk, P.M., Stalker, C.R., Field, N.J., Cayton, R.M. et al., Association between risk factors for coronary heart disease in schoolboys and adult mortality rates in the same localities, *Arch. Dis. Child.*, 65, 78, 1990.

734. Stewart, K.J., Brown, C.S., Hickey, C.M., McFarland, L.D., Weinhofer, J.J., and Gottlieb, S.H., Physical fitness, physical activity, and fatness in relation to blood pressure and lipids in preadolescent children. Results from the FRESH Study, *J. Cardiopulm. Rehabil.*, 15, 122, 1995.

735. Perrone, L., Marotta, A., Ponticiello, E., Palombo, G., Boccia, E., Calabro, C., Di Lascio, R., and Di Toro, R., Anthropometric indexes and risk factors for atherosclerosis in obesity, *Int. J. Obes. Relat. Metab. Disord.*, 22 (Suppl. 4), S25, 1998.

736. Guo, S.S., Huang, C., Chumlea, W.C., Roche, A.F., Wisemandle, W., and Siervogel, R.M., Long-term changes in BMI during growth in relation to adulthood obesity and cardiovascular risk factors, *Int. J. Obes. Relat. Metab. Disord.*, 22 (Suppl. 4), S25, 1998.

737. Ernst, N.D. and Obarzanek, E., Child health and nutrition: obesity and high blood cholesterol, *Prev. Med.*, 23, 427, 1994.

738. Tulio, S., Egle, S., and Greilly, B., Blood pressure response to exercise of obese and lean hypertensive and normotensive male adolescents, *J. Hum. Hypertens.*, 9, 953, 1995.

739. Anding, J.D., Kubena, K.S., McIntosh, W.A., and Brien, B., Blood lipids, cardiovascular fitness, obesity, and blood pressure: the presence of potential coronary heart disease risk factors in adolescents, *J. Am. Diet. Assoc.*, 96, 238, 1996.

740. Hypponen, E., Virtanen, S.M., Knip, M., and Akerblom, H.K., Obesity is associated with an increased risk of insulin-dependent diabetes mellitus in children, *Int. J. Obes. Relat. Metab. Disord.*, 22 (Suppl. 4), S22, 1998.

741. Whitaker, R.C., Pepe, M.S., Seidel, K.D., Wright, J.A., and Knopp, R.H., Gestational diabetes and the risk of offspring obesity. *Pediatrics*, 101, E9, 1998.

742. McCance, D.R., Pettitt, D.J., Hanson, R.L., Jacobsson, L.T., Bennett, P.H., and Knowler, W.C., Glucose, insulin concentrations and obesity in childhood and adolescence as predictors of NIDDM, *Diabetologie*, 37, 617, 1994.

743. Miyzaki, Y., Shimamoto, K., Ise, T., Shiiki, M., Higashiura, K., Hirata, A., Masuda, A., Nakagawa, M., and Iimura, O., Effects of hyperinsulinaemia on renal function and the pressor system in insulin-resistant obese adolescents, *Clin. Exp. Pharmacol. Physiol.*, 23, 287, 1996.

744. Molnár, D., Decsi, T., and Csábi, G., Multimetabolic syndrome in childhood obesity, *Int. J. Obes. Relat. Metab. Disord.*, 21 (Suppl. 2), S141, 1997.

745. Lusky, A., Barell, V., Lubin, F., Kaplan, G., Layani, V., Shohat, Z., Lev, B., and Wiener, M., Relationship between morbidity and extreme values of body mass index in adolescents, *Int. J. Epidemiol.*, 25, 829, 1996.

746. Kawasaki, T., Hashimoto, N., Kikuchi, T., Takahashi, H., and Uchiyama, M., The relationship between fatty liver and hyperinsulinaemia in obese Japanese children, *J. Pediatr. Gastroenterol. Nutr.*, 24, 317, 1997.

747. Bergoni, A., Lughetti, L., Corciulo, N., Peverelli, P., Cammareri, V., Grifi, G., Celi, F., Morino, G., Agnello, D., and DeLuca, F., Italian multicenter study of liver damage in pediatric obesity, *Int. J. Obes. Relat. Metab. Disord.*, 22 (Suppl. 4), S22, 1998.

748. Somerville, S.M., Rona, R.J., and Chinn, S., Obesity and respiratory symptoms in primary school, *Arch. Dis. Child.*, 59, 940, 1984.

749. Dietz, W.H., Gross, W.L., and Kirkpatrick, J., Blount's disease (tibia vara): Another skeletal disorder associated with childhood obesity, *J. Ped.*, 101, 735, 1982.

750. Le Veau, B.F. and Bernhardt, D.B., Developmental Biomechanics, *Phys. Ther.*, 63, 2, 1984.

751. Frost, H.M., *The Physiology of Cartilaginous, Fibrous and Body Tissue: Orthopedic Lectures*, Vol. 2, Charles C Thomas, Springfield, IL, 1972.

752. Frost, H.M., A chondral modeling theory, *Calcified Tissue Int.*, 28, 181, 1979.

753. Felson, D.T., Anderson, J.J., Naimark, A., Walker, A.M., and Meenan, R.F., Obesity and knee osteoarthritis, *Ann. Intern. Med.*, 109, 18, 1988.

754. Engel, G.M. and Staheli, L.T., The natural history of torsion and other factors influencing gait in childhood, *Clin. Orthop. Rel. Res.*, 99, 12, 1974.

755. Inman, V.T., Human Locomotion, *Can. Med. Assoc. J.*, 94, 1047, 1966.

756. Jahss, M., *Disorders of the Foot*, W. B. Saunders, Philadelphia, 1982.

757. Bar-Or, O., Obesity, in *Sports and Exercise for Children with Chronic Health Conditions*, Goldberg, B., Ed., Human Kinetics, Champaign, IL, 1995, Chap. 23.

758. Hills, A.P. and Parker, A.W., Gait characteristics of obese pre-pubertal children: effects of diet and exercise on parameters, *Int. J. Rehabil. Res.* 14 (4), 348, 1991.

759. Hills, A.P. and Parker, A.W., Locomotor characteristics of obese children, *Child: Care, Health Develop.*, 18, 29, 1992.

760. Hills, A.P., Locomotor characteristics of obese children, in *Exercise and Obesity*, Hills, A.P. and Wahlqvist, M.L., Smith-Gordon/London, 1994.

761. Boeck, M.A., Chen, C., and Cunningham-Rundles, S., Altered immune function in a morbidly obese pediatric population, *Ann. N.Y. Acad. Sci.*, 699, 253, 1993.

762. Pallaro, A., Barbeito, S., Taberner, P., Marino, P., Franchello, A., Strasnoy, I., Ramos, O., and Slobodianik, N., Total salivary IgA, serum C3c and IgA in obese children, *Int. J. Obes. Relat. Metab. Disord.*, 22 (Suppl. 3), S208, 1998.

763. Plagemann, A., Heindrich, I., Gotz, F., Rohde, W., and Dorner, G., Obesity and enhanced diabetes and cardiovascular risk in adult rats due to early postnatal overfeeding, *Exp. Clin. Endocrinol.*, 99, 154, 1992.

764. Pařízková, J., Effect of the interrelationships between diet and physical activity on aging, in *Ecology of Aging, J. Human. Ecol. Special Issue*, Siniarska, A. and Wolanski, N., Guest Eds., J., Kamla-Raj, New Delhi, 2000, Chap. 3.

765. Kozlov, V.I., *Long Living in Abkhasia*, Nauka, Moscow, 1987 (in Russian).

766. Ballor, D.L., Katch, V.L., Becque, M.D., and Marks, C.R., Resistance weight training during caloric restriction enhances lean body weight maintenance, *Am. J. Clin. Nutr.*, 47, 19, 1988.

767. Dietz, W.H. and Hartung, R., Changes in height velocity of obese preadolescents during weight reduction, *Am. J. Dis. Ch.*, 139, 705, 1985.

768. Nuutinen, O. and Knip, M., Long-term weight control in obese children: persistence of treatment outcome and metabolic changes, *Int. J, Obes. Relat. Metab. Disord.*, 16, 279, 1992.

769. Nuutinen, O. and Knip. M., Predictors of weight reduction in obese children, *Eur. J. Clin. Nutr.*, 16, 785, 1992.

770. Golan, M., Weizman, A., Apter, A., and Fainaru, M., Parents as exclusive agents of change in the treatment of childhood obesity, *Am. J. Clin. Nutr.*, 67, 1130, 1998.

771. Epstein, L.H., Valoski, A., Wing, R.R., and McCurley, J., Ten-year outcome of behavioral family-based treatment for childhood obesity, *Health Psychol.*, 13, 373, 1994.

772. Wabitsch, M., The obese child: the need for a specific approach; treatment compounds: an update, *Int. J. Obes. Relat. Metab. Disord.*, 21 (Suppl. 2), S139, 1997.

773. Rollnick, S., Behaviour change in practice: targeting individuals, *Int. J. Obes. Relat. Metab. Disord.*, 20 (Suppl. 2), S22, 1996.

774. Epstein, L.H., Exercise in the treatment of childhood obesity, *Int. J. Obes. Relat. Metab. Disord.*, 19 (Suppl. 4), S117, 1995.

775. Epstein, L.H., Valoski, A.M., Kalarchian, M.A., and McCurley, J., Do children lose and maintain weight easier than adults: a comparison of child and parent weight changes from six months to ten years, *Obes. Res.*, 3, 411, 1995.

776. Epstein, L.H., Wing, R.P., Penner, B.C., and Kress, M.J., Effect of diet and controlled exercise on weight loss in obese children, *J. Pediatr.*, 107, 358, 1985.

777. Bandini, L.G. and Dietz, W.H., Myths about childhood obesity, *Pediatr. Ann.*, 21, 647, 1992.

778. Zwiauer, K.F.M., Treatment of childhood obesity: which approach? *Int. J. Obes. Relat. Metab. Disord.*, 22 (Suppl. 4), S2, 1998.

779. Dietz, W.H. and Robinson, T.N., Assessment and treatment of childhood obesity, *Pediatr. Rev.*, 14, 337, 1993.

780. Davis, K. and Christoffel, K.K., Obesity in preschool and school-age children. Treatment early and often may be best, *Arch. Pediatr. Adolesc. Med.*, 148, 125, 1994.

781. Blecker, U., Sothern, M., Udall, J., von Almen, K., Schumacher, H., Hargis, J., and Suskind, R., Initial obesity level impacts long term weight maintenance in obese youth, *Int. J. Obes. Relat. Metab. Disord.*, 22 (Suppl. 3), S63, 1998.

782. Asayama, K., Uchida, N., Hayashibe, H., Dobashi, K., Nakane, T., Kodera, K., and Nakazawa, S., A new mode of therapy for obese children in Japan, *Int. J. Obes. Relat. Metab. Disord.*, 22 (Suppl. 3), S62, 1998.

783. Flanery, R.C. and Kirschenbaum, D.S., Dispositional and situational correlates of long-term weight reduction in obese children, *Addict. Behav.*, 11, 249, 1986.

784. Zanelli, R., Rebeggiani, A., Chiarelli, F., and Morgese, G., Hyperinsulinism as a marker in obese children, *Am. J. Dis. Child.*, 147, 837, 1993.

785. Pařízková, J., Food choices in Czechoslovakia, *Appetite*, 21, 299, 1993.

786. Epstein, L.H., Koeske, R., Wing, R.R., and Valoski, A., The effect of family variables on child weight change, *Health Psychol.*, 5, 1, 1986.

787. Epstein, L.H., Kuller, L.H., Wing, R.R., Valoski, A., and McCurley, J., The effect of weight control on lipid changes in obese children, *Am. J. Dis. Child.*, 143, 454, 1989.

788. Epstein, L.H., McCurley, J., Wing, R.R., and Valoski, A., Five-year follow-up study of family based behavioral treatments for childhood obesity, *J. Consult. Clin. Psychol.*, 58, 661, 1990.

789. Foreyt, J.P., Ramirez, A.G., Cousins, J.H., and Cuidando, E.C., A weight reduction intervention for Mexican Americans, *Am. J. Clin. Nutr.*, 53 (Suppl. 6), S1639, 1991.

790. Tsukuda, T. and Shiraki, K., Excessive food aversion, compulsive exercise and decreased height gain due to fear of obesity in a prepubertal girl, *Psychother. Psychosom.*, 62, 203, 1994.

791. Woolley, S.C. and Woolley, O.W., Should obesity be treated at all? In Conn, H.L., Jr., De Felice, E.A., and Kuo, P., Eds., *Health & Obesity*, Raven Press, New York, 1983, 185.

792. Kalker, U., Hovels, O., and Kolbe-Saborowski, H., Significance of gender of obese children and body weight of parents and siblings for the results of the treatment of obesity in childhood, *Monatschr. Kinderheilkd*, 139, 24, 1991 (in German).

793. Epstein, L.H., Wing, R.R., Koeske, R., and Valoski, A., Effect of parent weight on weight loss in obese children, *J. Consult. Clin. Psychol.*, 54, 400, 1986.

794. Epstein, L.H., Family-based behavioral intervention for obese children, *Int. J. Obes. Relat. Metab. Disord.*, 20 (Suppl. 1), S14, 1996.

795. Chen, W., Ku, F.D., and Wu, K.W., Parent-directed weight reduction program for obese children: model formulation and follow-up, *J. Formos. Med. Assoc.*, 92, 237, 1993 (in Chinese).

796. Epstein, L.H., Wing, R.R., Valoski, A., and DeVos, D., Long-term relationship between weight and aerobic-fitness change in children, *Health Psychol.*, 7, 47, 1988.

797. Wadden, T.A., Stunkard, A.J., Rich, L., Rubin, C.J., Sweidel, G., and McKinney, S., Obesity in black adolescent girls: a controlled clinical trial of treatment by diet, behavior modification, and parental support, *Pediatrics*, 85, 345, 1990.

798. Epstein, L.H., Valoski, A., and McCurley, J., Effect of weight loss by obese children on long-term growth, *Am. J. Dis. Child*, 147, 1076, 1993.

799. Flodmark, C.E., Ohlsson, T., Ryden, O., and Sveger, T., Prevention of progression to severe obesity in a group of obese schoolchildren treated with family therapy, *Pediatrics*, 91, 880, 1993.

800. Suttapreyasri, D., Suyhonta, N., Kanpoem, J., Krainam, J., and Boonsuya, C., Weight-control training models for obese pupils in Bangkok, *J. Med. Assoc. Thai.*, 73, 394, 1990.

801. Siegfried, W., Siegfried, A., Ziegler, A.and Hebebrand, J., Follow-up of severely obese adolescents after long-term inpatient treatment, *Int. J. Obes. Relat. Metab. Disord.*, 22 (Suppl. 3), S63, 1998.

802. Kemm, J.R., Eating patterns in childhood and adult health, *Nutr. Health*, 4, 205, 1987.

803. Pařízková, J., Early prevention and treatment of children's obesity, *Int. J. Obes. Relat. Metab. Disord.*, 22 (Suppl. 4), S30, 1998.

804. Schoeller, D.A., Bandini, l. G., Levitsky, L.L., and Dietz, W.H., Energy requirements of obese children and young adults, *Proc. Nutr. Soc.*, 47, 241, 1988.

805. Dietz, W.H., Childhood obesity: susceptibility, cause, and management, *J. Ped.*, 103, 676, 1983.

806. Saito, K. and Tatsumi, M., Effect of dietary therapy in a school health program for obese children, *Nippon Koshu Eisei Zasshi*, 41, 693, 1994 (in Japanese).

807. Satter, E.M., Internal regulation and the evolution of normal growth as the basis for prevention of obesity in children, *J. Am. Diet Assoc.*, 96, 860, 1996.

808. Bell, L., Chan, L., and Pencharz, P.B., Protein sparing diet for severely obese adolescents: design and use of an equivalency system for menu planning, *J. Am. Diet. Assoc.*, 85, 459, 1985.

809. Figueroa-Colon, R., von Almen, T.K., Franklin, F.A., Schuftan, C., and Suskind, R., M., Comparison of two hypocaloric diets in obese children, *Am. J. Dis. Child.*, 147, 160, 1993.

810. Stallings, V.A., Archibald, E.H., Pencharz, P.B., Harrison, J.E., and Bell, L.E., One-year follow-up of weight, total body potassium, and total nitrogen in obese adolescents treated with the protein sparing modified fast, *Am. J. Clin. Nutr.*, 48, 91, 1988.

811. Figueroa-Colon, Franklin, F.A., Lee, J.Y., von Almen, T.K., and Suskind, R.M., Possibility of a clinic-based hypocaloric dietary intervention implemented in a school setting for obese children, *Obes. Res.*, 4, 419, 1996.

812. Burniat, W. and Van Aelst, C., Evaluation of the food intake in 75 obese children successfully treated at least during 6 months, *Int. J. Obes. Relat. Metab. Disord.*, 17 (Suppl. 2), 34, 1993.

813. Schmidinger, H., Weber, H., Zwiauer, K., Weidinger, F., and Widhalm, K., Potential life-threatening cardiac arrythmias associated with conventional hypocaloric diet, *Int. J. Cardiol.*, 14, 55, 1987.

814. Zwiauer, K., Schmidinger, H., Klicpera, M., Mayr, H., and Widhalm, K., 24 hours electrocardiographic monitoring in obese children and adolescents during 3 weeks of low calorie diet (500 kcal), *Int. J. Obes.*, 13 (Suppl. 2), 101, 1989.

815. Peterson, S. and Sigman-Grant, M., Impact of adopting lower-fat food choices on nutrient intake of American children, *Pediatrics*, 100, E4, 1997.

816. Sigman-Grant, M., Zimmerman, S., and Kris-Etherton, P.M., Dietary approaches for reducing fat intake of preschool-age children, *Pediatrics*, 91, 955, 1993.

817. Kniazev, Iu. A., Turkina, T.I., Tsyvilskaia, L.A., and Pakhomova, V.M., Effect of diet therapy on indicators of lipid metabolism in obese children, *Voprosy pitan.*, Mar.-Apr., 1985 (in Russian).

818. Nuutinen, O., Long-term effects of dietary counselling on nutrient intake and weight loss in obese children, *Eur. J. Clin. Nutr.*, 45, 287, 1991.

819. Chang, F.T., Hu, S.H., and Wang, R.S., The effectiveness of dietary instruction in obese children in southern Taiwan, *Kao Hsiung I Hsueh Tsa Chin*, 14, 528, 1998 (in Chinese).

820. Stallings, V.A. and Pencharz, P.B., The effect of high protein low-calorie diet on the energy expenditure of obese adolescents, *Eur. J. Clin. Nutr.*, 46, 897, 1992.

821. Widhalm, K.M. and Zwiauer, K.F., Metabolic effects of a very low calorie diet in obese children and adolescents with special reference to nitrogen balance, *J. Am. Coll. Nutr.*, 6, 467, 1987.

822. Kimm, S.Y., The role of dietary fiber in the development and treatment of childhood obesity, *Pediatrics*, 96, 1010, 1995.

823. Williams, C.L., Importance of dietary fiber in childhood, *J. Am. Diet. Assoc.*, 95, 1140, 1995.

824. Molnár, D., Dober, I., and Soltesz, G., The effect of unprocessed wheat bran on blood glucose and plasma immunoreactive insulin levels during oral glucose tolerance test in obese children, *Acta Paediatr. Hung.*, 26, 75, 1985.

825. Vido, L., Faccchin, P., Antonello, I., Gobber, D., and Rigon, F., Childhood obesity treatment: double blind trial on dietary fibres (gluconnan) versus placebo, *Pediatr. Padol.*, 28, 133, 1993.

826. Di Toro, A., Marotta, A., Todisco, N., Ponticiello, E., Collini, R., Di Lascio, R., Perrone, C., Unchanged iron and copper and increased zinc in the blood of obese children after two hypocaloric diets, *Biol. Trace Elem. Res.*, 57, 97, 1997.

827. Archibald, E.H., Stallings, V.A., Pencharz, P.B., Duncan, W.J., and Williams, C., Changes in intraventricular septal thickness, left ventricular wall thickness and left ventricular volume in obese adolescents on a high protein weight reducing diet, *Int. J. Obes.*, 13, 265, 1989.

828. Pidlich, J., Pfeffel, F., Zwiauer, K., Schneider, B., and Schmidinger, H., The effect of weight reduction on the surface electrocardiogram: a prospective trial in obese children and adolescents, *Int. J. Obes. Relat. Metab. Disord.*, 21, 1018, 1997.

829. Weder, A.B., Torretti, B.A., Katch, V.L., and Rocchini, A.P., The antihypertensive effects of calorie restriction in obese adolescents: dissociation of effects on erythrocyte countertransport and cotransport, *J. Hypertens.*, 2, 507, 1984.

830. Rocchini, A.P., Key, J., Bondie, D., Chico, R., Moorehead, C., Katch, V., and Martin, M., The effect of weight loss on the sensitivity of blood pressure to sodium in obese adolescents, *N. Engl. J. Med.*, 31, 321, 1989.

831. Brambilla, P.D., Arcais, A.F., Guarneri, M.P., Rondanini, G., Righetti, F., Bosio, L., Cella, D., and Chiumello, G., Changes in dynamic respiratory volumes in obese children and adolescents related to weight loss and sex, *Minerva Pediatr.*, 44, 159, 1992 (in Italian).

832. Lecendreux, M., Frelut, M.L., Quera-Salva, M.A., Fromageot, C., Elbaz, M., De Lattre, J., Willig, T.N., Navarro, J., Gadjos, P., and Guilleminault, C., Weight loss reduces sleep associated breathing disorders in morbidly obese children, *Int. J. Obes. Relat. Metab. Disord.*, 21 (Suppl. 2), S141, 1997.

833. Knip, M. and Nuutinen, O., Long-term effects of weight reduction on serum lipids and plasma insulin in obese children, *Am. J. Clin. Nutr.*, 57, 490, 1993.

834. Zwiauer, K., Kerbl, B., and Widhalm, K., No reduction of high density lipoprotein 2 during weight reduction in obese children and adolescents, *Eur. J. Pediatr.*, 149, 192, 1989.

835. Zwiauer, K. and Widhalm, K., Effect of 2 different reducing diets on the concentration of HDL cholesterol in obese adolescents, *Klin. Pediatr.*, 199, 392, 1987 (in German).

836. Wabitsch, M., Blum, W.F., Muche, R., Heinze, E., Haug, C., Mayer, H., and Teller, W., Insulin-like growth factors and their binding proteins before and after weight loss and their associations with hormonal and metabolic parameters in obese adolescent girls, *Int. J. Obes. Relat. Metab. Disord.*, 20, 1073, 1996.

837. Holub, M., Zwiauer, K., Winkler, C., Dillinger-Paller, B., Schuller, E., Schober, E., Stockler-Ipsiroglou, S., Patsch, W., and Strobl, W., Relation of plasma leptin to lipoproteins in overweight children undergoing weight reduction, *Int. J. Obes. Relat. Metab. Disord.*, 23, 60, 1999.

838. Bueno-Lozano, M., Balsamo, A., and Cacciari, E., Diet-induced changes as risk factors in obese children: arterial pressure, glycoregulation and lipid profile, *An. Esp. Pediatr.*, 35, 335, 1991 (in Spanish).

839. Hoffman, R.P., Stumbo, P.J., Janz, K.F., and Nielsen, D.H., Altered insulin resistance is associated with increased dietary weight loss in obese children, *Hormon. Res.*, 44, 17, 1995.

840. Thomas-Dobersen, D.A., Butler-Simon, N., and Fleshner, M., Evaluation of a weight management intervention program in adolescents with insulin-dependent diabetes mellitus, *J. Am. Diet. Assoc.*, 93, 535, 1993.

841. Kravets, E.B. and Kniazev, Iu. A., The effect of a hypocaloric diet enriched with polyunsaturated fatty acids on various indicators of cellular immunity in obese children, *Vopr. Pitan.*, Nov.-Dec., 6, 13, 1989.

842. Garrow, J.S., Effect of exercise on obesity, *Acta. Med. Scand.*, Suppl 711, 67, 1986.

843. Walberg, J. and Ward, D., Physical activity and childhood obesity, *J. Phys. Educ., Recr., Dance*, 12, 82, 1985.

844. Bar-Or, O. and Baranowski, T., Physical activity, adiposity, and obesity among adolescents, *Pediatr. Exer. Sci.*, 6, 348, 1994.

845. Sallis, J.F., A commentary on children and fitness: A public health perspective, *Res. Q. Exer. Sp.*, 58, 326, 1987.

846. Stunkard, A.J., Obesity: risk factors, consequences and control, *Med. J. Aust.*, 148, S21, 1988.

847. Grant, A.M., Edwards, O.M., Howard, A.N., Challard, G.S., Wraight, E.P., and Mills, I.H., Thyroidal hormone metabolism in obesity during semi-starvation, *Clin. Endocrinol.*, 9, 227, 1978.

848. Blanchard, M.S., Thermogenesis and its relationship to obesity and exercise, *Quest*, 34, 2, 143, 1982.

849. Skinner, J.S., Exercise Testing and Exercise Prescription for Special Cases, Lea & Febiger, Philadelphia, 1987.

850. Davie, M.W.J., Abraham, R.R., Godsland, I., Moore, P., and Wynn, V., Effect of high and low carbohydrate diets on nitrogen balance during calorie restriction in obese patients, *Int. J. Obes.* 6, 457, 1982.

851. Howard, A.N., The historical development, efficiency and safety of very low calorie diets, *Int. J. Obes.*, 5, 195, 1981.

852. Stern, J.S., Is obesity a disease of inactivity?, in *Eating & Its Disorders*, Stunkard, A.J. and Stellar, E., Eds, Raven Press, New York, 1983.

853. Brownell, K.D. and Stunkard, A.J., Behavioral treatment of overweight children and adolescents, in *Obesity*, Stunkard, A.J., Ed., W.B. Saunders, Philadelphia, 1980.

854. Oscai, L.B., The role of exercise in weight control, in *Exercise and Sports Sciences Reviews*, Wilmore, J.H., Ed., Academic Press, New York, 1973, 103.

855. Wilmore, J.H., Body composition in sport and exercise. Directions for future research, *Med. Sci. Sports Exerc.*, 1521, 1983.

856. Gwinup, G., Effect of exercise alone on weight of obese women, *Arch. Int. Med.*, 135, 676, 1975.

857. Sothern, M.S., Hunter, S., Suskind, R.M., Brown, R., Udall, J.N., and Blecker, V., Motivating the obese child to move: the role of structured exercise in pediatric weight management, *South. Med. J.*, 92, 577, 1999.

858. Sothern, M.S., Loftin, J.M., Udall, J.N., Suskind, R.M., Ewing, T.L., Tang, S.C., and Blecker, U., Inclusion of resistance exercise in a multidisciplinary outpatient treatment program for preadolescent obese children, *South. Med. J.*, 92, 585, 1999.

859. Stock, M. and Rothwell, N., *Obesity and Leanness. Basic Aspects*, John Wiley, London, 1982.

860. Bray, G.A., Nutrient balance: new insights into obesity, *Int. J. Obes.*, 11 (Suppl. 3), 83, 1987.

861. Barbeau, P., Gutin, B., Litaker, M., Owens, S., Riggs, S., and Okuyama, T., Correlates of individual differences in body composition changes resulting from physical training in obese children, *Am. J. Clin. Nutr.*, 69, 705, 1999.

862. Blair, S.N., Kohl, H.W., Gordon, N.F., and Paffenberger, R.S., How much physical activity is good for health? *Ann. Rev. Publ. Health*, 13, 9, 1992.

863. Brownell, K.D., The psychology and physiology of obesity: Implications for screening and treatment, *J. Am. Diet. Assoc.*, 84, 4, 406, 1984.

864. Bar-Or, O., A commentary on children and fitness: a public health perspective, *Res. Q. Exer. Sp.*, 58, 304, 1987.

865. Hills, A.P. and Byrne, N.M., The promotion of physical activity and the prescription of exercise in the obese, *J. Physiol. Biochem.*, 55 (2), 107, 1999.

866. Tremblay, A., Doucet, E., and Imbeault, P., Physical activity and weight maintenance, *Int. J. Obes. Relat. Metab. Disord.*, 23 (Suppl. 3), S50, 1999.

867. Saris, W.H., Habitual physical activity in children: methodology and findings in health and disease, *Med. Sci. Sports. Exerc.*, 18, 253, 1986.

868. Pellegrini, A.D. and Smith, P.K., Physical activity play: the nature and function of a neglected aspect of playing, *Child Dev.*, 69, 607, 1998.

869. Shea, S., Basch, C.E., Gutin, B., Stein, A.D., Contento, I.R., Irigoyen, M., and Zybert, P., The rate of increase in blood pressure in children 5 years of age is related to changes in aerobic fitness and body mass index, *Pediatrics*, 94, 465, 1994.

870. Moore, L.L., Nguyen, U.S., Rothman, K.J., Cupples, L.A., Ellison., R.C., Pre-school physical activity level and change in body fatness in young children: The Framingham Children's Study, *Am. J. Epidemiol.*, 142, 982, 1995.

871. Deheeger, M., Rolland-Cachera, M.F., and Fontvieille, A.M., Physical activity and body composition in 10 year old French children: linkages with nutritional intake? *Int. J. Obes. Relat. Metab. Disord.*, 21, 372, 1997.

872. Pařízková, J., Longitudinal study of body composition and build development in boys with various physical activity from 11 to 15 years, *Human Biol.*, 40, 212, 1968.

873. Pařízková, J., Nutrition and work performance, in *Critical Reviews in Tropical Medicine*, Vol. 1., Chandra, R.K., Ed., Plenum Press, New York, 1982, 307.

874. Pařízková, J., Physical training and weight reduction in obese adolescents, *Ann. Clin. Res.*, 14 (Suppl. 34), 63, 1982.

875. Šprynarová, S., *Biological Basis of Physical Fitness*, Universita Karlova, Prague, 1984 (in Czech).

876. Owens, S., Gutin, B., Ferguson, M., Allison, J., Karp, W., and Le, N.A., Visceral adipose tissue and cardiovascular risk factors in obese children, *J. Pediat.*, 133, 41, 1998.

877. Pařízková, J. and Heller, J., Relationship of dietary intake to work output and physical performance in Czechoslovak adolescents adapted to various work loads, in Human Growth, Physical Fitness and Nutrition, Shephard, R.J. and Pařízková, J., Eds., *Med. Sport Sci.*, Vol. 31, Rager, Basel, 1991, 156.

878. Thompson, J.L., Energy balance in young athletes, *Int. J. Sport. Nutr.*, 8, 160, 1998.

879. Lopez-Benedicto, M.A., Nuviala-Mateo, K.J., Gomez-Diaz-Bravo, E., Sarria-Chueca, A., and Giner-Soria, A., Lipid, lipoproteins, apoproteins and physical exercise in young female athletes, *An. Esp. Pediatr.*, 28, 395, 1988 (in Spanish).

880. Hoppeler, H., Skeletal muscle substrate metabolism, *Int. J. Obes. Relat. Metab. Disord.*, 23 (Suppl. 3), S7, 1999.

881. Štich, V., de Glisezinski, I., Galitzki, J., Hejnová, J., Crampes, F., Rivière, D., and Berlan, M., Endurance training increases the β-adrenergic lipolytic response in subcutaneous adipose tissue in obese subjects, *Int. J. Obes. Relat. Metab. Disord.*, 23, 374, 1999.

882. Mayer, J., Marshall, N.B., Vitale, J.J. et al., Exercise, food intake and body weight in normal rats and genetically obese adult mice, *Am. J. Physiol.*, 177, 544, 1954.

883. Chin, M.K., Lo, A.Y.S., Li, X.H., Sham, M.Y., and Yuan, Y.W.Y., Obesity, diet, exercise and weight control? A current review, *J. Hong Kong Med. Assoc.*, 44, 181, 1992.

884. Scheuring, A.J.W., Ammar, A.A., Benthem, B., van Dijk, G., and Sodersen, P.A.T., Exercise and the regulation of energy intake, *Int. J. Obes. Relat. Metab. Disord.*, 23 (Suppl. 23), S1, 1999.

885. Pařízková, J. and Poupa, O., Some metabolic consequences of adaptation to muscular work, *Brit. J. Nutr.*, 17, 341, 1963.

886. Pařízková, J., Body composition and nutrition of different types of athletes, in *Proc. XIII Int. Congr. Nutr. 1985*, Taylor, T.G. and Jenkins, N.K., Eds., John Libbey, London, 1986, 309.

887. Kaplan, T.A., Obesity in a high school football candidate: a case presentation, *Med. Sci. Sports Exerc.*, 24, 406, 1992.

888. Jeszka, J., Regula, J., and Kostrzewa-Tarnowska, A., Effect of sex on the results of weight reduction program in obese adolescents, *Scand. J. Nutr.*, 43 (Suppl. 34), S43, 1999.

889. Pařízková, J. and Novák, J., Dietary intake and metabolic parameters in adult men during extreme work load, in *Impacts on Nutrition and Health*, Simopoulos, A.P., Ed., *World Rev. Nutr. Diet*, Vol. 65, Karger, Basel, 72, 1991.

890. Sallis, J.F., McKenzie, T.L., Alcaraz, J.E., Kolody, B., Hovell, M.F., and Nader, P.R., Project SPARK. Effects of physical education on adiposity in children, *Ann. N.Y. Acad. Sci.*, 699, 127, 1993.

891. Goran, M.I., Shewchuk, R., Gower, B.A., Nagy, T.R., Carpenter, W.H., and Johnson, R.K., Longitudinal changes in fatness in white children: no effect of childhood energy expenditure, *Am. J. Clin. Nutr.*, 67, 309, 1998.

892. Mo-suwan, L., Pongprapai, S., Junjana, Ch., and Puetpaiboon, A., Effects of controlled trial of a school-based exercise program on the obesity indices of preschool children, *Am. J. Clin. Nutr.*, 68, 1006, 1998.

893. Rippe, J.M. and Hesse, S., The role of physical activity in the prevention and management of obesity, *J. Am. Diet. Assoc.*, 90, S31, 1998.

894. Abrosimova, L.I., Baibikova, L.S., Simonova, L.A., Malova, N.A., and Fetisov, G.V., Effect of motor activity on the physical work capacity of schoolchildren with excessive body weight, *Gig. Sanit.*, 8 (Aug.), 29, 1984 (in Russian).

895. Bordi, D., Giorgi, G., Porqueddu Zacchello, G., Zanon, A., and Rigon, F., Obesity, overweight and physical activity in elementary school children, *Minerva Pediatr.*, 47, 521, 1995.

896. Booth, F.W. and Tseng, B.S., America needs to exercise for health, *Med. Sci. Sports Exerc.*, 27, 462, 1995.

897. Ding, Z., Exercise prescription for obese children, *Chung Hua I Hsueh Tsa Chih Taipei*, 72, 131, 1992 (in Chinese).

898. Gutin, B., Cucuzzo, N., Islam, S., Smith, C., Moffat, R., and Pargam, D., Physical training improves body composition of black obese 7- to 11-year-old girls, *Obes. Res.*, 3, 305, 1995.

899. Amador, M., Flores, P., and Pena, M., Normocaloric diet and exercise: a good choice for treating obese adolescents, *Acta Paediatr. Hung.*, 30, 123, 1990.

900. Gutin, B., Owens, S., Okuyama, T., Riggs, S., Ferguson, M., and Litaker, M., Effect of physical training and its cessation on percent fat and bone density of children with obesity, *Obes. Res.*, 7, 208, 1999.

901. Ferguson, M.A., Gutin, B., Owens, S., Barbeau, P., Tracy, R.P., and Litaker, M., Effects of physical training and its cessation on the hemostatic system in obese children, *Am. J. Clin. Nutr.*, 69, 1130, 1999.

902. Kahle, E.B., Zipf, W.B., Lamb, D.R., Horswill, C.A., and Ward, K.M., Association between mild, routine exercise and improved insulin dynamics and glucose control in obese adolescents, *Int. J. Sports Med.*, 17, 1, 1996.

903. Gutin, B., Ramsey, L., Barbeau, P., Camady, W., Ferguson, M., Litaker, M., and Owens, S., Plasma leptin concentrations in obese children, changes during 4-month period with and without physical training, *Am. J. Clin. Nutr.*, 69, 388, 1999.

904. Hayashi, T., Fujino, M., Shindo, M., Hiroki, T., and Arakawa, K., Echocardio-graphic and electrocardiographic measures in obese children after an exercise program, *Int. J. Obes.*, 11, 465, 1987.

905. Gutin, B., Owens, S., Slavens, G., Riggs, S., and Treiber, F., Effect of physical training on heart-rate variability in obese children, *J. Pediatr.*, 130, 938, 1997.

906. Blaak, E.E., Westerterp, K.R., Bar-Or, O., Wouters, L.J., and Saris, W.H., Total energy expenditure and spontaneous activity in relation to training in obese boys, *Am. J. Clin. Nutr.*, 55, 777, 1992.

907. Sasaki, J., Shindo, M., Tanaka, H., Ando, M., and Arakawa, K., A long-term aer-obic exercise program decreases the obesity index and increases the high density lipoprotein cholesterol concentration in obese children, *Int. J. Obes.*, 11, 339, 1987.

908. Pařízková, J., Obesity and physical fitness: an age-dependent functional and social handicap, in *Social Aspects of Obesity*, deGarine, I. and Pollock, N.J., Eds., Gordon and Breach Publishers, Australia, 1995, 163.

909. Epstein, L.H., Saelens, B.E., Myers, M.D., and Vito, D., Effects of decreasing sedentary behaviors on activity choice in obese children, *Health Psychol.*, 16, 107, 1997.

910. Sothern, M.S., von Almen, T.K., Schumacher, H., Zelman, M., Farris, R.P., Carlisle, L., Udall, J.N., and Suskind, R.M., An effective multidisciplinary ap-proach to weight reduction in youth, *Ann. N.Y. Acad. Sci.*, 699, 292, 1993.

911. Ulanova, L.N., Korchagin, G.K., Volodina, N.N., Zhakovskaia, R.I., and Sycheva, E.K., Role of therapeutic physical exercise in the combined treatment of children with obesity, *Pediatriia*, 4, 66, 1985 (in Russian).

912. Peja, M. and Velkey, L., The joint influence of diet and increased physical ac-tivity in obese children, *Acta Paediatr. Hung.*, 29, 373, 1988.

913. Korsten-Reck, U., Wolfarth, B., Berg, A., and Keul, J., Sports and nutrition. An outpatient program for obese children, *Int. J. Obes. Relat. Metab. Disord.*, 22 (Suppl. 3), S63, 1998.

914. Ylitalo, V.M., Treatment of obese schoolchildren, *Klin. Pediatr.*, 194, 310, 1982.

915. Epstein, L.H., Koeske, R., Zidansek, J., and Wing, R.R., Effects of weight loss on fitness in obese children, *Am. J. Dis. Child.*, 137, 654, 1983.

916. L'Allemand, D., Mundt, A., and Gruters, A., Physical activity improves the outcome of a pediatric weight control program, *Int. J. Obes. Relat. Metab. Disord.*, 22 (Suppl. 3), S9, 1998.

917. Amador, M., Ramos, L.T., Morono, M., and Hermelo, M.P., Growth rate reduc-tion during energy restriction in obese adolescents, *Exp. Clin. Endocrinol.*, 96, 73, 1990.

918. Pařízková, J., Consequences of reduction treatment of child obesity in adult age, in *Proc. 1ˢᵗ Int. Congr. Obes., Recent Advances in Obesity Research*, Howard, A., Ed., Human Publishing Ltd., London, 1975, 293.

919. Figueroa-Colon, R., Mayo, M.S., Aldridge, R.A., Winder, T., and Weinsier R.L., Body composition changes in obese children after a 10-week weight loss pro-gram using dual-energy X-ray absorptiometry measurements (DXA), *Int. J. Obes. Relat. Metab. Disord.*, 22 (Suppl. 4), S12, 1998.

920. Pařízková, J., Compositional growth in relation to metabolic activity, in *Proc. XIIᵗʰ Int. Congr. Pediatrics*, Opening Plenary Session, Mexico City, Dec. 2–7, 1968, Vol. I., 32.

921. Katch, V., Becque, M.D., Marks, C., Morehead, C., and Rocchini, A., Basal me-tabolism of obese adolescents: inconsistent diet and exercise effects, *Am. J. Clin. Nutr.*, 48, 565, 1988.

922. Rocchini, A.P., Katch, V., Anderson, J., Hinderliter, J., Becque, D., Martin, M., and Marks, C., Blood pressure in obese adolescents: effect of weight loss, *Pediatrics*, 82, 16, 1988.
923. Johnson, W.G., Hinkle, L.K., Carr, R.E., Anderson, D.A., Lemmon, C.R., Engler, L.B., and Bergeron, K.C., Dietary and exercise interventions for juvenile obesity: long-term effect of behavioral and public health models, *Obes. Res.*, 5, 257, 1997.
924. Hoerr, S.L., Nelson, R.A., and Essex-Sorlie, D., Treatment and follow-up of obesity in adolescent girls, *J. Adolesc. Health Care*, 9, 28, 1988.
925. Cezar, C., Lopez, F.A., Vitolo, R., and Daibes, A., Obese female adolescents in a follow up of intervention with physical exercise and nutritional education, isolated and combined, *Int. J. Obes. Relat. Metab. Disord.*, 22 (Suppl. 288), 1998.
926. Schwingshandl, J. and Borkenstein, M., Changes in lean body mass in obese children during weight reduction program: effect of short term and long term outcome, *Int. J. Obes. Relat. Metab. Disord.*, 19, 752, 1995.
927. Cohen, C.H., McMillan, C.S., and Samuelson, D.R., Long-term effects of a lifestyle modification exercise program on the fitness of sedentary, obese children, *J. Sports Med. Phys. Fitness*, 31, 183, 1991.
928. Pena, M., Bacallao, J., Barta, L., Amador, M., and Johnston, F.E., Fiber and exercise in the treatment of obese adolescents, *J. Adolesc. Health Care*, 10, 30, 1989.
929. Korsten-Reck, U., Bauer, S., and Keul, J., Sports and nutrition? An out-patient program for adipose children (long-term experience), *Int. J. Sports Med.*, 15, 242, 1994.
930. Berg, A., Halle, M., Bauer, S., Korsten-Reck, U., and Keul, J., Physical activity and eating behavior: strategies for improving the serum lipid profile of children and adolescents, *Wien Med. Wochenschr.*, 144, 138, 1994 (in German).
931. Hermelo, M.P., Alonso, A., Amador, M., and Alvarez, R., Changes in body composition and serum lipid fractions after four weeks of slimming treatment: results in nineteen obese male adolescents, *Acta Paediatr. Hung.*, 28, 29, 1987.
932. Sterpa, A., Pappini, A., Picciotti, M., Sommariva, D., and Chiumello, G., Changes of the lipid and protein profile in the obese child in diet therapy (with and without added fiber), *Pediatr. Med. Chir.*, 7, 419, 1985.
933. Hermelo, M.P., Amador, M., Alvarez, R., and Alonso, A., Slimming treatment and changes in serum lipid and lipoprotein in obese adolescents, *Exp. Clin. Endocrinol.*, 90, 347, 1987.
934. Endo, H., Takagi, Y., Nozue, T., Tuwahata, K., Uemasu, F., and Kobayashi, A., Beneficial effects of dietary intervention on serum lipid and apolipoprotein levels in obese children, *Am. J. Dis. Child.*, 146, 303, 1992.
935. Epstein, L.H., Coleman, K.J., and Myers, M.D., Exercise in treating obesity in children and adolescents, *Med. Sci. Sports Exerc.*, 28, 428, 1996.
936. Goran, M.I., Reynolds, K.D., and Lindquist, C.H., Role of physical activity in the prevention of obesity in children, *Int. J. Obes. Relat. Metab. Disord.*, 23 (Suppl. 3), S18, 1999.
937. Rychlewski, T., Szczesniak, L., Kasprzak, Z., Nowak, A., Banaszak, F., and Konys, L., Complex evaluation of body reaction in obese boys with systematic physical exertion and a low energy diet, *Pol. Arch. Med. Wewn.*, 96, 344, 1996 (in Polish).
938. Nichols, J.F., Bigelow, D.M., and Canine, K.M., Short-term weight loss and exercise training effects on glucose-induced thermogenesis in obese adolescent males during hypocaloric feeding, *Int. J. Obes.*, 13, 683, 1989.

939. Holub, M., Zwiauer, K., Winkler, C., Dillinger-Paller, B., Schuler, E., Patsch, W., and Strohl, W., Plasma leptin decreases in obese children undergoing weight reduction and binds to high-density lipoproteins, *Int. J. Obes. Relat. Metab. Disord.*, 22 (Suppl. 4), S28, 1998.

940. Kahle, E.B., Dorisio, T.M., Walker, R.B., Eisemann, P.A., Reiser, S., Cataland, S., and Zipf, W.B., Exercise adaptation responses for gastric inhibitory polypeptide (GIP) and insulin in obese children, *Diabetes*, 35, 579, 1986.

941. Gutin, B., Ferguson, M.A., Owens, S., Ngoc-Ahn, L, Litaker, M., Humphries, M., Okuyama, T., and Riggs, S., Effect of physical training and its cessation on components of the insulin resistance syndrome in obese children, *Int. J. Obes. Relat. Metab. Disord.*, 22 (Suppl. 4), S23, 1998.

942. Knip, M., Lautala, P., and Puukka, R., Reduced insulin removal and erythrocyte insulin binding in obese children, *Eur. J. Pediatr.*, 148, 233, 1988.

943. Lehingue, Y., Locard, E., Vivant, J.F., Mounier, A., and Mamelle, N., Restoration of GH in urine during an in-patient slimming course in obese children, enhanced by physical activity, *Int. J. Obes. Relat. Metab. Disord.*, 22 (Suppl. 4), S26, 1998.

944. Locard, E., Lehingue, Y., Vivant, J.F., Mounier, A., and Mamelle, N., Which anthropometric measurements are related with urine GH excretion restoration in obese children attending an in-patient slimming course? *Int. J. Obes. Relat. Metab. Disord.*, 22 (Suppl. 4), S26, 1998.

945. Guzzaloni, G., Grugni, G., Moro, D., Calo, G., Tonelli, E., Ardizzi, A., and Morabito, F., Thyroid-stimulating hormone and prolactin response to thyrotropin-releasing hormone in juvenile obesity before and after hypocaloric diet, *J. Endocrinol. Invest.*, 18, 621, 1995.

946. Pintor, C., Loche, S., Faedda, A., Fanni, V., Nurchi, A.M., and Corda, R., Adrenal androgens in obese boys before and after weight loss, *Horm. Metab. Res.*, 16, 544, 1984.

947. Ebbeling, C.B. and Rodriguez, N.R., Effects of exercise combined with diet therapy on protein utilization in obese children, *Med. Sci. Sports Exerc.*, 31, 378, 1999.

948. Frelut, M.L., Guibourdenche, J., Oberlin, F., Boulimane, N., Peres, G., Novo, R., and Navarro, J., Changes in bone mineral density and vitamin status in obese adolescents during weight loss, *Int. J. Obes. Relat. Metab. Disord.*, 22 (Suppl. 4), S33, 1998.

949. Madeiros-Neto, G.A., Should drugs be used for treating obese children? *Int. J. Obes. Relat. Metab. Disord.*, 17, 363, 1993.

950. Molnár, D., Torok, K., Erhardt, E., and Jeges, S., Effectivity and safety of Letigen (caffeine/ephedrine): the first double blind placebo-controlled pilot study in adolescents, *Int. J. Obes. Relat. Metab. Dis.*, 23 (Suppl. 5), S62, 117, 1999.

951. Rand, C.S. and MacGregor, A.M., Adolescents having obesity surgery: a 6-year follow-up, *South. Med. J.*, 87, 1208, 1994.

952. Malandry, D., Frelut, M.L., Werther, J.R., and Mitz, V., Interest in plastic surgery for weight loss sequellae in children, *Int. J. Obes. Relat. Metab. Disord.*, 22 (Suppl. 4), S33, 1998.

953. Bollen, P., De Schepper, J., Delanghe, K., Asselman, P., and Vandenplas, Y., Intragastric balloon in the treatment of morbid obesity in adolescents: alternative treatment or gadget? *Int. J. Obes. Relat. Metab. Disord.*, 22 (Suppl. 4), S33, 1998.

954. Huang, M.H., Yang, R.C., and Hu, S.H., Preliminary results of triple therapy for obesity, *Int. J. Obes. Relat. Metab. Disord.*, 20, 830, 1996.
955. Gadzhiev, A.A., Mugarab-Samedi, V.V., Isaev, I.I., and Rafieva, S.K., Acupuncture therapy of constitutional-exogenous obesity in children, *Probl. Endokrinol.*, (Mosk), 39, 21, 1993 (in Russian).
956. Turnin, M.C., Tauber, M.T., Couvaras, O., Jouret, B., Pene, C., Gayrard, M., Fabre, D., Rouzaud, A., and Tauber, J.P., Learning good eating habits by playing computer games at school: perspectives for education of obese children, *Int. J. Obes. Relat. Metab. Disord.*, 22 (Suppl. 3), S62, 1998.
957. Scaglioni, S., Radice, N., Usuelli, M., and Valenti, M., The role of childhood diet in preventing adult obesity, *Int. J. Obes. Relat. Metab. Disord.*, 23 (Suppl. 5), S6, 1999.
958. Sahota, P., Rudolf, M.C.J., Dixey, R., Hill, A.J., and Barth, J.H., Apples: a school-based intervention to reduce obesity risks, *Int. J. Obes. Relat. Metab. Disord.*, 22 (Suppl. 3), S62, 1998.
959. Vitolo, M.R., Perion, V., Oliviera, F.L., Andrade, T., Garofolo, A., Patin, R.V., and Ancona Lopez, F., Group treatment for post-pubertal obese adolescents, *Int. J. Obes. Relat. Metab. Disord.*, 22 (Suppl. 3), S257, 1998.
960. Kalvachová, B., Nováková, J., Schneiberg, F., Břicháček, V., Janda, B., and Strenaková, D., Summer-vacation hospitalization of obese children, *Česk. Pediatr.*, 41, 275, 1986.
961. Gately, P., Cooke, C.B., and Mackreth, P., A three-year follow up of an eight week diet and exercise programme on children attending a weight loss camp, in *Abstr., 8th Int. Congress of Obesity, Satellite Symposium Physical Activity and Obesity, Maastricht, Aug. 26–29*, 38, 1998.
962. Lebedkova, S.E., Belova, O.K., Batanova, I.E., and Maleeva, N.P., Effectiveness of treatment of obese children in a pioneer camp of a sanatorium type, *Pediatriia*, 8, 51, 1984 (in Russian).
963. Southam, M.A., Kirkley, B.G., Murchison, A., and Berkowitz, R.I., A summer day camp approach to adolescent weight loss, *Adolescence*, 19, 855, 1984.
964. Jirapinyo, P., Limsathayourat, N., Wongarn, R., Limsathayourat, N., Bunnag, A., and Chockvivatvanit, S., A summer camp for childhood obesity in Thailand, *J. Med. Assoc. Thai*, 78, 238, 1995.
965. Braet, C., Van Winckel, M., and Van Leuwen, K., Follow-up results of different treatment programs for obese children, *Acta Paediatr.*, 86, 397, 1997.
966. Donelly, J.E., Jacobsen, D.J., Whatley, J.E., Hill, J.O., Swift, L.L., Cherrington, A., Polk, B., Tran, Z.V., and Reed, G., Nutrition and physical activity program to attenuate obesity and promote physical and metabolic fitness in elementary school children, *Obes. Res.*, 4, 229, 1995.
967. Widdowson E.M., Nutritional individuality, *Proc. Nutr. Soc.*, 21, 121, 1962.
968. Mahan, L.K., Family-focused behavioral approach to weight control in children, *Pediatr. Clin. North Am.*, 34, 983, 1987.
969. Flodmark, C.E., How to influence the development of eating behaviors – implications for the prevention of obesity, *Int. J., Obes. Relat. Metab. Disord.*, 23 (Suppl. 5), S6, 1999.
970. Hills, A.P., Education for preventing obesity, *J. Int. Counc. Health, Phys. Ed. Recr. Dance*, 30, 1, 30, 1993.
971. Chalew, S.A., Lozano, R.A., Armour, K.M., and Kovarski, A.A., Reduction of plasma insulin levels does not restore integrated concentration of growth hormone to normal in obese children, *Int. J. Obes. Relat. Metab. Disord.*, 16, 459, 1992.

# Figure References

F1. Vol, S., Tichet, J., and Rolland-Cachera, M.F., Trends in the prevalence of obesity between 1980 and 1996 among French adults and children, *Int. J. Obes. Relat. Metab. Disord.*, 22 (Suppl. 3), S210, 1998.

F2. Rolland-Cachera, M.F. and Bellisle, F., No correlation between adiposity and food intake: why are working class children fatter? *Am. J. Clin. Nutr.*, 44, 779, 1986.

F3. Rolland-Cachera, M.F., Deheeger, M., Akrout, M., and Bellisle, F., Influence of macronutrients on adiposity development: a follow-up study of nutrition and growth from 10 months to 8 years of age, *Int. J. Obes. Relat. Metab. Disord.*, 19, 573, 1995.

F4. Prentice, A.M., Lucas, A., Vasquez-Velasquez, L., Davies, P.S., and Whitehead, R.G., Are current dietary guidelines for young children a prescription for overfeeding? *Lancet*, 2(8619), 1066, 1988.

F5. Rolland-Cachera, M.F., Obesity among adolescents: evidence for the importance of early nutrition, in *Human Growth in Context*, Johnson, F.E., Zemel, B., and Eveleth, P.B., Eds., Smith-Gordon, Tokyo, 1999, 245.

F6. Pařízková, J., *Body Fat and Physical Fitness: Body Composition and Lipid Metabolism in Different Regimes of Physical Activity*, Martinus Nijhoff B.V. Medical Division, The Hague, 1977.

F7. Taylor, R.W., Gold, E., Manning, P., and Goulding, A., Gender differences in body fat content are present well before puberty, *Int. J., Obes. Relat. Metab. Disord.*, 21, 1082, 1997.

F8. Pařízková, J., Obesity and physical activity, in *Nutricia Symposion on Nutritional Aspects of Physical Performance*, De Wijn, J.F., and Binkhorst, R.A., Eds., Nutricia Ltd., Zoetermeer, The Netherlands, 1972, 146.

F9. Pařízková, J., Obesity and its treatment by diet and exercise, in *Nutrition and Fitness in Health and Disease*, Simopoulos, A.P., Ed., Karger, Basel, 1993, 78.

F10. Molnár, D. and Schutz, Y., The effect of obesity, age, puberty and gender on resting metabolic rate in children and adolescents, *Eur. J. Pediatr.*, 156, 376, 1997.

F11. Maffeis, C., Schutz, Y., and Pinelli, L., Effect of weight loss on resting energy expenditure in obese prepubertal children, *Int. J. Obes. Relat. Metab. Disord*, 16, 41, 1992.

F12. Maffeis, C., Zoccante, L., Micciolo, R., and Pinelli, L., Meal induced thermogenesis in lean and obese prepubertal children, *Am. J. Clin. Nutr.*, 57, 481, 1993.

F13. Bandini, L.G., Schoeller, D.A., and Dietz, W.H., Energy expenditure in obese and nonobese adolescents, *Pediatr. Res.*, 27, 198, 1990.

F14. Salbe, A.D., Fonteinvielle, A.M., Harper, I.T., and Ravussin, E., Low levels of physical activity in 5-year-old children, *J. Pediatr.*, 131, 423, 1997.

F15. Maffeis, C., Zaffanello, M., and Schutz, Y., Relationship between physical inactivity and adiposity in prepubertal boys, *J. Pediatr.* 131, 288, 1997.

F16. Maffeis, C., Zaffanello, M., Pinelli, L., and Schutz, Y., Total energy expenditure and patterns of activity in 8- to 10-year-old obese and nonobese children, *J. Pediatr. Gastroenterol. Nutr.*, 23, 256, 1996.

F17. DeLany, J.P., Harsha, D.W., Kime, J.C., Kumler, J., Melancon, L., and Bray, G., Energy expenditure in lean and obese prepubertal children, *Obes. Res.*, 3 (Suppl. 1), 67, 1995.

F18. Pařízková, J., Interaction between physical activity and nutrition early in life and their impact on later development, *Nutr. Res. Rev.*, 11, 71, 1998.

F19. Maffeis, C., Schena, F., Zafanello, M., Zoccante, L., Schutz, Y., and Pinelli, L., Maximal aerobic power during running and cycling in obese and non-obese children, *Acta Pediatr.*, 83, 113, 1994.

F20. Pařízková, J., Hainer, V., Štich, V., Kunešová, M., and Ksantini, M., Physiological capabilities of obese individuals and implications for exercise, in *Exercise and Obesity*, Wahlquist, M. and Hills, A.P., Eds., Gordon & Smith, London, 1995, 131.

F21. McMurray, R.G., Harrel, J.S., Levine, A.A., and Gansky, S.A., Childhood obesity elevates blood pressure and total cholesterol independently of physical activity, *Int. J. Obes. Relat. Metab. Disord.*, 19, 881, 1995.

F22. Pařízková, J., *Nutrition, Physical Activity, and Health in Early Life*, CRC Press, Boca Raton, 1996.

F23. Greco, M., Croci, M., Tufano, A., Sassano, G., Panigoni, G., Costa, M., Morricone, L., Longari, V., Mazzochi, M., and Caviezel, F., Caloric intake and distribution of the main nutrients in a population of obese children, *Minerva Endocrinol.*, 15, 257, 1990.

F24. Nguyen, N.V., Larson, D.E., Johnson, R.K., and Goran, M.I., Fat intake and adiposity in children of lean and obese parents, *Am. J. Clin. Nutr.*, 63, 507, 1996.

F25. Maffeis, C., Schutz, Y., and Pinelli, L., Postprandial thermogenesis in obese children before and after weight reduction, *Eur. J. Clin. Nutr.*, 46, 577, 1992.

F26. Salas-Salvado, J., Barenys-Manent, M., Recasens Gracia, M.A., Marti-Henneberg, C., Influence of adiposity on the thermic effect of food and exercise in lean and obese adolescents, *Int. J. Obes. Relat. Disord.*, 17, 717, 1993.

F27. Maffeis, C., Pinelli, L., and Schutz, Y., Increased fat oxidation in prepubertal obese children: a metabolic defence against further weight gain? *J. Pediatr.*, 126, 15, 1995.

F28. Ferrer-Gonzales, J., Belda Galiana, I., Segarra Aznar, F.M., Fenollosa Entrena, B., and Dalmau Serra, J., The development of lipid and anthropometric parameters in the treatment of pre-pubertal obese patients, *An. Esp. Pediatr.*, 48, 267, 1998 (in Spanish).

F29. Hoffman, R.P. and Armstrong, P.T., Glucose effectiveness, peripheral and hepatic insulin sensitivity, in obese and lean prepubertal children, *Int. J. Obes. Relat. Metab. Disord.*, 20, 521, 1996.

F30. Lahlou, N., Landais, P., De Boissieu, D., and Bougeners, P.F., Circulating leptin in normal children and during the dynamic phase of juvenile obesity: relation to body fatness, energy metabolism, caloric intake, and sexual dimorphism, *Diabetes*, 46, 989, 1997.

F31. Williamson, D.A., *Assessment of Eating Disorders. Obesity, Anorexia, and Bulimia Nervosa*, Pergamon Press, Elmsford, New York, 1990.

F32. Byrne, N.M. and Hills, A.P., An evaluation of body image assessment protocols with implications for age and gender differences, *Proc. Australasian Soc. Study Obes.*, Melbourne, 1993.

F33. Zwiauer, K., Schmidinger, H., Klicpera, M., Mayr, H., and Widhalm, K., 24-hr electrocardiographic monitoring in obese children and adolescents during 3-week low calorie diet (500 kcal), *Int. J. Obes.*, 13 (Suppl. 2), 101, 1989.

F34. Archibald, E.H., Stallings, V.A., Pencharz, P.B., Duncan, W.J., and Williams, C., Changes in intraventricular septal thickness, left ventricular wall thickness and left ventricular volume in obese adolescents on a high protein weight reducing diet, *Int. J. Obes.*, 13, 265, 1989.

F35. Pidlich, J., Pfeffel, F., Zwiauer, K., Schneider, B., and Schmidinger, H., The effect of weight reduction on the surface electrocardiogram: a prospective trial in obese children and adolescents, *Int. J. Obes. Relat. Metab. Disord.*, 21, 1018, 1997.

F36. Deheeger, M., Rolland-Cachera, M.F., and Fontvieille, A.M., Physical activity and body composition in 10-year-old French children: linkages with nutritional intake? *Int. J. Obes. Relat. Metab. Disord.*, 21, 372, 1997.

F37. Pařízková, J., Age trend in fatness in normal and obese children, *J. Appl. Physiol.*, 16, 173, 1961.

F38. Pařízková, J., The impact of age, diet and exercise on man's body composition, *Ann. N.Y. Acad. Sci.*, 110, 661, 1963.

F39. Pařízková, J., Longitudinal study of body composition and body build development in boys of various physical activity from 11 to 15 years of age, *Human Biol.*, 40, 212, 1968.

F40. Pařízková, J., Longitudinal study of the relationship between body composition and anthropometric characteristics in boys during growth and development, *Glasnik Antropol. Drusstvo Jugoslav.*, 7, 33, 1970.

F41. Pařízková, J., Growth and growth velocity of lean body mass and fat in adolescent boys, *Pediatric Res.*, 10, 647, 1976.

F42. Gutin, B., Owens, S., Slavens, G., Riggs, S., and Treiber, F., Effect of physical training on heart period variability, *J. Pediat.*, 130, 938, 1997.

F43. Pařízková, J., Compositional growth in relation to metabolic activity, in *Proc. XIIth Int. Congr. Pediatr.*, Opening Plenary Session, Mexico City, Dec. 2–7, 1968, Vol. I, 32.

F44. Pařízková, J., Consequences of reduction treatment of child obesity in adult age, in *Proc. 1st Int. Congr. Obes., Recent Advances in Obesity Research*, Howard, A., Ed., Human Publishing, London, 1975, 293.

F45. Endo, H., Takagi, Y., Nozue, T., Tuwahata, K., Uemasu, F., and Kobayashi, A., Beneficial effects of dietary intervention on serum lipid and apolipoprotein levels in obese children, *Am. J. Dis. Child.*, 146, 303, 1992.

F46. Lisková, S., Hošek, P., and Stožický, F., The metabolic syndrome and cardiovascular risk factors in obese children, *Int. J. Obes. Relat. Metab. Disord.*, 22 (Suppl. 4), S25, 1998.

F47. Kratzsch, J., Dehmel, B., Pulzer, F., Keller, E., Englaro, P., Blum, W.F., and Wabitsch, M., Increased serum GHBP levels in obese pubertal children and adolescents: relationship to body composition, leptin and indicators of metabolic disturbances, *Int. J. Obes. Relat. Metab.*, 21, 1130, 1997.

# Table References

T1. Pařízková, J., Obesity and physical activity, in *Nutricia Symposium on Nutritional Aspects of Physical Performance*, De Wijn, J.F. and Binkhorst, R.A., Eds., Nutricia Ltd., Zoetermeer, The Netherlands, 1972, 146.

T2. World Health Organization, *Energy and Protein Requirements, Report of a Joint FAO/WHO/UNU Expert Consultation*, Rome 1981, World Health Organization, Techn. Rep. series No. 724, WHO Geneva, 1985, 180.

T3. James, W.P.T. and Schofield, E.C., *Human Energy Requirements*, Oxford Medical Publ., Oxford University Press, Oxford, 1990.

T4. Šonka, J., Kostiuk, P., Hilgertová, J., Limanová, Z., and Drozdova, V., Hormonal and metabolic adaptation to a reducing regimen in children, *Acta Univ. Carolinae*, 39, 33, 1993.

# Index

## A

# Y